# FIRST AID FOR THE®
# MATCH

## FIFTH EDITION

**TAO LE, MD, MHS**
Assistant Clinical Professor of Medicine and Pediatrics
Section of Allergy and Clinical Immunology
University of Louisville

**VIKAS BHUSHAN, MD**
Diagnostic Radiologist

**CHRISTINA SHENVI, PhD, MD**
Resident, Department of Emergency Medicine
University of North Carolina in Chapel Hill

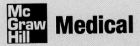 **Medical**

NEW YORK  CHICAGO  SAN FRANCISCO  LISBON  LONDON  MADRID  MEXICO CITY
MILAN  NEW DELHI  SAN JUAN  SEOUL  SINGAPORE  SYDNEY  TORONTO

**First Aid for the® Match, Fifth Edition**

1 2 3 4 5 6 7 8 9 0   WDQ/WDQ   14  13  12  11  10

ISBN 978-0-07-170289-8
MHID 0-07-170289-X
ISSN 1090-364X

**Notice**

Medicine is an ever-changing science. As new research and clinical experience broaden our knowledge, changes in treatment and drug therapy are required. The authors and the publisher of this work have checked with sources believed to be reliable in their efforts to provide information that is complete and generally in accord with the standards accepted at the time of publication. However, in view of the possibility of human error or changes in medical sciences, neither the authors nor the publisher nor any other party who has been involved in the preparation or publication of this work warrants that the information contained herein is in every respect accurate or complete, and they disclaim all responsibility for any errors or omissions or for the results obtained from use of the information contained in this work. Readers are encouraged to confirm the information contained herein with other sources. For example and in particular, readers are advised to check the product information sheet included in the package of each drug they plan to administer to be certain that the information contained in this work is accurate and that changes have not been made in the recommended dose or in the contraindications for administration. This recommendation is of particular importance in connection with new or infrequently used drugs.

This book was set in Goudy by Rainbow Graphics.
The editors were Catherine A. Johnson and Christine Diedrich.
The production supervisor was Phil Galea.
Project management was provided by Rainbow Graphics.
The designer was Mary McKeon.
World Color Dubuque was printer and binder.

This book is printed on acid-free paper.

McGraw-Hill books are available at special quantity discounts to use as premiums and sales promotions, or for use in corporate training programs. To contact a representative please e-mail us at bulksales@mcgraw-hill.com.

# DEDICATION

To the contributors of this and past editions, who took time to share their experience, advice, and humor for the benefit of future physicians.

And

To our families, friends, and loved ones, who supported us in the task of assembling this guide.

# CONTENTS

**Fellowship Training**

*Selected Medical Specialties*

*Selected Surgical Specialties*

## CHAPTER 5 INTERNATIONAL MEDICAL GRADUATES AND THE MATCH PROCESS ........ 113

## CHAPTER 6 GETTING RESIDENCY INFORMATION AND APPLICATIONS ........ 133

## CHAPTER 7 THE APPLICATION ........ 153

# AUTHORS

Sundeep Bhat, MD
Resident, Division of Emergency Medicine
Stanford University

Justin Brent Cohen, MD
Resident, Department of Plastic and
Reconstructive Surgery
Washington University in St. Louis
Barnes-Jewish Hospital

Bryan Hong, MD
Resident, Department of Ophthalmology
University of Southern California
Doheny Eye Institute

Mina Safain, MD
Resident, Department of Neurosurgery
Tufts Medical Center

Mark Schlangel, MD
Resident, Department of Anesthesiology
Columbia University
New York Presbyterian Hospital

# FACULTY REVIEWERS

Laura Bontempo, MD
Assistant Professor of Emergency Medicine
Residency Program Director
Yale University School of Medicine

Stephen Huot, MD, PhD
Professor of Medicine and Nephrology
Primary Care Residency Program Director
Yale University School of Medicine

C. Robert Bernardino, MD
Associate Professor of Opthalmology
Residency Program Director
Yale University School of Medicine

Karen Jubanyik, MD
Assistant Professor of Emergency Medicine
Academic Advisor
Yale University School of Medicine

Jamal Bokhari, MD
Associate Professor of Diagnostic Radiology
Residency Program Director
Yale University School of Medicine

# PREFACE

With the fifth edition of *First Aid for the® Match*, we continue our commitment to providing students and international medical graduates (IMGs) with the most useful and up-to-date information to help guide them through the residency application and interview process and obtain a residency position in the specialty of their choice. The fifth edition represents a thorough revision and includes:

- The latest insider advice from students who have successfully made it through the 2009 National Residency Matching Program (NRMP) Match

- Up-to-date information and statistics from the NRMP Match, including the latest trends in each of the specialty fields

- A revised and expanded chapter on advice for IMGs

- Updated specialty coverage, including specialty trends in education, research, and clinical practice

- An expanded guide to the Electronic Residency Application Service (ERAS)

- Top residency application mistakes and how to avoid them

- A revised, in-depth travel advice section, with detailed information on discount airfares and hotel lodging, as well as descriptions of many unique online travel and lodging sites

- An extensive compilation of commonly asked interview questions, broken down by specialty

The fifth edition would not have been possible without the help of dedicated students and faculty members, who contributed their feedback and suggestions. We invite both students and faculty to share their thoughts and ideas to help us continue to improve *First Aid for the® Match* in the future. (See How to Contribute, p. xv.)

| | |
|---|---|
| *Louisville* | Tao Le |
| *Los Angeles* | Vikas Bhushan |
| *Durham* | Christina Shenvi |

# ACKNOWLEDGMENTS

This has been a collaborative project from the start. We gratefully acknowledge the thoughtful comments and advice of the residents, international medical graduates, and faculty who have supported the authors in the development of *First Aid for the® Match*.

For support and encouragement throughout the process, we are grateful to Thao Pham and Jonathan Kirsch. We owe a special thanks to Selina Franklin and Louise Peterson for their administrative assistance during this revision. We thank Steven Abramowitz for his contributions to Chapters 8 and 9. Thanks to our publisher, McGraw-Hill, for the valuable assistance of their staff. For enthusiasm, support, and commitment to this challenging project, thanks to our editor, Catherine Johnson. For outstanding editorial work, we thank Susan Brownstein. A special thanks to Rainbow Graphics for remarkable production work.

We gratefully acknowledge the input of the following physicians, residents, and fellows who wrote or reviewed the sections pertaining to their specialty in Chapter 4. The tips, advice, critiques, and insight from these contributors, who have all been highly successful in their field, is what allows us to present each specialty from an insider's perspective. Thank you to Adam Schoenfeld, Benjamin Sherman, Brian Whang, Casius Chaar, Charles Sun Dela Cruz, Daniel Paik, Diane George, Dirk Johnson, Douglas Housman, Douglas Wallad, Eomonn Mahoney, Felix Knauf, Francis Chan, Guy Manetti, James Wu, Jeffrey Bigelow, Juan Carlos Cleves-Bayon, Kusum Mathews, Loren Berman, Madison Cuffy, Maxwell Laurens, Mina Xu, Misaki Kiguchi, Omar Chaudhary, Paras Bhatt, Ranee Lleva, Robert Turelli, Ronnie Klein, Samit Joshi, Scott Nishikawa, Stella Lee, Stephanie Massaro, Tracy Rabin, and Vikram Reddy.

| | |
|---|---|
| *Louisville* | Tao Le |
| *Los Angeles* | Vikas Bhushan |
| *Durham* | Christina Shenvi |

# HOW TO CONTRIBUTE

*First Aid for the* ® *Match* incorporates many contributions and changes from students and faculty. We invite you to participate in this process. In addition, we offer **paid internships** in medical education (please see below). Please send us:

- Strategies for applying and interviewing in your specialty

- Your personal statement and CV (feel free to edit or mask for privacy)

- Anecdotes of your application and interviewing experiences

- Your medical school's guide to the Match

- Corrections and clarifications

Personalized contributions (ie, anecdotes and personal statements), if used, will be altered to protect the identity of the contributor. For entries incorporated into the next edition, you will receive an Amazon.com gift certificate and personal acknowledgment in the next edition. Significant contributions will be compensated at the discretion of the authors.

The preferred way to submit suggestions and corrections is via electronic mail, addressed to:

firstaidteam@yahoo.com

Otherwise, you can send entries, neatly written or typed or on disk (Microsoft Word), to:

**First Aid Team**
**914 North Dixie Avenue, Suite 100**
**Elizabethtown, KY 42701**
**Attention: Match Contributions**

All entries become property of the authors and are subject to editing and reviewing. Please verify all data and spellings carefully. In the event that similar or duplicate entries are received, only the first entry received will be used. Please follow the style, punctuation, and format of this edition if possible.

# INTERNSHIP OPPORTUNITIES

The author is pleased to offer part-time and full-time paid internships in medical education and publishing to motivated medical students and physicians. Internships may range from two to three months (eg, a summer) up to a full year. Participants will have an opportunity to author, edit, and earn academic credit on a wide variety of projects, including the popular *First Aid* series. Writing/editing experience, familiarity with Microsoft Word, and Internet access are desired. For more information, e-mail a résumé or a short description of your experience along with a cover letter to **firstaidteam@yahoo.com.**

# The Match

## INTRODUCTION

Preparing for the Match is a time to celebrate! Graduation is on the horizon, and opportunities abound. With this wide variety of opportunities, however, comes responsibility. Choosing a residency position is likely to be more complicated than choosing a university or medical school. Many view postgraduate education as more of an uncharted sea, as paths diverge widely. More than 37,000 students will compete in the Match, and there will be over 25,000 rank-order lists (ROLs) submitted for approximately 22,400 residency spots. You will therefore need to plan your senior year carefully and be prepared to make decisions on a strict, strategic timetable. Once you have chosen your specialty, you must obtain program information and applications. In addition, senior electives must be scheduled to coincide with the application and interview process, and a personal statement and curriculum vitae (CV) must be written in conjunction with advisor meetings. A well-thought-out plan of action for the senior year will maximize your likelihood of success. Fortunately, faculty, colleagues, and advisors have seen the process evolve year after year, sharing in students' successes and remembering their mistakes. Presented below are the suggestions, advice, and experience of students, residents, and deans. We look forward to helping you chart this great sea of opportunity called the Match.

Students' two biggest fears are (1) not matching at any program; and (2) ending up in a program that is not right for them. Approximately 5.7% of U.S. students and 49.6% of non-U.S. foreign graduates in the National Resident Matching Program (NRMP) went without a matched position on the big day in 2009. Conversely, almost 4.8% of available NRMP positions remained unfilled. Detailed data from past years' Matches is available online (www.nrmp.org/data). However, try to avoid getting bogged down by numbers and worries, and instead focus your energy on making sure you have the best application possible!

## COMMON MISTAKES

> Most mistakes that students make during the residency application process can be easily avoided.

A number of common mistakes that medical students make year after year result in an unmatched or a poor-choice position. This guide will help students avoid mistakes such as:

- **Not understanding the details of the Match for a particular specialty.** For example, for some specialties, a preliminary year must be secured along with the specialty program. Some programs have their own match process as well as an earlier timetable for each step of the senior-year plan.

- **Starting the application process too late.** One step follows another, and a late start can result in more interviews in the later months than can actually be accomplished.

- **Applying to or ranking too few programs to ensure a match.** By the time a student realizes that he or she has been invited to only a few interviews, it may be too late to add program applications. Always err on the side of applying to more programs rather than fewer! There is a small fee for applying to more programs, but it is money well invested if you avoid going unmatched. This is particularly true in the more competitive specialties.

- **Not seeking adequate counseling and advice.** No student is an island in the Match process. Independent thinking and individualism may be admired in the medical profession, but the residency Match requires input from a variety of sources, including publications (such as the one you wisely picked up today!), advisors, colleagues, and word of mouth.

- **Inadequately preparing for and understanding the role of interviews, personal statements, and CVs.** Learn about these instruments through the eyes of those who use them to rank students.

- **Having unclear goals and expectations.** Most students have the necessary credentials for acceptance into excellent programs. However, students must work to find the right programs, focus on the programs of choice, and define what they are really looking for in a residency program.

- **Becoming overly confident during the application process.** Many programs will be very positive about the applicant. Some candidates, however, will misinterpret compliments about their record as a guarantee of a match.

- A small number of students who do not match may miss out on many opportunities that are briefly available during "Scramble Day." These students need intense assistance and counseling at that strategic time in the process.

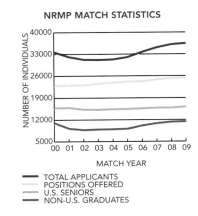

**NRMP MATCH STATISTICS**

TOTAL APPLICANTS
POSITIONS OFFERED
U.S. SENIORS
NON-U.S. GRADUATES

**FIGURE 1-1.**

ERAS, SF Match, URMP, and NRMP are separate entities. Know which ones apply to you.

## WHAT IS THE MATCH?

Although there are actually several matches, most people know the NRMP as the Match. While the NRMP offers positions in a wide range of specialties, a handful of specialties use their own match (see Table 1-1). With more than 90% of all graduating U.S. and Canadian medical students participating, along with a surprisingly high number of international medical graduates (IMGs), the NRMP is the largest match by far (see Figure 1-1).

The basic modus operandi of the Match is as follows: After the interview season, residency training programs submit a list of applicants in the order in which they would offer acceptances, and students enter lists of programs in the order in which they would accept offers. Both students and programs then submit their rankings to the NRMP. Subsequently, in a matter of minutes, a computer program matches each student to the highest program on his or her list that offered a position. The Match usually occurs in late February, and its results are announced simultaneously across the country on "Match Day" in mid-March. In 2009, 29,890 applicants enrolled in the Match, and of the 25,808 applicants who submitted ROLs, 21,340 received offers (see Figure 1-2).

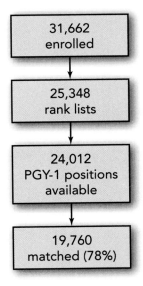

31,662 enrolled

25,348 rank lists

24,012 PGY-1 positions available

19,760 matched (78%)

**FIGURE 1-2.** Flowchart of the NRMP Match, based on 2009 NRMP Match data.

If you are a U.S. medical student, you will automatically receive information about the NRMP Match through your school during the spring of your third year. However, the NRMP can be contacted directly for more information at:

National Resident Matching Program
2450 N Street, N.W.
Washington, D.C. 20037-1127
(202) 828-0566 for applicants calling from outside the U.S.
(866) 617-5838 for toll-free calls in the U.S.
www.nrmp.org, nrmp@aamc.org

## WHY IS THERE A MATCH?

The Match exists in the form that we know it today to provide a semblance of order to an otherwise seemingly chaotic process of matching thousands of medical graduates with residency programs across the spectrum of specialties. Before a formal matching process was instituted in 1952, both applicants and programs were not given a fair opportunity to explore all of their options. Less competitive programs tried to get a head start by asking applicants to commit to their programs early in the fourth and sometimes even third year of medical school. Students were forced to gamble—that is, to decide whether to accept an early offer from a less competitive program, thereby forfeiting a later shot at better programs, or to pass up the early offer and risk not being accepted in a better program that offered positions after sifting through a larger pool of applicants. Residency directors faced a similar dilemma in that if they filled their positions too quickly, they would not be able to offer spots to more attractive applicants. The 1952 Match was a huge success; for the first time, applicants and programs were able to rank each other on the basis of desirability without being forced to make hasty decisions. The algorithm used to match applicants with programs has remained largely unchanged over the years (see Chapter 12).

## WHAT OTHER MATCHES ARE THERE?

Although the NRMP is the largest matching program available to U.S. medical students and IMGs, there are other matches as well, including some that operate independently of the NRMP.

### SPECIALTIES WITH THEIR OWN MATCHES

Some specialties have their own match processes and different match days.

The San Francisco Match is used by ophthalmology, child neurology, neurotology, and certain plastic surgery programs. Since these specialties require preliminary training in medicine, pediatrics, or surgery prior to beginning the residency-training program, applicants also match through the NRMP for one or two years of preliminary training.

## TABLE 1-1
### Specialties with Their Own Matches

| Specialty | Matching Program | Month of Match Day | Web Site |
|---|---|---|---|
| **Child Neurology & Neurodevelopmental Disabilities** | Child Neurology/NDD Matching Program<br>SF Match<br>655 Beach Street<br>San Francisco, CA 94109<br>(415) 447-0350<br>Fax: (415) 561-8535 | January of senior year | www.sfmatch.org<br><br>help@SFmatch.org |

The Child Neurology Matching Program (CNMP) supplements the matching services of the NRMP Pediatrics Match. It is timed to allow U.S. senior applicants to know their PGY-3 placement in Child Neurology/NDD before they submit their rank lists for PGY-1 prerequisite training.

| Specialty | Matching Program | Month of Match Day | Web Site |
|---|---|---|---|
| **Neurotology** | Neurotology Matching Program<br>SF Match<br>655 Beach Street<br>San Francisco, CA 94109<br>(415) 447-0350<br>Fax: (415) 561-8535 | October of senior year | www.sfmatch.org<br><br>help@SFmatch.org |

There is no centralized application service available for neurotology residencies. Applicants should contact each program individually for application materials and procedures.

| Specialty | Matching Program | Month of Match Day | Web Site |
|---|---|---|---|
| **Ophthalmology** | Ophthalmology Matching Program<br>SF Match<br>655 Beach Street<br>San Francisco, CA 94109<br>(415) 447-0350<br>Fax: (415) 561-8535 | January of senior year | www.sfmatch.org<br><br>help@SFmatch.org |

Applicants must also participate in the NRMP Match after submitting materials through ERAS to secure a preliminary training spot for their PGY-1 years.

| Specialty | Matching Program | Month of Match Day | Web Site |
|---|---|---|---|
| **Urology** | Urology Residency Matching Program<br>1000 Corporate Boulevard<br>Linthicum, MD 21090<br>(866) RING AUA (1-866-746-4282), ext. 3913<br>Fax: 410-689-3939 | January of senior year | www.auanet.org<br><br>resmatch@AUAnet.org |

Rank lists for residency in urology are processed through the Urology Match, which also has an earlier timeline than the NRMP. However, application materials are distributed through the Electronic Residency Application Service (ERAS), and applicants must contact programs to request application forms for those programs not participating in ERAS.

| Specialty | Matching Program | Month of Match Day | Web Site |
|---|---|---|---|
| **Plastic Surgery (noncombined)** | Plastic Surgery Residency Matching Program<br>SF Match<br>655 Beach Street<br>San Francisco, CA 94109<br>(415) 447-0350<br>Fax: (415) 561-8535 | May, after satisfactory completion of 3–4 years of approved surgical residency training; NOT open to senior medical students | www.sfmatch.org<br><br>help@SFmatch.org |

This is one of two routes into plastic surgery residency. The other, more common way is to go through the regular NRMP Match during senior year of medical school. Check with individual programs for prerequisite training requirements.

Urology holds a separate match specifically for urology residencies through the URMP, although applications are distributed through the Electronic Residency Application Service (ERAS) or through direct correspondence, depending on the preference of the individual program.

## NRMP COUPLES MATCH

In the Couples Match, the NRMP allows any two people to be matched with residency programs in the same geographic area if they so desire. Any two people can apply as a couple. Partners apply and interview separately at programs in the same geographic region. They then submit an ROL of pairs of programs in the order in which they would accept offers. Because couples are often limited by geographic constraints, they frequently submit more applications to maximize the likelihood of achieving a successful match. To help matters, the ROL gives a couple the option of seeking matches in separate locations or allowing one partner to go unmatched in the event that a Couples Match is not possible.

Some residency directors and deans believe that many couples do better together in the Match than they would if they applied and matched separately. Couples tend to be viewed as more stable and less likely to leave residency programs; on the other hand, couples matching in the same specialty may prove to be more difficult than matching in different specialties. Given the hassles involved in moving again after residency, especially with kids, couples are also regarded as more likely to contribute to the faculty pool of the institution in which they trained. Nevertheless, the results of the Couples Match can be unpredictable, especially when both people are applying to competitive programs. In addition, couples tend to seek reassurance from their interviewers that everything will turn out well and may thus be particularly prone to misinterpret encouragement as a guarantee about the match result. For more information about the Couples Match, consult the section on "Special Cases" in your NRMP Handbook for Students or consult the NRMP Web site (www.nrmp.org/res_match/special_part/us_seniors/couples.html).

## SHARED-SCHEDULE MATCH

A few programs in the Match offer shared-residency positions. This is rare, however, and may not be an option at most programs or in all fields. Shared-schedule positions in the NRMP Match allow two people to share the duties and responsibilities of one residency position. An applicant enrolls individually in the NRMP Match and then pairs up with a partner by completing a Shared Residency Pair Form, due in the fall preceding Match Day. The pair shares one NRMP applicant code, applies and interviews together, and submits a single ROL. Although each person will spend less than full time working (eg, alternate months on rotation), both will spend more time in residency and will eventually do as much work as, if not more work than, a full-time resident. Applicants may seek shared-schedule positions because of family responsibilities or research, among other reasons. When a pair is matched to a position, both are bound to accept it. With the enforcement of

> Any two people can apply as a couple in the Couples Match.

80-hour workweeks, such paired programs may become even less common. Consult "Special Cases" in your NRMP Handbook for Students for more information or consult the NRMP Web site (www.nrmp.org/res_match/special_part/inst_officials/about.html).

## CANADIAN MATCH

The Canadian Resident Matching Service (CaRMS) was founded in 1970. Like its U.S. counterpart, the CaRMS Match is an orderly approach toward matching applicants to their top choices and residency programs to their preferred applicants. In fact, the CaRMS uses the same matching algorithm as the NRMP, although its Match Day is in mid-February. Approximately 1400 Canadian students apply for roughly 1500 slots annually offered through the Canadian Match. The CaRMS is an eight-month process that includes an application cycle, an interview period, a ranking period, and match result announcements. The CaRMS is open to U.S. seniors, although few apply. In September, applicants are sent a unique token by e-mail to initiate their application by the Applicant Webstation. Most graduating Canadian medical students participate in the First Iteration Match. In addition, 700 "independent" applicants compete for approximately 200 positions available in the Second Iteration Match. Independent applicants include former graduates of Canadian medical schools, U.S. students, and graduates of international medical schools. For more information, contact:

Canadian Resident Matching Service

171 Nepean Street

Suite 300

Ottawa, ON K2P 0B4

(613) 237-0075

Fax: (613) 563-2860

www.carms.ca/eng

help@carms.ca

## OSTEOPATHIC MATCH

The AOA Intern/Resident Registration Program, the osteopathic version of the Match, is run by the National Matching Services Inc. (NMS). All osteopathic graduates are required to take a one-year osteopathic rotating internship approved by the American Osteopathic Association (AOA) before entering an osteopathic residency. Applicants interview in late summer and fall, submit an ROL by late January, and await results on the osteopathic Match Day in mid-February.

Approximately 2200 osteopathic internships and 1100 residency positions are offered through the osteopathic match every year. Osteopathic residency directors have recently had more difficulty filling their positions, as osteopathic graduates have gained wider acceptance in allopathic residency programs, and the AOA has relaxed its restrictions on osteopathic graduates pursuing allopathic training through the NRMP Match. The AOA opportunities database of internship and residency positions is available on the AOA's Web site at www.do-online.org (select the option for students and residents). For more information, contact:

American Osteopathic Association
Department of Education
142 East Ontario Street
Chicago, IL 60611
(800) 621-1773, ext. 7426
Fax: (312) 202-8200

National Matching Services
P.O. Box 1208
Lewiston, NY 14092-8208
www.do-online.org
info@osteotech.org
(716) 282-4013
Fax: (716) 282-0611

National Matching Services
20 Holly Street, Suite 301
Toronto, Ontario, Canada M45 3B1
(416) 977-3431
Fax: (416) 977-5020

## ARMED FORCES MATCH

Army, Navy, and Air Force residencies conduct their own matching process early in the senior year, several months before the NRMP Match takes place. Applicants usually have military service obligations (eg, graduates of the Uniformed Services University of the Health Sciences School of Medicine and participants in the Health Professions Scholarship Program). After senior-year applicants have been interviewed, the military programs convene in late November and early December each year to match programs and applicants in a weeklong affair known as "Selection Boards." Many students apply to both matches using the NRMP as a fallback, particularly when a competitive military program is sought. Students who do not match successfully in a military program can usually begin interviewing late as long as initial applications have been completed. All medical graduates of the Uniformed Services University are preferentially placed through an Armed Forces match. If you match with a military residency program, you are obliged to withdraw from the NRMP Match or from any other civilian match. Applicants should be cautioned about applying in a specialty with an early match (ophthalmology) and the military match. If they match in both, they can place the civilian program in jeopardy.

For more information on the Army military match, contact the regional Army Medical Department (AMEDD) counselor.

For more information on the Air Force military match, contact:

Headquarters AFPC/DPAME

550 C Street West, Suite 27

Randolph Air Force Base, TX 78150-4729

(800) 531-5800

DSN 487-6331

For more information on the Navy military match, contact:

Bureau of Medicine and Surgery

2300 E Street, N.W. Washington, D.C. 20372-5300

(202) 653-1318

medicine.creighton.edu/MMSA/match

## WHAT ARE MY CHANCES OF SUCCESS IN THE MATCH?

In general, U.S. seniors do well in the NRMP Match. Roughly 85% of U.S. seniors obtain one of their top three choices each year (see Table 1-2). The U.S. senior nonmatch rate has held steady at 6–7% for the past ten years and was 5.7% in 2009. In contrast, other applicants fare rather poorly (see Table 1-3). In the 2009 Match, only 44.6% of U.S. graduates (as opposed to U.S. seniors) and 41.6% of IMGs in the NRMP were successfully matched. IMGs, whether U.S. citizens or not, generally fare the worst.

## TABLE 1-2

| Success of U.S. Seniors in the NRMP Match in Percentage | | | | | |
| --- | --- | --- | --- | --- | --- |
| Choice Obtained | 2005 | 2006 | 2007 | 2008 | 2009 |
| First | 62.5 | 50.4 | 58.6 | 59.9 | 56.5 |
| Second | 15.0 | 19.1 | 15.7 | 15.8 | 16.2 |
| Third | 8.7 | 11.2 | 9.5 | 8.9 | 9.2 |
| Fourth | 4.7 | 6.8 | 5.5 | 5.0 | 5.3 |
| > Fourth | 9.1 | 10.7 | 10.7 | 10.4 | 12.8 |

## TABLE 1-3

### PGY-1 NRMP Match Rate (%)

| Applicant Type | 2005 | 2006 | 2007 | 2008 | 2009 |
|---|---|---|---|---|---|
| U.S. seniors | 93.7 | 93.7 | 93.4 | 94.2 | 93.1 |
| U.S. graduates | 44.3 | 45.2 | 45.4 | 44.0 | 44.6 |
| Osteopaths | 68.6 | 67.9 | 68.8 | 71.6 | 69.9 |
| Canadian students | 72.9 | 60.9 | 64.5 | 62.2 | 71.4 |
| U.S. citizen foreign graduates | 54.7 | 50.6 | 50.0 | 51.9 | 47.8 |
| Non-U.S. citizen foreign graduates | 55.6 | 48.9 | 45.5 | 42.4 | 41.6 |

## HOW DO I REGISTER FOR THE NRMP MATCH?

### U.S. SENIORS

A U.S. senior is defined as one who has attended a Liaison Committee on Medical Education (LCME)-accredited school and is on schedule for graduation the year of the Match. Registration occurs online through the NRMP Web site, www.nrmp.org/res_match. The system uses the Association of American Medical Colleges (AAMC) ID along with a password that can be assigned during registration. Students are asked to review the terms of the Match Agreement and the policies of the NRMP.

Payment of the registration fee of $50 also occurs online through use of a credit card number. As stated by the NRMP, registration entitles the user to access to the NRMP site, the processing of up to 20 program ranks and 20 ranks on the supplemental ROLs (SROLs), and access to a restricted Web site that lists unfilled positions. An additional $30 is assessed for each program added to your ROL after you have selected 20 programs. Remember, while the Match is run through the NRMP, the actual application is through ERAS, which has its own fees. ERAS is discussed in detail in Chapter 7.

### INDEPENDENT APPLICANTS

The category of "independent applicant" includes several groups: previous graduates of a U.S. medical school, Canadian students/graduates, osteopathic students/graduates, students of a fifth-pathway program, and IMGs. Registration is online and follows the same method as that for U.S. seniors. You will be asked to select the correct category of application. The NRMP will collect information to verify eligibility, including the United States Medical Licensing Examination/Educational Commission for Foreign Medical Graduates (USMLE/ECFMG) identification number in the case of IMGs.

The NRMP requires that foreign graduates pass all exams necessary for ECFMG certification, including the Clinical Skills Assessment. Independent applicant names should be exactly the same as those used by ERAS and the ECFMG.

Payment is also online, and registration entitles independent applicants to the same benefits as U.S. seniors.

## WHAT ABOUT THE OTHER MATCHES?

If you are a U.S. medical student, information pamphlets and registration materials for specialties outside the NRMP Match should be available at your dean's office. Otherwise, you can contact the specialty match programs directly for information and registration forms (see Table 1-1). To register for the armed forces match, contact your military branch's medical personnel counselor or your local armed forces recruitment officer. **Don't forget to register for the NRMP Match regardless of what other matches you enroll in.**

Nothing prevents you from enrolling in multiple matches; you just can't accept more than one appointment. Many non-NRMP Matches require a preliminary transitional year obtained through the NRMP Match. In addition, many of these matches are highly competitive, and the NRMP Match is a nice backup. While you lose the registration fee, that is preferable to running the risk of not matching in the earlier match and being unable to participate in the NRMP at all.

## NRMP PUBLICATIONS

The NRMP offers a wealth of valuable publications that few students know about and fewer still take the time to read. A handbook and the NRMP Directory are provided online in the Register/Log-in area to registered participants. The rest can be ordered from the NRMP by calling (202) 828-0416 or by filling out the NRMP publications order form found in the back of the NRMP Directory and mailing it to:

Attention: Membership and Publication Orders
National Resident Matching Program
2450 N Street, N.W.
Washington, D.C. 20037-1127

> Always enroll in the NRMP Match as a backup regardless of what other matches interest you.

You can also order NRMP publications through the NRMP Web site (www.nrmp.org). Each NRMP publication is listed below.

### NRMP HANDBOOK FOR STUDENTS

The NRMP Handbook for Students is available free of charge through U.S. medical schools and is aimed at U.S. seniors and sponsored graduates. Read it from cover to cover, as it thoroughly describes the NRMP and its role in the residency application process. You will be able to decipher the NRMP philosophy despite the stilted prose. The handbook includes current details for registering for the Match and describes the Couples Match and shared-residency positions. It also supplies concise explanations for ROLs and SROLs. However, some of the juiciest information in the handbook can be found in its appendices, which include selected statistics from the previous Match, NRMP policy statements, and an explanation of the Match algorithm. Finally, the handbook's back cover lists key dates applicable to the Match process.

> Have a look at the NRMP data. The results may surprise you!

## NRMP HANDBOOK FOR INDEPENDENT APPLICANTS

Like the NRMP Handbook for Students, this free publication from the NRMP is a must-read for independent applicants. You can get a copy by calling the NRMP at (202) 828-0566. The version for independent applicants covers the same topics as the general student handbook. In addition, the Handbook for Independent Applicants contains guidelines for the verification of credentials for Match eligibility, an NRMP publications order form, and Match dates for specialties covered in the NRMP's Specialties Matching Services.

## NRMP DIRECTORY/HOSPITALS AND PROGRAMS PARTICIPATING IN THE MATCHING PROGRAM

The NRMP Directory is a catalog of residency programs participating in the Match. Part I of the directory organizes the programs by hospital. Use this section to see what other specialty training programs are offered at the hospitals you're interested in. For example, since the presence of an internal medicine program typically means a lower caliber of training for family practice residents, family practice applicants may want to find hospitals without internal medicine programs. Part II lists programs by specialty type and is much more useful. You should receive the edition for the previous Match at no cost upon registration. You will also receive a revised edition for your Match year late in the fall.

## NRMP PROGRAM RESULTS/LISTING OF FILLED AND UNFILLED PROGRAMS FOR THE MATCH

If you want to find out which programs in your specialty were not filled last year, this is the book to get. It's like going through someone's dirty laundry. The NRMP Program Results book is distributed on Unmatch Day to unmatched applicants, who must then enter the Scramble. Part II lists programs that did not fill all their spots. This can be a real eye-opener and can also give you a better feel for regional trends in competitiveness. If you are a marginal candidate applying in a competitive specialty, you may want to consider applying to several of the programs that went unfilled last year. But be forewarned—these programs probably went unfilled for good reason. Although this publication is supposedly available free of charge only to applicants who failed to find placements in the previous Match, you can check your school's student affairs office for a copy.

## NRMP DATA

The NRMP Web site has a wealth of information, with exhaustive data on the previous year's Match and trends over the last several years. It tracks Match trends and puts you and your target specialty into perspective in terms of the ratio of number of applicants to positions. The data report also lists each specialty within each individual hospital, with the number of positions they have and the number that remained unfilled in the Match. The central Web site for NRMP data and statistics contains several publications that are worth perusing (www.nrmp.org/data/). The data and results file for the 2009 Match are also available online (www.nrmp.org/data/resultsanddata2009.pdf).

The NRMP also tracks outcomes of the Match based on the credentials of the applicant. This publication is listed on their main data page and is called "Charting Outcomes in the Match." It shows, for example, the average USMLE Step 1 score for applicants who matched or did not successfully match in each specialty. Again, do not let yourself get lost or overwhelmed by all the data. Instead, use it as a tool to candidly assess how competitive you are for a given specialty. The statistics should help guide your decisions about how many programs to apply to, and whether to apply in a second field in which you might have better chances of matching.

## UNIVERSAL APPLICATION FOR RESIDENCY AND PROGRAM DESIGNATION CARD

Programs that use ERAS or are under the SF Match do not use the Universal Application; however, some programs (eg, those in neurotology) will accept this application in lieu of their own forms. You get one or two Universal Applications free when you sign up for the Match. There should be no need to purchase additional copies. Because you send a photocopy of the Universal Application to the few programs that accept it, simply photocopy your application if you need more copies (ie, as a worksheet). For detailed advice on completing the Universal Application, see Chapter 7.

You will also receive one free program designation and acknowledgment card with your Universal Application. This self-addressed card to acknowledge receipt of your application is a bit useless, as it has no space for the program secretary to acknowledge receipt of other materials, such as letters of recommendation and medical school transcripts. You can easily design a more useful acknowledgment card yourself (see application status postcard, p. 000).

## REFERENCES

National Resident Matching Program. *Advanced Copy of Results and Data, 2009 Match.* Washington, D.C., 2009.

National Resident Matching Program. *Handbook for U.S. Medical Students, 2009 Match.* Washington, D.C., 2009.

National Resident Matching Program. *NRMP Data and Statistics: 2009.* Washington, D.C., 2009.

National Resident Matching Program Web site (www.nrmp.org/data/).

AAMC Newsroom Web site (www.aamc.org/newsroom/pressrel/2009/090319.htm).

# Setting Up the
# Senior Year

The senior year of medical school is an exciting, busy year! After years of training, you are almost a doctor. There are many things to learn and do in order to transition to the next stage as resident. Despite what you have heard from friends and colleagues, the fourth year of medical school is full of events and deadlines, so it is important to stay organized and avoid procrastination. In arranging the senior year, you need to arm yourself with tools to navigate the residency application process from start to finish. For a maximally fulfilling and successful senior year, you must also take advantage of the resources that surround you at your medical school and beyond. The first step is finding an advisor.

## HOW DO I PICK AN ADVISOR?

> An advisor should be both counselor and advocate.

During your first three years of medical school, you may have identified or have been assigned an academic advisor who shepherded you through a variety of situations, from surviving gross anatomy to helping you choose a medical specialty. If your advisor is an internist and you want to go into internal medicine, you may already be in great shape. However, if you choose a field that differs from that of your advisor, or if your advisor does not closely monitor your application and matching process, you will need someone else to provide you with additional advice.

In selecting an advisor, you should seek someone who is savvy about a wide variety of factors regarding your career choice and the Match (see Figure 2-1). Your advisor should be able to keep you informed of both academic and economic trends as well as training and job opportunities in your chosen field. He or she should be familiar with the strong and weak points of your candidacy and should know you well enough to offer personal, honest advice. You should also seek an advisor who is familiar with the programs in which you are interested. For example, an advisor who trained on the East Coast may not be familiar with West Coast programs. Similarly, if you are interested in academic medicine, you should not choose an advisor who is primarily involved in private practice (or vice versa). Your advisor should be able to answer a range of questions about the application process, from matters of fact (What are the requirements for this residency program?) to advice (Whom should I ask for recommendations? How many schools should I apply to?). Some students even advocate a dual-advisor system: one advisor to assist you with the "nuts and bolts" of the process and another, more senior, well-known faculty member whose connections and telephone lobbying might open more doors for you.

How do you find such an advisor? Start by asking students in the class ahead of you about outstanding faculty members in your discipline. Your current medical school advisor may also have some suggestions. The dean of students can often guide you to the appropriate advisors. Ask the department chair or the residency director at your school whom they would recommend. The best advisors are faculty members who are involved in residency selection and who have advised applicants in previous years. In the process of identifying your ideal advisor, however, you should be aware of the following potential pitfalls:

- **Advisor overload:** A person who counsels so many students that you're left with little attention (this can also be a problem with faculty who write many recommendation letters each year).

## ✓ checklist

- ○ Help direct you toward potential research opportunities, or recommend academic conferences to attend.
- ○ Provide overall view of the application process, highlighting aspects specific to your field.
- ○ Review and critique your application (eg, personal statement, CV).
- ○ Discuss any trends in the specialty, such as locations of practice (academic vs. private), economic trends, important areas of research, etc.
- ○ Offer an honest assessment of your competitive standing.
- ○ Offer advice about the number of programs you should apply to, interview at, and rank (remember to get opinions from several people on this, such as your dean of students, program director, or department chair!).
- ○ Conduct a mock interview. This may be with a different adviser, depending on whether your school already has a program in place for assigning students to mock interviewers.
- ○ Meet with you after interview season to discuss your impressions and review your rank order list.
- ○ Make a key phone call to one (and only one) program that is your top choice in support of your application and to communicate your excitement about their program. At some medical schools it is the program director or chair of the department who makes these phone calls.

**FIGURE 2-1** Checklist for the career adviser.

- **Advisor oversight:** A person who tends to misjudge a student's competitiveness or the competitiveness of the field.

- **Advisor nostalgia:** A faculty member who remembers what it was like in your field many years ago but who no longer has an accurate perception of the Match.

- **Advisor bias:** One who gives all students the same "pet" list of programs to apply to regardless of their personal career goals, their geographic constraints, or the strength of their candidacy.

Some students also make the mistake of sticking with a mentor with whom they worked on a research project during the first two years of medical school. Often, this choice is made out of fear that your former mentor will be insulted if he or she is excluded from your residency plans. Such faculty members, however, may or may not be the best advisors for you, especially if they are not actively involved in the residency application process at your school. So bear in mind that a mentor does not always make the best advisor, just as racecar drivers don't always make the best driving instructors.

> Start looking for an advisor early, as they are often pressed for time.

# WHEN SHOULD I SCHEDULE MY ACTING INTERNSHIPS?

There is a checklist/timeline on the inside front cover of this book for organizing Match activities during your senior year of medical school. Conventional wisdom says that you should do at least one acting internship (or AI, also called a subinternship, externship, junior internship, or senior clerkship) in your target specialty early in your fourth year (or late in your third year at some schools). Your evaluation during this rotation is one of the most influential factors considered by the selection committee. In addition, a strong letter of recommendation from an attending physician on this rotation is usually critical to a competitive application. Some programs will expect at least one letter of recommendation from an AI (if you did one) as part of your application. Verify with the dean's office the last rotation block that will show up in your dean's letter and on your transcript (usually September).

Given the importance of this rotation, many students like to do a "warm-up" rotation before going all out on the AI. Students interested in internal medicine, for example, often rotate on cardiology, infectious disease, or emergency medicine before beginning an internal medicine AI. This warm-up rotation allows you to acquire the experience, knowledge, and skills (both interpersonal and intellectual) that are necessary for success on your AI. The rotation also ensures that you will enter the AI refreshed and enthusiastic. Don't relax too much, however, as strong grades or evaluations within electives of your target specialty are also highly regarded by selection committees. Students interested in surgical specialties (eg, orthopedics, neurosurgery) often elect to do a general surgery AI before beginning an AI in their specific interest in order to hone their floor management and operating room skills.

If you choose to do a second AI, either by requirement or by desire, note that there are good reasons for doing them early as well as for postponing them. If you do the second AI early, it offers you a chance at a strong letter of recommendation (especially if third-year performance was weak). The evaluation would also go in your dean's letter. Some advantages to doing the second AI later are that the evaluation won't be included in the dean's letter, so there is less pressure for you to perform at 110% every day. Also, it would spread out the tougher rotations more evenly over fourth year to prevent having two or three months of intense AIs in a row.

Know if your specialty requires an in-house subinternship. If so, schedule it early, as these tend to book quickly!

## SHOULD I DO AUDITION ROTATIONS?

Early in the fourth year, many students do audition rotations (away rotations or externships) at other schools in their target specialties either to find out more about a specific program or to improve their chances of entering that program. Be careful. An away rotation is a double-edged sword—you can stumble as well as shine. Remember that you will probably be compared with medical students at that institution who are already familiar with the hospital environment and its faculty. On the positive side, many programs will grant visiting students a "courtesy interview" at the end of an audition rotation. In fact, some programs in certain competitive specialties, such as orthopedic surgery or emergency medicine, take only "known quantities"—students who have done rotations on site.

An additional factor to consider is that several specialties—most notably surgical subspecialties such as neurosurgery and orthopedics—effectively require an "in-house" rotation if a student is to be considered at that program. See Chapter 4 for the trends in each specialty. For the rest of you, consider doing away rotations only if you are aiming for a long-shot program in which you would not otherwise have a chance. If people from your medical school have matched at the program you are considering, keep in mind that the program likely has a positive impression of your medical school, so an away rotation may actually diminish your candidacy. If no one from your school has ever matched at that program, an audition rotation may give you that "foot in the door" as long as you do an excellent job. In evaluating the potential benefits of an audition rotation, you must size up whether you come across better in person or on paper. If you simply want to find out more about a program at a specific institution, consider doing an away rotation there, but not in your target specialty (eg, emergency medicine at an institution whose surgery program interests you). Otherwise, you risk exposing yourself to unnecessary scrutiny.

> Away subinternships can hurt as much as they help.

> Use the fourth year to learn new things and have fun, not to reproduce your internship.

## WHAT ABOUT OTHER ELECTIVES?

Your fourth year is a fantastic opportunity to fulfill your intellectual and personal curiosity by sampling all that medicine has to offer. Don't waste it! Although it's wise to take an elective or two that will prepare you for internship (see Table 2-1), do not try to duplicate your internship during your fourth year—you'll get more than enough experience during your residency training. In addition, you might consider taking some electives that may not be available to you again. Your career advisor should have some good suggestions for fourth-year electives, as will students in the class ahead of you. Some options to consider are to travel abroad and do an international elective. You may never see those strange parasitic diseases you learned so much about in the second year here in the United States, but they are out there! Research electives can give you insight into the direction in which your field is headed. This might be interesting for you on a personal level and will provide excellent conversation for those low points in the interview.

> A national meeting can be fun, but don't go too far out of your way to attend.

> Your school may finance a trip to a national meeting if you present.

## TABLE 2-1

**Recommended Fourth-Year Electives by Specialty**

| Specialty | Recommended Electives for Internship | Related Electives |
|---|---|---|
| Anesthesiology | Surgical ICU | Radiology, emergency medicine, medical ethics |
| Dermatology | Infectious disease, medicine subinternship, pathology | Emergency medicine, ophthalmology, pediatric subinternship |
| Emergency medicine | ICU, radiology, gynecology, trauma surgery | Cardiology, dermatology, psychiatry crisis center, toxicology |
| Family practice | Cardiology, emergency medicine, gastroenterology, orthopedics | Dermatology, ophthalmology, overseas elective, radiology, sports medicine |
| Internal medicine | Cardiology, emergency medicine, infectious disease, pulmonary | Dermatology, orthopedics, OB/GYN, otolaryngology, overseas elective |
| Neurology | Psychiatry subinternship, radiology, geriatrics | Neurosurgery, emergency medicine |
| Obstetrics and gynecology | Maternal/fetal medicine, pediatrics, surgery subinternship, urology | Emergency medicine, family practice, endocrinology |
| Orthopedics | Emergency medicine, trauma surgery | ICU, rheumatology, radiology, sports medicine |
| Otolaryngology | Emergency medicine, neurology, surgery subinternship | Dermatology, pulmonary medicine |
| Ophthalmology | Emergency medicine, neurology | Dermatology, medicine consult |
| Pathology | Clinical anatomy, radiology | Laboratory medicine, infectious disease, hematology |
| Pediatrics | Emergency medicine, dermatology, pediatric infectious disease, pediatric intensive care medicine | Child psychiatry, medicine consult, radiology, pediatric surgery |
| Psychiatry | Endocrinology, neurology subinternship, medicine consult | Emergency medicine, toxicology, substance abuse |
| Radiology | Clinical anatomy, anatomic pathology | Informatics, orthopedics, emergency medicine |
| Surgery | Emergency medicine, ICU, trauma surgery, clinical anatomy | Medicine consult, surgical pathology, anesthesiology |

## WHEN SHOULD I SCHEDULE VACATION?

Don't forget to take time for yourself. Some students take a light rotation during September of their fourth year or take two weeks off during that period so that they can attend to residency applications. Remember that once residency starts, you will be limited to two to five weeks of vacation per year—and you can probably forget holidays such as Christmas, Hanukkah, and Thanksgiving.

Consider spending part of your vacation at a major national meeting in one or two of your top specialty choices, either late in your third year or early in your fourth year. This is especially true if the meeting is nearby or if your advisor is planning to go. A list of national meetings is published regularly in *JAMA* as well as on specialty organization Web sites (see Table 2-2). Most of these conferences have special reduced registration rates for medical students. Some students submit abstracts based on clinical cases, which may enable them to obtain travel and registration funding from the department and/or dean's office. Your career advisor can provide more detailed information about the best ones to attend. At these meetings, you can meet the field's celebrities, find out what's hot, hear about problems and politics, and scope out the turf wars. You can preview programs in the specialty by looking at research posters or by listening to scheduled faculty talks. Spending time at a major meeting will provide you with valuable insights and perspectives and can also make you a more knowledgeable and interesting candidate during interviews.

You may want to take one of two approaches to vacation during the fourth year. Those students applying to ten or more programs should probably use at least some of their vacation time for interviews in December and January, as described above. Alternatively, those students who are applying to fewer programs might want to do all their interviews "on the fly" during clinical rotations in the fourth year. This will allow you to finish your fourth-year requirements and take a sizable (two-month) vacation, right after Match Day. Also consider vacation for taking the USMLE Step 2 CK if your USMLE Step 1 performance was poor.

## TABLE 2-2
### Partial List of Specialty Organizations

| Specialty | Organization/Contact Information | Web Site |
|---|---|---|
| General | American Medical Women's Association (AMWA)<br>100 North 20th Street, 4th Floor<br>Philadelphia, PA 19103<br>Phone: (215) 320-3716 or (866) 564-2483<br>Fax: (215) 564-2175<br>E-mail: info@amwa-doc.org | www.amwa-doc.org |
| | American Medical Association (AMA)<br>515 N. State Street<br>Chicago, IL 60654<br>Phone: (800) 621-8335 | www.ama-assn.org |
| | American Medical Student Association<br>1902 Association Drive, Reston, VA 20191<br>Phone: (703) 620-6600<br>Fax: (703) 620-5873<br>E-mail: amsa@amsa.org | www.amsa.org |
| Anesthesiology | American Society of Anesthesiologists (ASA)<br>520 N. Northwest Highway, Park Ridge, IL 60068-2573<br>Phone: (847) 825-5586<br>Fax: (847) 825-1692<br>E-mail: mail@asahq.org | www.asahq.org |

*(continued)*

| | | |
|---|---|---|
| Dermatology | American Academy of Dermatology (AAD)<br>P.O. Box 4014 Schaumberg, IL 60168-4014<br>Phone: (866) 503-SKIN (7546)<br>International: (847) 240-1280<br>Fax: (847) 240-1859 | www.aad.org |
| Emergency medicine | American College of Emergency Physicians (ACEP)<br>P.O. Box 619911<br>Dallas, TX 75261-9911<br>Phone: (800) 798-1822<br>Fax: (972) 580-2816 | www.acep.org |
| | Society for Academic Emergency Medicine (SAEM)<br>901 North Washington Avenue<br>Lansing, MI 48906-5137<br>Phone: (517) 485-5484<br>Fax: (517) 485-0801 | www.saem.org |
| | American Academy of Emergency Medicine (AAEM)<br>555 East Wells Street, Suite 1100<br>Milwaukee, WI 53202<br>Phone: (800) 884-2236<br>Fax: (414) 276-3349 | www.aaem.org |
| Ophthalmology | Academy of Ophthalmology (AAO)<br>P.O. Box 7424<br>San Francisco, CA 94120<br>Phone: (415) 561-8500<br>Fax: (415) 561-8533 | www.aao.org |
| Orthopedics | American Academy of Orthopaedic Surgeons (AAOS)<br>6300 North River Road Rosemont, IL 60018-4262<br>Phone: (847) 823-7186<br>Fax: (847) 843-8125 | www.aaos.org |
| Otolaryngology | American Academy of Otolaryngology—Head and Neck Surgery (AAO-HNS)<br>One Prince Street<br>Alexandria, VA 22314<br>Phone: (703) 836-4444 | www.entnet.org |
| Pathology | College of American Pathologists (CAP)<br>325 Waukegan Road Northfield, IL 60093<br>Phone: (800) 323-4040 or (847) 832-7000<br>Fax: (847) 832-8000 | www.cap.org |
| | American Society for Clinical Pathology (ASCP)<br>2100 West Harrison Street<br>Chicago, IL 60612-3798<br>Phone: (312) 738-1336 or (800) 621-4142<br>Fax: (312) 738-1619 | www.ascp.org |
| Pediatrics | American Academy of Pediatrics (AAP)<br>141 Northwest Point Boulevard<br>Elk Grove Village, IL 60007<br>Phone: (847) 434-4000<br>Fax: (847) 434-8000 | www.aap.org |
| Physical medicine and rehabilitation | American Academy of Physical Medicine and Rehabilitation (AAPM&R)<br>330 North Wabash Avenue, Suite 2500<br>Chicago, IL 60611-7617<br>Phone: (312) 464-9700<br>Fax: (312) 464-0227 | www.aapmr.org |

| Psychiatry | American Psychiatric Association (APA)<br>1000 Wilson Boulevard, Suite 1825<br>Arlington, VA 22209-3901<br>Phone: (888) 357-7924 or (703) 907-7300<br>E-mail: apa@psych.org | www.psych.org |
| | American Academy of Child and Adolescent Psychiatry (AACAP)<br>3615 Wisconsin Avenue, N.W.<br>Washington, D.C. 20016<br>Phone: (202) 966-7300<br>Fax: (202) 966-2891 | www.aacap.org |
| Radiology | American College of Radiology (ACR)<br>1891 Preston White Drive<br>Reston, VA 20191-4397<br>Phone: (703) 648-8900 or (800) 227-5463<br>E-mail: info@acr.org | www.acr.org |
| | ACR-LINE Radiological Society of North America (RSNA)<br>820 Jorie Boulevard<br>Oak Brook, IL 60523-2251<br>Phone: (630) 571-2670 or (800) 381-6660<br>Fax: (630) 571-7837 | www.rsna.org |
| Radiation oncology | American College of Radiation Oncology (ACRO)<br>5272 River Road<br>Bethesda, MD 20816<br>Phone: (301) 718-6515<br>Fax: (301) 656-0989 | www.acro.org |
| | American Society for Therapeutic Radiology and Oncology (ASTRO)<br>8280 Willow Oaks Corporate Drive, Suite 500<br>Fairfax, VA 22031<br>Phone: (703) 502-1550<br>Fax: (703) 502-7852 | www.astro.org |
| Surgery | American College of Surgeons (ACS)<br>633 N. St. Clair Street<br>Chicago, IL 60611<br>Phone: (312) 202-5000 or (800) 621-4111<br>Fax: (312) 202-5001<br>E-mail: postmaster@facs.org | www.facs.org |
| | American College of Chest Physicians (ACCP)<br>3300 Dundee Road<br>Northbrook, Illinois 60062<br>Phone: (847) 498-1400 or (800) 343-2227 | www.chestnet.org |
| | American Society of Colon and Rectal Surgeons (ASCRS)<br>85 W. Algonquin Rd., Suite 550<br>Arlington Heights, IL 60005<br>Phone: (847) 290-9184<br>Fax: (847) 290-9203<br>E-mail: ascrs@fascrs.org | www.fascrs.org |
| Urology | American Urological Association (AUA)<br>1000 Corporate Boulevard<br>Linthicum, MD 21090<br>Phone: (866) 746-4282<br>Fax: (410) 689-3800 | www.auanet.org |

## WHEN SHOULD I SCHEDULE TIME FOR INTERVIEWS?

For the majority of students, interview dates run from November to early February. Students participating in "early matches" (eg, child neurology, urology, ophthalmology) should leave time for interviews as early as mid-October through early December, while keeping in mind that interviews for the preliminary- or transitional-year programs can run through early February. Most students take a month off for interviews starting right before or after the winter break. However, unless you are considering a smaller number of programs in a limited geographic area, a two-week winter break is usually not enough. That said, you should keep in mind that with the exception of your AI, most of your fourth year will consist of elective time. These rotations expect a degree of absenteeism from fourth-year medical students. Attendings were students once, too, and recognize the hassles involved in interviewing across the country. Most will understand if you miss a day or two here and there.

Students who interview in January may have a slight advantage over those who interview earlier. Because these students' interviews occur after the holidays, committee members may be more likely to remember their applications and to push for them during highly charged ranking sessions. In addition, it may be hard for you to remember the specifics of a program you visited in December when making your rank-order list (ROL) in February. If you interview early, consider revisiting programs that you plan to rank highly both to refresh your memory and to reiterate your interest to the selection committee; however, make sure that your preferred programs allow revisits, as some programs frown upon it.

If you plan to visit many programs in the Northeast or upper Midwest, however, January may be a bad month because of winter traveling conditions. During the first week of January, one of us got stranded at a subway stop in a blizzard while visiting a program in Cleveland. A half-hour trip from the airport to the university thus turned into a two-and-a-half-hour ordeal. So allow extra time during snow season for visiting programs in these areas.

As a final note, try to schedule some fun into each interview trip; otherwise, the burden of schlepping from one city to the next gets overwhelming. See that big arch in St. Louis, eat some chowdah in Boston, and try and make it to the beach in January in San Diego! In addition to having a good time, you will learn what each city is like at its best, which will help you when you return home to make ROL-related decisions.

## SHOULD I STICK AROUND MY SCHOOL ON MATCH DAY?

The month featuring Match Day (March for most applicants) is generally not a good time to be vacationing or doing electives outside the country. A certain percentage of U.S. medical students and international medical graduates (IMGs) will not be placed on Match Day and will have to enter the Scramble. If you do not match and have to enter the Scramble or if there is a problem with your ROL, you'll need to be in close communication with your dean and your advisor, either in person or by phone. This is especially true if you are trying to match in a competitive specialty. So if you feel the need to flee, try to choose another time. If you must be out of the country, make contingency plans with your dean and advisor, and get access to a fax machine. The WebROLIC system will allow you to find out if and where you matched via the Internet—but keep in mind that many students will be logging in on Match Day, and it may be easier to call your dean's office.

Finally, there is only one Match Day, when you get to celebrate with your classmates. Do not miss out on this opportunity to enjoy the fruits of your labor with your classmates. This is even true if you matched early; it is not a day to be missed.

> Play it safe: Try to be in the country on Match Day.

## REFERENCES

American Academy of Child and Adolescent Psychiatry Web site (www. aacap.org).

American Academy of Dermatology Web site (www.aad.org).

American Academy of Emergency Medicine Web site (www.aaem.org).

American Academy of Family Physicians Web site (www.aafp.org).

American Academy of Neurology Web site (www.aan.com).

American Academy of Ophthalmology Web site (www.aao.org).

American Academy of Orthopaedic Surgeons Web site (www.aaos.org).

American Academy of Otolaryngology—Head and Neck Surgery Web site (www.entnet.org).

American Academy of Pediatrics Web site (www.aap.org).

American Academy of Physical Medicine and Rehabilitation Web site (www.aapmr.org).

American Association of Neurological Surgeons Web site (www.aans.org).

American College of Chest Physicians Web site (www.chestnet.org).

American College of Emergency Physicians Web site (www.acep.org).

American College of Obstetricians and Gynecologists Web site (www.acog.org).

American College of Physicians Web site (www.acponline.org).

American College of Preventive Medicine Web site (www.acpm.org).

American College of Radiation Oncology Web site (www.acro.org).

American College of Radiology Web site (www.acr.org).

American College of Surgeons Web site (www.facs.org).

American Geriatrics Society Web site (www.americangeriatrics.org).

American Medical Association Web site (www.ama-assn.org).

American Medical Student Association Web site (www.amsa.org).

American Medical Women's Association Web site (www.amwa-doc.org).

American Psychiatric Association Web site (www.psych.org).

American Society for Therapeutic Radiology and Oncology Web site (www.astro.org).

American Society of Anesthesiologists Web site (www.asahq.org).

American Society of Colon and Rectal Surgeons Web site (www.fascrs.org).

American Society for Clinical Pathology Web site (www.ascp.org).

American Urological Association Web site (www.auanet.org).

College of American Pathologists Web site (www.cap.org).

Emergency Medicine Residents' Association Web site (www.emra.org).

Fellowship and Residency Electronic Interactive Database (FREIDA) American Medical Association Web site (freida.ama-assn.org/Freida/user/viewProgramSearch.do).

National Resident Matching Program Web site (www.nrmp.org).

Radiological Society of North America Web site (www.rsna.org).

Reference directories. *JAMA* 273(21):1652, 1995.

Society for Academic Emergency Medicine Web site (www.saem.org).

Wagoner NE, Suriano R, Stoner JA. Factors used by program directors to select residents. *J Med Educ* 61(1):10–21, 1986.

# 3

# Choosing and Matching in Your Specialty

Choosing a specialty may be one of the most difficult decisions a student encounters during medical school. Ironically, this life decision comes at an early time during your medical education. The beginning of the fourth year, when third-year experiences are still clear in your mind, is the best time to choose a career and residency type. There are fewer exams and call nights, leaving ample time to contemplate this critical decision. Schedules are also flexible at this time, allowing you to choose elective rotations that can aid in decision making. These are the critical months during which you can reflect on your own interests and experiences during medical school, discuss your ideas with family, friends, and mentors, and evaluate your career aspirations.

Although some students confidently know their specialty calling by the end of the third year, many students are left undecided or are attracted to more than one specialty. The spring and summer months before the fourth year allow time to further explore career options with electives and subinternships. Rotations at an away site during this time may provide an important new perspective by allowing you to work with different faculty members in a novel environment. Scheduling these rotations and electives to occur early in the fourth year will help you make a specialty decision sooner and allow you more time to optimize your application.

As the end of summer approaches, you should have finalized your decision about the type of specialty you wish to pursue. Any lingering indecision could have a negative impact on the application process that fully begins in September. By late summer before your fourth year, you will be expected to write a personal statement that reflects your commitment to a particular area of medicine, choose faculty to write letters of recommendation (based in part on career choice), and begin to prepare for interviews.

Nonetheless, some students need additional time to explore their options. There are three major reasons that some students fail to make a choice of specialty by the fall of the fourth year:

1. One or more specialties appear very attractive, making it difficult for students to choose among several opportunities.

2. No single career choice stands out above the others.

3. Late or inadequate exposure to the specialty.

> Picking a specialty can feel like deciding who to marry after the first date.

## WEIGHING YOUR OPTIONS

If you are undecided, it is important to ask yourself questions about your personal and professional needs. In order to answer these questions, you must be honest with yourself. Only then will you be able to let your innate values, goals, and expectations guide you toward an appropriate specialty choice. Some questions to ponder include:

- What were your original goals when you decided to become a physician? Are they still valid? If not, what has changed and why?

- What part of a physician's role do you value the most? Is it the long-standing patient relationships, the ability to immediately help others, the intellectual challenge, the prestige, or using the newest technology to help patients?

- What type of doctor-patient relationship do you find the most rewarding?

- Are you interested in incorporating nonclinical aspects of medicine—research, medical education, or administration—into your career?

- What personal strengths do you feel you can offer to medicine? What skills (interpersonal, communication, technical, analytical, etc.) do you value most in yourself and hope to highlight during your career?

- What situations make you uncomfortable? In which types of patient encounters do you feel that you are not reaching your full potential?

- On which rotations did you feel most at ease and most excited to go back the next day? With which group of resident and attending physicians did you feel inspired, feel part of the group, and most enjoy working?

If you have identified and explored more than one career option, it is likely that you could excel in either choice. In addition to thinking about the questions listed above, it may also be helpful to review the categories that are commonly used in choosing a specialty; you may even elect to use a list or spreadsheet format to relate each item as a pro or con for the specialties you are considering. Such categories usually include:

- Personal satisfaction

- Family issues

- Prestige factor

- Salary

- Working conditions

> Family and lifestyle are increasingly considered to be critical factors.

While simple, honest reflection may be sufficient for some students to make this important decision, others may desire additional resources providing some concrete facts. Reviewing the Fellowship and Residency Electronic Interactive Database Access System (FREIDA) online physician workforce information to compare hours, salaries, and job satisfaction data from among the various specialties is a good idea. Each specialty has national societies and academic organizations, some of which may provide useful information on Web sites, brochures, or interest groups regarding choosing their particular field. In addition, these societies sometimes hold residency fairs at national meetings or specific meetings for medical students interested in the field. For students in U.S. medical schools, registering with the Association of American Medical Colleges (AAMC) Careers in Medicine Web site (services.aamc.org/careersinmedicine/) will provide you free access to a number of tools designed to help you identify which specialty might be the best match for you; these resources include a Myers Briggs Type Indicator, interest and values checklists, and a specific exercise on choosing your specialty. There is also information covering a range of different typical and atypical career paths, as well as detailed statistics and demographic information for each specialty.

Some medical schools also offer students access to the Glaxo Pathway Evaluation Program for Medical Professionals. This questionnaire allows you to rank values and interests related to medicine and then informs you how well your answers match with members who are part of particular specialties. If you need more help, additional references are listed at the end of the chapter. Throughout the process of choosing a specialty, however, you should always remember: reading current literature and data about specialty choices can be helpful, but do not let it distract you from the heart of this very personal decision.

For students who remain undecided at the "last hour," emphasis on personal satisfaction is key. Such students should ask the question, "What would make me most happy?" or "What would give me the most job satisfaction?" Most physicians would agree that enjoying the day-to-day work of the profession is critical to success and that all other considerations are secondary. So when time has run out and a decision must be made in order for the matching process to proceed, you should determine what you most enjoy doing and then go for it! It may be that excessive concerns about the opinion of a relative or spouse, an advisor's assessment of a particular field, or workload or salary issues are precisely what led to your indecision in the first place. If you are content with what you are doing, factors such as salary, workload, and prestige will usually become secondary.

## WHAT IF I STILL CAN'T DECIDE?

The profession of medicine offers an incredible variety of opportunities, so students should have found an attractive choice by the fall of their fourth year. If the fall of your fourth year has arrived and you still have no attractive specialty choice in sight, good counseling is imperative. Meetings with your senior advisor and associate dean of students should be scheduled immediately if they have not already taken place. This is the time to return to square one and take on candid self-reflection, to refocus on your own goals, and to receive honest feedback from mentors and deans. There are several scenarios that may describe students who find themselves lost in choosing a specialty by October or November of their fourth year.

In some cases, students may be committed to a primary care field but have trouble deciding among the primary care specialties. A student attempting to choose between medicine and family medicine, for example, might compare the diversity of experiences in family medicine to the more frequent diagnostic challenges and fellowship opportunities found in medicine. Some students with an interest in obstetrics and primary care may seek to discover more about opportunities to practice obstetrics within the field of family medicine.

For other students, career preferences may meet up with the harsh realities of competition. For example, a student may realize in the fall of senior year that he or she is unlikely to match in programs such as dermatology, orthopedics, or plastic surgery. Such students should seek good counseling, not only to optimize their chances of selection within the field of their first choice, but also to help them choose from among alternate fields. This choice of alternatives should be based on the student's attraction to the competitive fields. For example, after discussions with deans, they may seek to apply to programs within both their most desired field, such as plastic surgery, and the more broad area of general surgery.

These situations are in no way all encompassing, and regardless of which position you find yourself in, some decision about the following year must be made by October of the fourth year, whether it be a final choice of specialty or an alternate option. It should be noted, however, that few educators will recommend that students take a year away from medicine completely, since such a hiatus may lead students to stray from their career choice despite the considerable investment they have already made in both time and effort. However, if a specialty decision can absolutely not be made, there are a few other solutions to consider. One excellent choice may be a year dedicated to medical research, particularly if you are interested in pursuing an academic career or are preparing for a competitive residency. You may even find sources of funding for yearlong projects through the Howard Hughes Medical Institute Training Fellowship, the National Institutes of Health (NIH), national associations, or sometimes through medical school research grants. Many have found that this type of productive research year can significantly bolster their curriculum vitae (CV) and improve one's ability to compete for residency positions. Some schools may also provide an opportunity to pursue a joint degree program, such as a master's in public health or master's in business administration degree. Another possibility, if you are unable to select a specialty, is to pursue a transitional-year or a preliminary-year residency position. A yearlong training program may allow you to explore a specialty you are considering, can sometimes be counted toward your residency program once it is chosen, and will keep you involved in clinical medicine. Matching into a transitional or preliminary year, however, may require you to reapply for a categorical residency position during the next match cycle.

> Some schools may allow for an extra year, but early planning with the dean's office is essential.

**Preliminary year.** The preliminary year differs from a categorical position in that a preliminary year is a one-year position meant for people going into a specialty (anesthesia, radiology, etc.) that requires one year of another specialty first, or for people who are undecided or unmatched in the specialty of their choice. It counts toward one's residency training (versus the transitional year, which often does not) in terms of board-exam eligibility, but the program is under no obligation to grant the next year of training. A categorical position is one in surgery, medicine, or any other specialty that ensures a position for the full time course of the resident's training.

A preliminary year may be a better option than a transitional year for the undecided student. The preliminary year of medicine or surgery can be used to guide a student's choice of specialty, particularly if he or she is leaning toward either field. A preliminary year might also eliminate the need to repeat an internship and may be used as a prerequisite for such fields as radiology, anesthesiology, radiation oncology, and rehabilitation medicine. Some programs will offer up to four months of elective time that may be used to obtain additional experiences and hence facilitate the decision-making process.

A preliminary year in one's own medical school is usually advisable if the year is needed for specialty decision making. Some program directors for these programs will enthusiastically support tailoring the year for this purpose. However, it could be challenging to find appropriate spots in residency programs after completion of the preliminary year. For example, if you have completed a preliminary year in internal medicine and wish to continue and complete the internal medicine residency, you would need to apply for and be accepted into a program with an open second-year spot.

**Transitional year.** The transitional year of residency is an internship year designed to expose new physicians to several fields of medicine, usually including internal medicine, surgery, primary care, and some elective time. They are often more competitive positions and are often designed for and filled by individuals needing to complete an internship year before continuing onward to an advanced categorical residency such as radiology or anesthesiology. A transitional year could be beneficial for specialty decision making if you are considering several fields or if you truly have no clue as to which specialty you may eventually prefer. However, most transitional programs will allow only limited time working in each specialty and therefore may only frustrate students who could not choose a specialty under the much more favorable circumstances of their fourth year. Because transitional years rarely afford an individual enough experience in any one field, they will usually result in essentially two years of internship—a formidable task for even the most enthusiastic student.

When time has run out and a career decision must be made, take solace in knowing that all the facts and experiences you need are already in your mind. Choose the area of medicine that has appealed to you most! Do not delay decision making. Do not carve out another year of indecision. Do not try to find someone to make the choice for you. Remember why you wanted to become a physician in the first place. If you have lost confidence in yourself with exposure to so many other talented colleagues, reclaim that confidence. The right amount of confidence and passion will lead you to the right decision.

> A preliminary or transitional year can buy more time to decide on a specialty.

## OK, I'VE DECIDED—WHAT NEXT?

While the process of actually choosing a specialty can be extremely nerve-racking, once the decision is made, your work is far from over. Now begins the process of applying for and matching into your chosen specialty. In much the same way that different fields of medicine have their own particular culture and practices, the application processes for individual specialties can vary, having their own nuances and sometimes emphasizing different aspects of the application, such as letters of recommendation or the personal statement. Nonetheless, there are some overarching objective measures that will help every student understand how to have a competitive application. In a survey of program directors from several medical specialties, researchers identified several common criteria that were highly important in selecting residents:

- Grades in required clerkships
- USMLE Step 1 and USMLE Step 2 CK scores
- Number of honors grades
- Grades in senior electives and subinternships

> Objective standards such as your test scores are one way to gauge how competitive you are for a given field.

While this list reemphasizes the importance for students to excel in clinical performance, it is important to understand that you will be evaluated holistically, using other factors to complement these core aspects of the application. Some students may have achieved academic honors, such as awards or admittance into the Alpha Omega Alpha (AΩA) society. Other students may have completed a research project related to the field of interest, or they might have presented research in a publication or poster format. Others may have helped organize events for a medical school chapter of the specialty's interest group or helped mentor fellow preclinical students. All of these aspects of medical education, beyond the basic test scores and letters, will enhance your overall application and help make you more competitive when it comes to rankings for the Match.

> Information from your CV can be added to ERAS before your specialty choice is made.

The summer and fall of the fourth year will move quickly and will require organization and constant effort toward preparing the application. Start the process early once the important choice of specialty is made. Schedule meetings with advisors or faculty members from that department so that they can appropriately guide you and help you focus your application. Forming these relationships early in the process will help you as the application season moves along—these same mentors can later help you practice interviews, suggest strong programs, and perhaps even contact faculty members at your most desired program. You should begin researching programs within the specialty, drafting the personal statement, and seeking letter writers as soon as possible. You should update your CV, making sure to include information on awards, publications, and meaningful activities from medical school. In addition, you may want to consider your own USMLE Step 1 scores and determine when you will take the subsequent portions of the licensing examination, Step 2 CK and Step 2 CS. Planning the timing of Step 2 exams is especially important for those considering early match specialties. By staying organized, following the guidance of mentors in your chosen field, and preparing for the interview process, you can help make yourself more competitive for the Match process.

## REFERENCES

AAMC Careers in Medicine Web site (www.aamc.org/students/cim/).

AMA FREIDA Online Database (freida.ama-assn.org/Freida/user/viewProgram-Search.do).

AMA List of National Specialty Society Web sites (www.ama-assn.org/ama/pub/about-ama/our-people/the-federation-medicine/national-medical-specialty-society-websites.shtml).

Green M, Jones P, Thomas JX Jr. Selection criteria for residency: Results of a national program directors survey. *Acad Med* 84(3):362–367, 2009.

Howard Hughes Medical Institute: Research Training Fellowships for Students Web site (www.hhmi.org/grants/individuals/medfellows.html).

National Institutes of Health Student Training Opportunities Web site (www.training.nih.gov/student/).

Pathway Evaluation Program for Medical Professionals Web site (medpathway.wustl.edu/intro.htm).

# Your Specialty and the Match

Each specialty calls for a different approach toward preparing a successful application and interview. For example, psychiatry residency directors expect and appreciate in-depth personal statements with a thorough exploration of an applicant's background and motives for entering the specialty. Other specialties, such as orthopedics and neurosurgery, are heavily influenced by audition rotations.

In this chapter, we briefly profile selected specialties and subspecialties to highlight some of these core approaches. We have organized the information and advice for each specialty under the following headings:

- **Overview:** The specialty in terms of recent trends in the medical career market.

- **Application Tips:** Advice and guidance for the application process specific to each specialty.

- **Interview Tips:** Advice and guidance for the interview visit specific to that specialty.

- **For More Info:** A collection of essential career and residency application resources for each specialty.

- **Fellowship Training Opportunities:** This is a list of some (though not all, as the opportunities for sub- and sub-subspecialization are almost limitless) of the major fellowships available to residents in each field. Many fields offer research fellowships that provide the opportunity for dedicated research time in a large number of different topics related to the field.

- **Top 5 Most Frequently Encountered Diseases or Conditions**

Of special note, the **Overview** contains a brief description of the specialty itself, a glance at its socioeconomic trends and a summary of student, resident, and faculty observations. It is not intended as a basis for the complex and critical process of specialty selection. For more in-depth information about the specialty, consult the following resources:

- Faculty and house staff in the field.

- Brochures from the academic or certifying society in the field (listed under "For More Info").

- The Glaxo Pathway Evaluation Program, a free half-day seminar sometimes offered by the dean's office that helps you match your interests to different specialties. These seminars feature the Glaxo Medical Specialties Survey (1991), a catalog of medical specialties and subspecialties that includes descriptions, practitioner profiles, and anecdotal "picks and pans." Contact your student affairs office for details.

- Iserson KV, *Iserson's Getting into a Residency*, 7th ed., Tucson, AZ: Galen Press, 2006.

The trends in Match data are plotted for each specialty. One graph shows the yearly trends in number of positions offered and the number filled, which gives a sense of the competitiveness of the field. (Specialties that have high fill rates tend to be more competitive.) There is also a graph showing the percentage of positions filled overall and the percentage filled by U.S. seniors. The difference between these two numbers is the percentage of spots filled by independent applicants, who are primarily international medical graduates (IMGs). Fields that tend to have higher percentages of IMGs include family medicine and primary care. A graph showing the yearly unmatch rate is also shown. Note that this represents the unmatch rate for U.S. seniors who ranked only one specialty. However, it is not uncommon for students applying in the more competitive specialties to apply to a second field as a backup, rather than risk going unmatched. For example, students applying in plastic surgery frequently also apply in general surgery and rank the general surgery programs below the plastic surgery programs. Finally, a graph of the median income over several years is shown.

## REFERENCES

National Resident Matching Program, Results and Data. National Resident Matching Program, Washington, D.C., 2000-2010 (www.nrmp.org/data/index.html).

Physician Compensation and Production Survey 2009. Medical Group Management Association, Englewood, CO, 2009.

Medical Group Management Association (MGMA). Physician Compensation and Production Survey, 1999 to 2009.

American Association of Medical Colleges Careers in Medicine Web site. Careers in Medicine Specialty Pages, and top five most encountered conditions (services.aamc.org/careersinmedicine).

San Francisco Match data and statistics (www.sfmatch.org).

Washington University School of Medicine Residency Web site (residency.wustl.edu/medadmin/resweb.nsf).

## ANESTHESIOLOGY

Anesthesiologists are involved in many aspects and phases of patient care, and their footprints can be found in every area of the hospital. It is the anesthesiologist's primary goal to ensure the patient's well-being and safety at all times before, during, and after surgery. This begins with the preoperative evaluation, extends through the intraoperative management, and continues in the postanesthesia care unit, as well as potentially in the intensive care unit and pain management centers. Anesthesiologists function as highly trained consultants and are held in high regard for their extensive knowledge of physiology and pharmacology and for their technical skills.

> A good understanding of pharmacology, as well as the ability to make rapid decisions under pressure, are important in anesthesiology.

The desirable aspects of the practice of anesthesiology include intense hands-on care of patients, brief but positive doctor-patient interactions, a vast range of patient ages and health, career mobility, and above-average incomes. The consul-

# Quick Stats

## ANESTHESIOLOGY

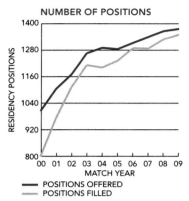

NUMBER OF POSITIONS

— POSITIONS OFFERED
— POSITIONS FILLED

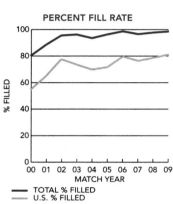

PERCENT FILL RATE

— TOTAL % FILLED
— U.S. % FILLED

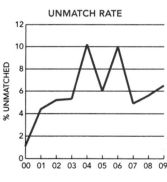

UNMATCH RATE

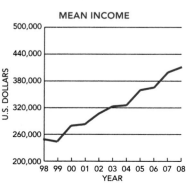

MEAN INCOME

tant role provides relatively predictable hours but frequent night shifts and call responsibilities. Although job opportunities are not as lucrative as in prior years, there is no shortage of job opportunities for new graduates. ACGME-accredited fellowship training in cardiothoracic anesthesia, pediatric anesthesia, critical care, or pain management is available and competitive.

## APPLICATION TIPS

Anesthesiology residency positions are becoming increasingly competitive. Most prestigious programs emphasize strong clerkships scores, above average USMLE scores, high medical school class standing, and strong letters of evaluation. Demonstration of an interest in physiology and pharmacology, either through strong basic science scores or research projects, is appealing. In addition, because anesthesiologists manage a multitude of medical conditions intraoperatively, strong clerkship grades in internal medicine are considered important.

Many anesthesiology programs are transitioning from a preliminary year plus three years of anesthesiology training to an integrated four-year program. Be sure to research each program to determine if you will need to apply for a preliminary year, and depending on the program, inquire whether interviews for separate preliminary positions can be made during the same visit.

## INTERVIEW TIPS

Interviews begin in November and continue into January. Ideal candidates commonly demonstrate strong interpersonal skills and proactive learning style, and have a passion in areas of life outside of medicine. Most resident education occurs during one-on-one interactions with an attending; therefore, candidates who can portray themselves as affable, organized, articulate, and quick-minded tend to be ranked higher. The ideal candidate also asks insightful questions about the residency program, such as the strength of the surgery department and its relationship with the anesthesiology department, board pass rates of graduates, research opportunities, exposure to subspecialties within anesthesiology, and the types of positions that graduates are offered.

Anesthesiologists view their jobs as stressful, requiring extreme vigilance and adaptability. It would be wise to save questions regarding call schedules, vacation, and lifestyle for the informal sessions with current residents. Programs in which candidates do not have ample opportunity to meet with residents should raise suspicions.

## FOR MORE INFO . . .

**American Society of Anesthesiologists, Medical Student Section**
www.asahq.org/msd/national.htm

*American Society of Anesthesiologists Information Packet.* This free career information packet includes general articles (of marginal value) on the specialty itself, a directory of anesthesiology training programs as listed in the Graduate Medical Education Directory, and a directory of fellowships for specialized training in pain management. The packet can be obtained by contacting:

**American Society of Anesthesiologists (ASA)**
520 North Northwest Highway
Park Ridge, IL 60068
(847) 825-5586
www.asahq.org

**Global Anesthesiology Server Network**
anestit.unipa.it/HomePage.html

## DERMATOLOGY

Dermatology is a specialty that focuses on only one organ—the skin—but encompasses a diverse range of fields, such as rheumatology, oncology, infectious disease, and pathology. Dermatology residents are trained to diagnose and treat both adult and pediatric patients. They see patients with malignant and benign disorders of the skin, as well as patients who present with the skin manifestations of systemic diseases. In addition, they are trained in specific surgical techniques used in dermatology and in dermatopathology. The field involves a combination of medicine, immunology, infectious disease, surgery, and pathology. It is this breadth of training that attracts many physicians.

Training in dermatology requires one year of internship followed by three years of residency. A strong preliminary medicine year is recommended since dermatology has a heavy emphasis on internal medicine, but any training involving clinical patient care, such as surgery or a transitional medicine year, may be acceptable. Be sure to check with individual programs to see which types of preliminary-year training they will accept. A small number of programs offer dermatology residency positions combined with a preliminary year in internal medicine. These are listed as categorical positions in the Electronic Residency Application Service (ERAS), and in 2009, 28 of these positions were offered.

While the dermatology residency is not overwhelmed with in-hospital hours, it requires a lot of studying. After completing internship, most of the first year of residency is spent learning the vocabulary, patterns, and morphology of skin lesions. After the first year, much time is spent on sharpening one's skills and gaining a deeper knowledge of the field. More specifically, residents learn about the vast number of genodermatoses (genetic dermatologic diseases) and rare cutaneous and systemic entities, while honing surgical skills (flaps, grafts, Mohs procedures) and expanding their understanding of dermatopathology. Depending on the program, one to two months each year are spent doing inpatient consultations, while the remainder of the time is spent at outpatient clinics, surgical centers, dermatopathology rotations, and electives. Most dermatology residency programs are extremely focused on teaching and have built-in academic time for resident learning.

Dermatology, more so than some other fields, is extremely patient oriented. As such, a good resident must be perceptive, detail oriented, conscientious, and kind. Most programs recommend that residents read approximately one hour per night on weeknights and devote one-half weekend day each week to studying dermatology. Since most dermatology programs are small, teamwork and respect for attendings, coresidents, nursing, and administrative staff is crucial. Self-motivation,

### TABLE 4-1

**Top Five Most Frequently Encountered Conditions in Anesthesiology**

1. Orthopedic procedures
2. Obstetrical and gynecologic procedures
3. Pain conditions
4. Cardiothoracic procedures
5. Abdominal procedures

### TABLE 4-2

**Selected Fellowship Training Opportunities in Anesthesiology**

Cardiac anesthesiology: 1 year

Critical care medicine: 1 or 2 years

Pain management: 1 year

Pediatric anesthesiology: 1 year

> Dermatology is heavily reliant on the physical examination, so residents must hone their skills in this area.

# Quick Stats

## DERMATOLOGY

### NUMBER OF POSITIONS

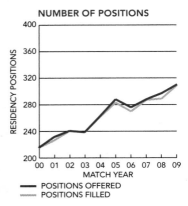

POSITIONS OFFERED
POSITIONS FILLED

### PERCENT FILL RATE

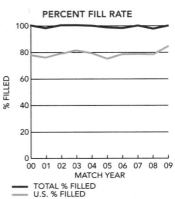

TOTAL % FILLED
U.S. % FILLED

### UNMATCH RATE

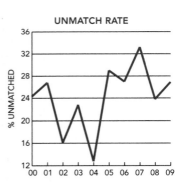

### MEAN INCOME

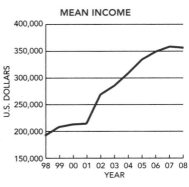

thorough history taking, creative approaches to patient issues, and evidence-based practice are all essential traits of a good dermatology resident.

Most dermatologists love their job and do not regret their choice of fields. The range of options they have after residency is one of the attractions often cited. There is flexibility in both the type of clinical practice environment and the number of hours worked. People in this specialty tend to rate the following values highly: independence, sufficient time off, variety, and working with people. Dermatologists in the United States today enjoy one of the most pleasant working environments of any specialty. They work the lowest number of hours per week on average while getting paid more than any other nonsurgical specialty. They also have a typically healthy patient population and are, to a large extent, immune to the increasing number of HMO-dictated regulations, as many patient visits are paid for out-of-pocket. One of the drawbacks is the lack of evidence-based medicine for many of the rare dermatological diseases. This can mean that treatment of these conditions may tend to be anecdotal, which can be frustrating. The field also suffers from a poor distribution of physicians: Most urban centers are saturated, while openings in more rural areas remain unfilled.

The choice of an academic career or a private practice is the biggest determinant of lifestyle after residency. Academia enables ample research opportunities, complicated patient cases, and continued learning. In academia, many institutions require clinical or basic science research combined with teaching and clinical practice. In contrast, private dermatology practices—like any other specialty—are businesses. Most appointments are scheduled in 5- to 15-minute blocks and efficiency is a necessity. Nonetheless, most private dermatologists average three to four workdays a week.

## APPLICATION TIPS

Given the competitive nature of dermatology, all aspects of the residency application are important. Dermatology programs screen applicants intensively before offering interviews to prospective residents. Many use AΩA status, at least three honors in clinical rotations, high board scores, and a top-notch Medical Student Performance Evaluation (MSPE) as preliminary considerations. Competitive programs often use the USMLE Step 1 score to screen applications, and research in dermatology is highly recommended. A glowing evaluation in the dermatology subinternship/elective and supportive letters of recommendation are vital as well. Applicants need to demonstrate more than just academic excellence.

Perhaps the most important aspect of the application in this field is the number of programs to apply to. All applicants, regardless of their curriculum vitae (CV), should apply to, interview at, and rank as many programs as they can (without violating the two rules of ranking outlined in Chapter 12). Be prepared to spend more than the national average on application and travel expenses. In 2009, there were 338 positions and a total of 567 applicants. It is not uncommon to apply in a second specialty as a backup plan.

## INTERVIEW TIPS

Be prepared to wait; most programs don't begin offering interviews until around Thanksgiving. Many interview dates will be during the months of December ("early" interviews), January, and February. Dermatology applicants have several things in common: stellar board scores, shining letters of recommendation, and impressive research experience. Therefore, program directors rely heavily on interviews to identify those few who will be ranked. Dermatology programs usually offer interviews to only 10–15% of their applicants. Many conduct multiple interviews per day (up to 12 to 15 interviews), each lasting anywhere from 8 to 30 minutes, so be prepared for a lot of questioning. Depending on the program, interviews may be conducted by individual faculty members or by a panel consisting of three or more interviewers.

Interviews are designed to measure applicants' interest in the specialty, to gauge the potential of each to contribute to the field, and to find out whether applicants would get along with the other people in the department. Applicants are rarely "pimped" but will be expected to discuss any prior research or involvement in dermatology both intelligently and in detail. If it doesn't work out the first time around, there are many "back door" entrances to dermatology, mainly through one- to two-year research fellowships, where, upon completing your research time, you have a very good chance of securing a spot in the residency program. Bottom line: If you want it badly enough, you can probably make it happen regardless of your board scores and medical school grades.

### FOR MORE INFO . . .

**American Academy of Dermatology**
www.aad.org/index.html

## REFERENCES

Rubenstein DS, Blauvelt A, Chen SC, Darling TN. The future of academic dermatology in the United States: report on the resident retreat for future physician-scientists, June 15–17, 2001. *J Am Acad Dermatol* 47(2):300–303, 2002.

Todd MM, Miller JJ, Ammirati CT. Dermatologic surgery training in residency. *Dermatol Surg* 28(7):547–549, 2002.

> There is a shortage of dermatologists in many rural areas in the United States.

> A track record in dermatology research is considered a big plus.

### TABLE 4-3

**Top Five Most Frequently Encountered Conditions in Dermatology**

1. Acne
2. Eczema
3. Skin cancer
4. Psoriasis
5. Warts

### TABLE 4-4

**Selected Fellowship Training Opportunities in Dermatology**

Dermatopathology: 1 year

Pediatric dermatopathology: 1 or 2 years

## EMERGENCY MEDICINE

Emergency medicine (EM) focuses on the triage, diagnosis, and implementation of potentially life-sustaining measures in acute illnesses and injury. EM physicians typically work in shifts and do not provide longitudinal care; rather, they quickly diagnose and stabilize patients with emergent physical and psychological conditions until the patients can receive definitive care in the ED or elsewhere, or can be safely discharged with appropriate follow-up. EM physicians have a broad base

# Quick Stats

## EMERGENCY MEDICINE

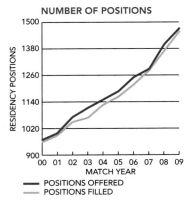

**NUMBER OF POSITIONS**

POSITIONS OFFERED
POSITIONS FILLED

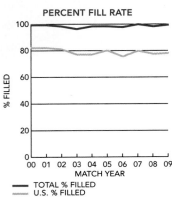

**PERCENT FILL RATE**

TOTAL % FILLED
U.S. % FILLED

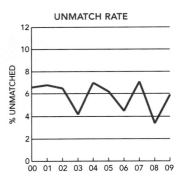

**UNMATCH RATE**

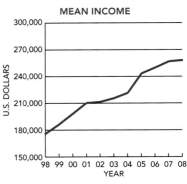

**MEAN INCOME**

of medical knowledge since they can encounter literally any disease on a given day. They are also the gatekeepers to the hospital, as a large proportion of hospital admissions come through the ED.

Residency programs in EM are unique in that they require either three or four years of total training. There has been talk in the past about standardizing the amount of training required, but this has yet to materialize. Both the three- and four-year programs must meet basic requirements to be accredited, and residents trained in both types of programs are competent physicians upon completion of the residency. The main difference often comes in the amount of elective time—one or two months in three-year programs and up to six months in four-year programs. In most cases, the internship year is integrated with the main EM training, which follows a traditional model of graduated responsibility. A few programs, called PGY 2–4 programs, do not have an integrated internship year, and require a separate preliminary year in medicine, surgery, or transitional medicine (although you do not have to do this at the same hospital). If you apply to hospitals that have PGY two- to four-year programs, be sure to apply separately for a preliminary or transitional year, and find out what type of training is preferred or required at your programs of interest! If you are considering a three-year program, make sure that program offers the number of patients and level of acuity you will need to acquire an adequate education in the three-year period. Also, if you are planning to pursue a fellowship afterwards, try to find out if the three-year program gives you enough exposure in your area of interest.

The bulk of EM training time is spent in emergency rooms, learning resuscitation techniques and treating both medical and trauma-related illnesses. However, residents also rotate through specialties such as medicine, pediatrics, OB/GYN, surgery, anesthesiology, orthopedic surgery, and the intensive care units. Different programs place "off-service" rotations in different years throughout the residency. Once you have interviewed at various programs, several factors will determine which programs you will rank more favorably. A recent study of residents just completing the EM match process revealed that the top five factors that they considered when choosing a program included friendliness (95%), environment (87%), perception of the program during the interview day (81%), academics (76%), and location (74%).

EM physicians require confidence and strength of character, but more importantly, they should have genuine concern for their patients. Patients who come to the ED are often having the worst day of their lives, whether it is due to a serious illness, a myocardial infarction, a motor vehicle collision, a self-inflicted wound, or a drug overdose. Not surprisingly, the ability to communicate well with patients is essential.

EM can certainly be challenging. It can be difficult to keep emotions in check during stressful situations, and it can be frustrating not to have enough time to completely treat or accurately diagnose a patient during their short time in the ED. It can sometimes require a high tolerance level for people yelling at you or becoming frantic and desperate for your help. A cool, calm, and collected personality is best suited for this field, along with a strong stomach. Diversity, unpredictability, and the demand for a quick and accurate diagnosis are frequently mentioned as attractions of this field. An advanced rotation is imperative to figure out if this field is for you. If your medical school has the opportunity, try to see emergency departments at multiple hospitals, including those that run like clockwork and those that are overpopulated and understaffed.

Over the past ten years, a number of hospitals and academic centers have added EM departments to their services, and many of these departments house residencies. Historically, EM is infamous for a high burnout rate. However, it is the youngest board-certified specialty (primary board status was not granted until 1989), so it is difficult to determine whether physicians who were trained in EM more recently will show the same burnout rate in future years. The ED can be stressful and night shifts can drag on, but the EM resident's mantra is that he or she can always go home at the end of the shift.

> EM is a field for those who love the constant activity and fast pace of the ED.

EM has enjoyed considerable growth in popularity over the past few years, and with good reason. Relatively abundant free time, high pay, and the ability to integrate medicine with surgical procedures all add to this field's appeal. Postresidency academic pursuits and fellowships can range from the exotic (international health, disaster/rescue medicine, and hyperbaric medicine) to the more commonplace (ultrasound, pediatrics, and toxicology). EM is one of the only specialties in which a graduating resident may have a chance at an attending position straight out of residency.

> Burnout has historically been high in EM, though this may be changing.

## APPLICATION TIPS

Given the competitive nature of EM, all aspects of the residency application are important. It is especially crucial to do well in an EM rotation and to ask for strong letters of recommendation from one of the attending physicians. EM has adopted the use of a standardized letter of recommendation (SLOR), typically completed by the residency program director for each student applying in EM. Having a standardized letter allows programs to more easily and rapidly evaluate and compare students. The SLOR contains various criteria by which the student is graded, such as personality, clinical capability, and commitment to EM. A copy of the SLOR can be downloaded from www.cordem.org/slor.htm. It is a good idea to look through it to see the kind of things program directors will be evaluating. Letters from surgery, medicine, pediatrics, or OB/GYN are also well regarded, but your application should contain at least one very strong EM letter.

EM remains a relatively close-knit field, especially at the attending level, so personal contact between attendings can be very helpful. If your program director or an attending is willing to "go to bat for you," consider having him or her make a phone call to your top program after you have finished interviewing. Remember, he or she can make only one phone call, so make sure it is to the program that you are ranking first.

To improve your chances at a highly competitive program, consider doing an externship at that institution, especially if you are not particularly strong on paper—and be prepared to excel during that externship. Some competitive programs are known to use the USMLE Step 1 score to screen applications. Any research, especially in EM, should be highlighted, and the physician with whom you did the research should write the "nonclinical" letter for your application.

Your application should also reflect your outside interests. In EM, perhaps

## TABLE 4-5

**Top Five Most Frequently Encountered Conditions in Emergency Medicine**

1. Acute trauma/injury/fractures
2. Angina/chest pain/coronary disease
3. Infectious diseases
4. Abdominal pain
5. Musculoskeletal pain

## TABLE 4-6

**Selected Fellowship Training Opportunities in Emergency Medicine**

Disaster medicine: 1 or 2 years

Emergency ultrasound/imaging: 1 or 2 years

EMS/pre-hospital: 1 or 2 years

Medical toxicology: 2 years

Pediatric EM: 2 years

Sports medicine: 1 or 2 years

Undersea and hyperbaric medicine: 1 to 3 years

International medicine: 1 year

Wilderness medicine: 1 year

Palliative care: 1 year

Internal medicine critical care: 2 years

more than in many other fields, camaraderie is crucial during long shifts. People want to know that the resident with whom they are working is relatively fun and interesting. So let that show through in your application. All applications and supporting material except for the MSPE should be submitted by late September. Your MSPE will be automatically added in early November, but some programs offer interviews before receiving the MSPE. The optimal number of applications to submit depends on the candidate's strength, but many suggest that 25 to 30 applications be submitted to yield 10 to 15 interviews. Timing of the interviews does not appear to affect selection committee rankings.

As with other fields, it is important for you to decide what type of program best fits your interests. Whether you are at an academic or county program, whether the program is three or four years, at a small or large institution, will have a significant impact on your training. If you are very interested in a program but are not invited to interview, it is acceptable to call or e-mail that program and express your level of interest. Often, the program will review your application with your level of interest in mind to see if they can accommodate you, especially when interview spots open up later in the interview season.

## INTERVIEW TIPS

On your interview day, expect three to four interview sessions typically lasting 15 to 30 minutes each. Interviews are conducted by residency directors, other attendings, and occasionally by residents. At one or two of the larger county programs a charge nurse may conduct interviews as well. In general, EM interviewers are relaxed, friendly, and genuinely interested both in giving information about their programs and in learning more about the applicant's personality and their life outside of medicine.

You should also come up with as many specific questions as you can regarding the hospital at which you are interviewing, as you will repeatedly be asked, "So, do you have any questions?" Interviewers will also ask what other programs you are applying to. Answer politely and honestly, and remember that the world of EM is small, so do not "trash talk" other programs even if your interviewer does so. Be sure to write thank-you notes when you get home from the interview unless you were specifically asked not to.

## FOR MORE INFO . . .

*ACEP Student Information Packet.* This packet includes a directory of emergency medicine training programs. To obtain a copy, write or call:

**American College of Emergency Physicians**
P.O. Box 619911
Dallas, TX 75261-9911
(972) 550-0911
(800) 798-1822
www.acep.org

**Emergency Medicine Residents' Association (EMRA).** In addition to the general information packet, you may wish to have a student membership in EMRA. A $45 annual fee provides you with a subscription to *Annals of Emergency Medicine*, *ACEP News* (a monthly newsletter), *EM Resident* (a bimonthly newsletter), and access to specialty meetings and conferences. Since the medical student affiliate (MSA) branch of EMRA was created in 1992, most information has been geared toward residents. To enroll, contact:

**Emergency Medicine Residents' Association**
1125 Executive Circle
Irving, Texas 75038-2522
(972) 550-0920
www.emra.org

**Society for Academic Emergency Medicine (SAEM)**
901 North Washington Avenue
Lansing, MI 48906-5137
(517) 485-5484
www.saem.org

**American Academy of Emergency Medicine (AAEM)**
555 East Wells Street Suite 1100
Milwaukee, WI 53202
(800) 884-2236
www.aaem.org

Delbridge TR. *Emergency Medicine in Focus: A Handbook for Medical Students and Prospective Residents.* A compact guide to the emergency medicine residency application process, it is available to EMRA/MSA members for $15. To order, call ACEP Publications, (800) 798–1822.

Koscove EM. An applicant's evaluation of an emergency medicine internship and residency. *Ann Emerg Med* 19:774, 1990. This article offers an exhaustive collection of factors to consider when applying for and interviewing at EM training programs.

## REFERENCES

DeSantis M and Marco CA. Emergency medicine residency selection: Factors influencing candidate decisions. *Acad Emerg Med* 12(6):559–561, 2005.

Gallagher EJ. Evolution of academic emergency medicine over a decade (1991–2001). *Acad Emerg Med* 9(10):995–1000, 2002.

Martin-Lee L, Park H, Overton DT. Does interview date affect match list position in the emergency medicine national residency matching program match? *Acad Emerg Med* 7(9):1022–1026, 2000.

## FAMILY MEDICINE

Family medicine (also called family practice) embraces the biopsychosocial model in its treatment of individuals and of the family as a whole. It is one of the few fields that allows you to treat patients of all ages and to provide care for medical, surgical, gynecological, obstetric, and psychiatric problems. Students entering fam-

# Quick Stats

## FAMILY MEDICINE

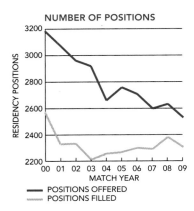

NUMBER OF POSITIONS

— POSITIONS OFFERED
— POSITIONS FILLED

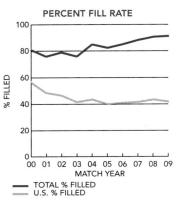

PERCENT FILL RATE

— TOTAL % FILLED
— U.S. % FILLED

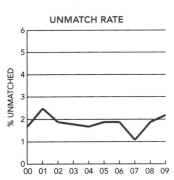

UNMATCH RATE

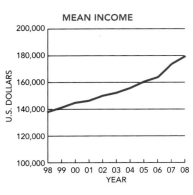

MEAN INCOME

ily practice have a strong commitment to primary care and enjoy the wide variety of patients and clinical problems encountered in this specialty. They usually enjoy forming long-term relationships with patients, working with people, and seeing a range of patients and diseases, primarily in the outpatient setting.

Family medicine graduates enjoy good job prospects throughout the country. This specialty has historically been popular among IMGs. In one recent comprehensive study, 42.8% of 2723 family medicine physicians stated that they were very satisfied with their career. This compares favorably to internal medicine, where 36.5% were very satisfied, and is similar to pediatrics, in which 48.1% were very satisfied.

In an academic center, the family practice graduate can often be an attending physician right out of residency. In some academic centers, the family physician is well respected for his or her breadth of knowledge and commitment to primary patient care. In other settings, the family physician may not be afforded due respect. Although subspecialty opportunities are limited, sports medicine and geriatrics are possible areas of further training. Geriatric medicine has a high career satisfaction rate, and opportunities in this area can only increase with the aging population. However, declining Medicare reimbursement rates may be an overriding negative for this specialty.

After residency, family medicine doctors have some flexibility and can tailor their practice somewhat to suit their interests. They can choose to see more adult or pediatric patients and can choose whether or not to care for obstetric patients. While family practitioners who perform obstetrics tend to have slightly higher income, their malpractice insurance premiums also tend to be higher.

In family medicine, there is relatively little consensus about the "best" programs to approach. You will generally be able to identify only the most "popular" programs, which depends on geographic region and setting—university versus community versus rural. Note that curricula vary with geography, especially in the amount of obstetrics taught. The most formal training and education are afforded by a university setting; however, family practice may be negatively affected by strong internal medicine and specialty programs. Community-based programs that are the only residency in a particular hospital may offer some advantages; however, specialty training and didactic teaching often suffer.

## APPLICATION TIPS

Graduates with strong academic credentials will receive the red-carpet treatment in family medicine residency programs. This is especially true in academic medical centers, where good family medicine residents are valued as role models for students. Programs want to see a strong commitment to family medicine, and they particularly value a mature, well-rounded personality. Some programs may be sensitive to your reasons for choosing family practice over internal medicine (especially primary care internal medicine) and will want to see a demonstrated interest in OB/GYN and pediatrics.

## INTERVIEW TIPS

Interviews are likely to be upbeat and supportive. Applicants have a particularly difficult task in information gathering, as assessment of the departments of pediatrics and OB/GYN is also important. The student needs to express the joy of patient care in and of itself, regardless of whether a particular case is "interesting."

Over 50% of residency spots have been filled by IMGs in recent years.

### FOR MORE INFO . . .

**American Academy of Family Physicians (AAFP)**
11400 Tomahawk Creek Parkway
Leawood, KS 66211-2672
(913) 906-6000
(800) 274-2237
www.aafp.org

**AAFP student membership.** For a one-time fee of $15 you can become a student member of the AAFP. The AAFP has a number of publications, many complimentary, aimed at medical students considering family practice. These include *Facts About Family Practice*. Geared toward number crunchers, this book includes detailed statistics about family practice.

**TABLE 4-7**

**Top Five Most Frequently Encountered Conditions in Family Medicine**

1. Hypertension
2. Diabetes
3. Upper respiratory infection
4. Anxiety/depression
5. Hypercholesterolemia/ hyperlipidemia

## REFERENCES

Koehn NN, Fryer GE, Phillips RL, Miller JB, Green LA. The increase in international medical graduates in family medicine residency programs. *Fam Med* 34(6):429–435, 2002.

Leigh JP, Kravitz RL, Schembri M, Samuels SJ, Mobley S. Physician career satisfaction across specialties. *Arch Intern Med* 162:1577–1584, 2002.

**TABLE 4-8**

**Selected Fellowship Training Opportunities in Family Medicine**

| |
|---|
| Geriatric medicine: 1 year |
| Sports medicine: 1 year |

## GENERAL SURGERY

A residency in general surgery provides training in a broad array of surgical techniques and fields. General surgeons primarily treat diseases of the abdomen, breasts, skin, neck, and vasculature. They care for a range of patients, from those who are relatively healthy to those who have experienced major trauma, such as gunshot wounds or motor vehicle accidents, and those who are critically ill. In addition to intraoperative expertise, general surgeons must know how to evaluate patients preoperatively and manage them postoperatively, including those patients who require intensive care.

General surgery abounds with both positive and negative attributes, all of which influence students' thinking about a career in the field. The specialty boasts a number of benefits: the chance to apply technical and procedural skills toward the quick resolution of medical problems, gratification from having a dramatic impact on patients' health, good doctor-patient relationships, and relatively high income. Drawbacks include long hours, rigorous training, increasing paperwork, and the intrusion of prickly nonclinical issues such as malpractice liability, government regulations, and third-party payers.

Apply in general surgery only if you truly love to be in the operating room.

# Quick Stats

## GENERAL SURGERY

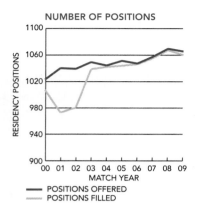

NUMBER OF POSITIONS

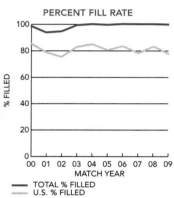

PERCENT FILL RATE

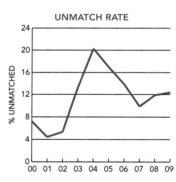

UNMATCH RATE

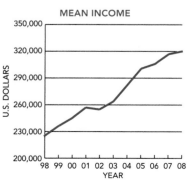

MEAN INCOME

It is often challenging for residents to balance their commitment to work and life outside the hospital. Surgery, by its very nature, is extremely demanding—both physically and emotionally—although this is also why the field is so rewarding. Generally, most surgeons remain highly satisfied with their work, notwithstanding the changes they have been forced to make in their practices to accommodate HMOs and other complications.

Above and beyond anything else, to thrive as a surgeon you have to love being in the operating room. You also have to be a hard worker, be able to function without much sleep, and work well under pressure. People who panic easily are not well suited for a career in surgery. You have to be confident and resourceful, but also know your own limits and know when to ask for help.

Surgical residencies require a minimum of five years of training, with some programs requiring as many as three additional research years. These often come in the middle or latter portion of the residency, at a time when residents can also moonlight. General surgery residents should expect to work the full 80-hour workweek and take in-house call for the entire duration of the residency. After completing general surgery residency, it is possible to go into practice right away without further specialization. However, it is becoming more and more common for general surgery residency graduates to pursue fellowship training.

The "bread and butter" general surgery cases include appendectomies, cholecystectomies, hernia repairs, breast surgeries, colon surgeries, and exploratory laparotomies. Some general surgeons may do more advanced oncologic cases or vascular surgery, depending upon the variety of specialists available where they practice.

As an attending, the type of patients you will be caring for and the hours you will keep are hugely variable, depending upon whether you decide to specialize and whether you are in academic or private practice. Academic practice carries with it the extra responsibilities of participating in research and teaching. General surgeons tend to take care of many emergencies, which means it is difficult to have a regular schedule. Even in a group practice, you will to be called upon to evaluate and care for patients at all hours. Certain subspecialties within general surgery, such as breast or endocrine surgery, tend to have few emergencies and therefore allow more predictable lifestyles.

## APPLICATION TIPS

Surgeons are hands-on people; they know things by seeing them. Applicants are no different. General surgery, like many surgical subspecialties, places great currency in the subinternship. It is therefore strongly recommended that applicants who are examining competitive programs consider doing an away rotation at that location. Before applying, you should think about whether you would be happier in a clinical or a research-oriented program, bearing in mind that the length of training can vary from one type of program to the other. Most academic programs are seven years in length, and community programs are five years.

Strong evaluations in the senior surgical rotations are generally essential to successful applications. The pièce de résistance would be a strong letter from the chief of the surgery department. Programs with an academic slant will definitely consider the applicant's research background fundamental to the evaluation process, whereas those with a clinical focus will attempt to determine the applicant's potential from that standpoint.

In a recent retrospective study, the most important applicant attributes were found to be enthusiasm, work ethic, and ability. It is helpful to find a mentor who is well known in the field and can advocate for you and advise you. As with other competitive residencies, early completion of application material is important. Although the desired number of applications depends on the applicant's quality, the average ranges from 15 to 20, with a goal of obtaining at least 10 to 12 interviews.

## INTERVIEW TIPS

The field of surgery is infamous for having some of the most colorful personalities in medicine. However, while the brilliant attending transplant surgeon may well be revered for his skill and feared for his outbursts of temper, no one is looking for the latter quality in a resident. Although interview committees often have a good idea of how they are going to rank you before they even meet you, the interview is an essential part of the process, if only to eliminate interpersonally challenged applicants.

Uniquely, surgical interview days are usually held on Saturdays, making it difficult for applicants to schedule more than one interview in a single trip. Interviews often consist of two to three sessions lasting 30 to 45 minutes each. Occasionally, an applicant is asked to present a clinical case or to discuss how to deal with the stress of a surgical residency. You should have a prepared answer to this latter question in particular. Interviews are often laid back, with little or no pimping. However, academic programs tend to opt for more pointed questions and may inquire about your research background as well as any current projects. Try to learn something about the program's reputation for research before your interview day.

### FOR MORE INFO . . .

Johansen K, Heimbach DM. *So You Want to Be a Surgeon: A Medical Student Guide to Finding and Matching with the Best Possible Surgery Residency.* This book includes a brief but very helpful discussion of surgical residency applications. The greater part of the book is devoted to descriptions of most of the surgery programs in the United States and Puerto Rico. The authors attempt to classify programs by the caliber of the house staff. The book can be accessed online at www.facs.org/residencysearch/. The book is also in some medical bookstores and can also be ordered for about $12 from:

**Educational Clearinghouse**
Department of Surgery
Southern Illinois University
School of Medicine
P.O. Box 19230
Springfield, IL 62794
(217) 785-3835

> Attitude and enthusiasm go a long way in surgery.

## TABLE 4-9

**Top Five Most Frequently Encountered Conditions in General Surgery**

1. Breast disease
2. Gall bladder disease
3. Hernias
4. Gastrointestinal cancer
5. Acute abdomen or appendicitis

## TABLE 4-10

**Selected Fellowship Training Opportunities in General Surgery**

Breast surgery: 1 year

Cardiothoracic surgery: 2–3 years

Colorectal surgery: 1 year

Critical care medicine: 1 or 2 years

Hand surgery: 1 year

Minimally invasive surgery: 1 year

Pediatric surgery: 2 years

Surgical critical care: 1 year

Surgical oncology: 1 or 2 years

Transplant surgery: 1 or 2 years

Vascular surgery: 1 or 2 years

*The Surgical Career Handbook.* This glossy booklet provides an overview of surgery and profiles its subspecialties. However, the information is often too general to be useful. This publication is available for $7 from:

**American College of Surgeons (ACS)**
633 North Saint Clair Street
Chicago, IL 60611
(312) 202-5000
www.facs.org

## REFERENCES

Dunnington GL, Williams RG. Addressing the new competencies for residents' surgical training. *Acad Med* 78(1):14–21, 2003.

Gilbart MK, Cusimano MD, Regehr G. Evaluating surgical resident selection procedures. *Am J Surg* 18(3):221–225, 2001.

Mayer KL, Perez RV, Ho HS. Factors affecting choice of surgical residency training program. *J Surg Res* 98(2):71–75, 2001.

## INTERNAL MEDICINE

> Internal medicine remains the most popular residency choice among U.S. medical students and IMGs.

Internal medicine physicians are typically the main medical practitioners in the United States. They focus on providing longitudinal, personalized, and comprehensive care for adults of all ages. Internists must be adept at diagnosing, managing, and treating a wide variety of acute and chronic medical conditions, from the very common to the unusual and complicated. Therefore, internal medicine requires a broad understanding of all organ systems and provides the opportunity of working in a hospital setting, an office practice, or both.

Internists also serve an essential function in promoting disease prevention and men's and women's health maintenance, typically through disease screening and regular physical examinations. Because of the lasting relationships formed, internists frequently help patients with substance abuse and mental health issues. Internal medicine physicians coordinate care and refer patients to specialists when appropriate and often are able to help patients navigate the health care system.

> Traditional internal medicine programs and primary care programs differ primarily in the amount of time spent treating ambulatory patients. Both paths can lead to subspecialty training.

Students are often attracted to internal medicine because of the opportunity for extensive patient contact and continuity of care while still leaving the door open for further subspecialty training. Internists often identify with characteristics such as compassion, a genuine interest in patients and medicine, diligence, good judgment, and the ability to synthesize information quickly and correctly. As there are inevitably difficult times when practicing medicine, it helps to have a sense of humor as well.

> Internal medicine offers a broad spectrum of subspecialty possibilities.

In many ways, too, internal medicine requires the regular use of skills that brought students to medical school in the first place: decision making, a vast knowledge base, and a commitment to patient care. However, this can also be a drawback as some residents cite this ever-expanding knowledge base as one of the field's challenges. In a career satisfaction survey conducted by Leigh et al., only 36.5% of internists described themselves as very satisfied with their field;

specialists were more satisfied. Specialties with the highest satisfaction rates, such as geriatrics (59.6% very satisfied), medical oncology (50.5% very satisfied), and infectious disease (50.0% very satisfied), actually ranked higher than orthopedic surgery, ophthalmology, and plastic surgery. Although it has lost some popularity among U.S. graduates, internal medicine is still by far the most commonly chosen residency program.

Internal medicine programs are usually three years in length and are divided into categorical ("traditional") programs and primary care programs. Traditional medicine offers more of an inpatient focus plus electives for sampling different subspecialties. Residents in primary care medicine have more outpatient experience and often receive additional training in gynecology and pediatrics. However, this distinction is blurring as traditional programs increasingly require significant ambulatory care training. Students going into primary care internal medicine are typically committed to primary care but are not as interested in the obstetrics, pediatrics, and surgical assisting experience offered by family practice. That said, many residents from traditional programs enter primary care, and conversely, many from primary care programs enter a subspecialty.

More than half of those who choose internal medicine continue their training in one of the many fellowships available (see Table 4-12). Hence, there is enormous flexibility in internal medicine, with areas of practice including primary care ambulatory careers, highly technical specialties such as interventional cardiology, and purely hospital-based practices without ambulatory patient management. Internal medicine training can be combined with other specialties. Combined programs include medicine–pediatrics, medicine–psychiatry, medicine–rehabilitation, medicine–preventive medicine, and medicine–emergency medicine.

## APPLICATION TIPS

U.S. graduates do not typically have a difficult time matching into one of the numerous excellent programs available. At the same time, there is considerable variability among program directors and committees with regard to which part of the application is weighted most heavily. Very competitive programs value high grades in medical clerkships and subinternships, as well as high class rank. Interest or accomplishments in research are highly regarded in academic programs. Internal medicine residents must also be good teachers of medical students if they are to make medicine clerkships work well, so an interest in teaching is always welcome!

If there is a particular program that is of special interest to you, it might be worthwhile to arrange an away elective to solidify your interest and demonstrate your capability. Many advisors suggest that students opt for a subspecialty elective rather than a subinternship, as it may be easier to make a good impression in a less rigorous and perhaps more academic subspecialty experience. It is reasonable to apply to at least 10 to 15 programs. However, depending on the strength of your application, you may wish to apply to more than this in order to improve your chances of matching.

# Quick Stats

## INTERNAL MEDICINE

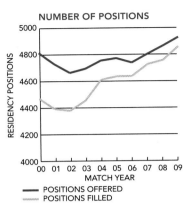

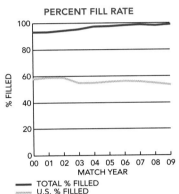

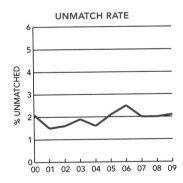

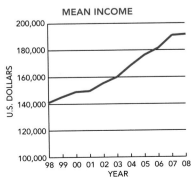

> Being a team player is an important characteristic of a good medicine resident.

## TABLE 4-11

### Top Five Most Frequently Encountered Conditions in Internal Medicine

1. Diabetes mellitus
2. Hypertension
3. Heart disease
4. Hyperlipidemias
5. Upper respiratory infections

## TABLE 4-12

### Selected Fellowship Training Opportunities in Internal Medicine

Cardiac electrophysiology: 1 year

Cardiology: 3 years

Critical care medicine: 1 or 2 years

Endocrinology: 2 years

Gastroenterology: 3 years

Geriatric medicine: 2 years

Hematology: 2 years

Hematology and oncology: 3 years

Infectious disease: 2 years

Interventional cardiology: 1 year (following a cardiology fellowship)

Medical genetics: 2 to 4 years

Nephrology: 2 years

Oncology: 2 years

Pulmonary disease: 2 years

Pulmonary disease and critical care medicine: 3 years

Rheumatology: 2 years

Sports medicine: 1 year

## INTERVIEW TIPS

There are no typical schedules or interview days in internal medicine. Several interviews lasting 15 to 30 minutes each is the common format. Time is often spent giving applicants information about the strengths of the particular program. It is very rare for applicants to present cases or be asked factual questions. However, program directors will almost always want to know about your choice of internal medicine versus various specialties. There is no "right answer" to these questions, just make sure your answer is well thought out. Be prepared to discuss your career interests, why you are interested in a particular program, and, in a nonegocentric fashion, talk about your personal strengths. An excellent work ethic is a quality that all program directors will value.

## FOR MORE INFO . . .

**American College of Physicians (ACP)**
190 North Independence Mall
West Philadelphia, PA 19106-1572
(800) 523-1546, ext. 2600
(215) 351-2600
www.acponline.org

**American College of Preventive Medicine (ACPM)**
1307 New York Avenue, N.W., Suite 200
Washington, D.C. 20005
(202) 466-2044
www.acpm.org

**American Geriatrics Society (AGS)**
Empire State Building
350 Fifth Avenue, Suite 801
New York, NY 10118
(212) 308-1414
www.americangeriatrics.org

**American Gastroenterological Association**
4930 Del Ray Avenue
Bethesda, MD 20814
(301) 654-2055
www.gastro.org

## REFERENCE

Leigh JP, Kravitz RL, Schembri M, Samuels SJ, Mobley S. Physician career satisfaction across specialties. *Arch Intern Med* 162:1577–1584, 2002.

## INTERNAL MEDICINE–PEDIATRICS

Internal medicine–pediatrics (med-peds) training and practice integrate the disciplines of both internal medicine and pediatrics. Similar to family medicine training, med-peds physicians care for patients throughout their lives in inpatient and outpatient settings. Therefore, a comprehensive breadth of knowledge concerning acute and chronic diseases afflicting anyone from newborns to geriatric patients is necessary. This remarkable versatility allows practitioners to follow many career options, such as researcher, hospitalist, specialist, outpatient practitioner, public health advocate, or hospital administrator.

Internal medicine–pediatrics is a growing field in medicine. This combined program began in 1967 (even before the first family medicine residency) and currently has more than 4500 practitioners nationwide and 1500 residents. This field is sought by those who find continuity of care and close, long-term doctor-patient relationships rewarding. Residents often enter this field because there are too many things that they love about being a physician to be able to narrow the choice to one specialty or patient population.

Two key characteristics needed to succeed in a med-peds residency are the ability to communicate well with patients and families and a love of clinical practice. While communication skills are essential to all specialties, it is important to recognize that there are nuances to being able to work effectively with both sick children and their parents, as well as sick adults and their children (who may be serving as caretakers). Med-peds residents learn to smoothly function with a foot in both worlds as they move from integrated clinics where a newborn weight check may be followed by a routine follow-up for a middle-aged adult with diabetes and hypertension, to the inpatient floors, emergency department, and a variety of critical care settings. They especially have a niche in caring for chronic "pediatric" health conditions that continue to affect a patient into adulthood (eg, congenital heart disease and cystic fibrosis).

Although many med-peds practitioners describe this variety as an attraction to the field, it can also be challenging to constantly enter new environments. Each ward within the hospital typically has its own culture and way of functioning, and residents can feel overwhelmed trying to navigate the transitions from week to week. Additionally, a common complaint among second- and third-year med-peds residents is that they feel academically behind when they compare themselves to categorical colleagues, whose knowledge and experience base will necessarily grow faster. Although this discrepancy tends to even out during the fourth year of training, it is often a source of angst up until that point.

The four-year med-peds residency, unlike family medicine residency, does not include any formal obstetrical or surgical training; instead, it provides more thorough training in adult and pediatric medicine. The resident schedules need to meet the requirements of both the internal medicine and pediatrics licensing boards. As a result, med-peds schedules tend to be weighted more toward floor and ICU rotations, with a lot of overnight call time and a minimum of electives. Once the four-year residency is complete, med-peds physicians are board eligible in both internal medicine and pediatrics. On average, board pass rates are greater than or equal to categorical internal medicine or pediatric physicians.

Med-peds graduates have the ability to fill unique niches in the health care community. According to the National Med-Peds Resident Association (NMPRA), the top three postresidency career paths are primary care (approximately 50% of graduates), fellowship/subspecialty (approximately 25% of graduates), and the hospitalist track (approximately 15% of graduates). Of those who enter primary care, more than 75% will choose to care for both adults and children, and nearly half will have some type of academic affiliation as well. For those

## Quick Stats

### INTERNAL MEDICINE– PEDIATRICS

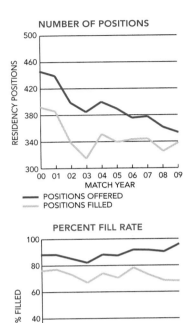

NUMBER OF POSITIONS

POSITIONS OFFERED
POSITIONS FILLED

PERCENT FILL RATE

TOTAL % FILLED
U.S. % FILLED

> Med-peds allows you to have great breadth of learning.

who enter fellowship training, there are opportunities to train in either adult- or pediatric-specific subspecialties, or to participate in a combined med-peds subspecialty training program.

No surveys have been done to determine the mean income for med-peds physicians, but it is estimated to be similar to that of other generalists (ie, pediatrics, internal medicine, and family practice). Following residency, a broad range of fellowships is available. Many fellowships offer training in both the adult and pediatric field; for example, you could pursue an integrated adult/pediatric infectious disease fellowship. Alternatively, you could pursue training in just the adult or pediatric realm.

## APPLICATION TIPS

In general, the limited number of med-peds positions nationally makes these programs more competitive than their parent categorical programs. Even so, most determined applicants do not have a problem obtaining a position. Students generally apply to 15 to 20 programs and hope for a comfortable 10 interviews. However, the number of programs you should apply to depends highly on the strength of your application. Programs will want to sense your desire to work with both children and adults. Extracurricular activities and your personal statement are perfect places in which to emphasize this desire. In addition, strong grades in both pediatric and internal medicine clerkships as well as excellent letters of support from faculty members in both fields are essential. Finding the time to successfully complete a subinternship in internal medicine, pediatrics, is also important.

## INTERVIEW TIPS

During the interview process, you will interview with both the internal medicine and pediatrics departments at each institution, which usually makes the interview a two-day event. Programs will want to see well-rounded, dedicated candidates with a strong desire to work with both children and adults. Candidates should be able to confidently explain why they chose to pursue med-peds training instead of family practice. In addition, as with all generalist fields in medicine, excellent communication skills are highly favored. Make sure you schedule enough time between interviews at different institutions to keep yourself from getting burned out. The two-day interviews can be tiring, and you want to be your best on each day.

> During the interview, make sure you are prepared to explain your choice of med-peds over pediatrics, medicine, or family practice.

## FOR MORE INFO . . .

**National Med-Peds Residents' Association (NMPRA)**
www.medpeds.org

**Guidelines for Combined Internal Medicine/Pediatrics Residency Training**
www.acgme.org/acWebsite/RRC_sharedDocs/sh_medPedREq.pdf

**American Academy of Pediatrics (AAP) Med-Peds Section**
www.aap.org/sections/med-peds/

## REFERENCE

NMPRA. *Introduction to Med-Peds Pamphlet, November 2008.* (medpeds.org/medpeds/NMPRApamphlet.pdf).

# NEUROLOGICAL SURGERY

A neurological surgeon provides the operative treatment for disorders of the central, peripheral, and autonomic nervous systems, along with the relevant ancillary structures and vasculature. However, neurosurgeons also give more comprehensive care by being involved in the evaluation, critical care, and rehabilitation of patients with neurosurgical conditions. The brain is what makes us uniquely human. Neurosurgery allows a unique view into this complicated organ, and new technology allows treatment of neurological disease in previously unimagined ways. The dynamic nature of this field as well as the rising prevalence of neurological disease makes neurosurgery an exciting field to explore.

> Neurosurgery requires a lifestyle choice as well as a professional one.

Training in neurological surgery begins with a one-year internship, which is typically split between general surgery and neurology, followed by five to six years of residency in neurosurgery. Neurosurgical ICU and floor management usually begins during the second year of residency. A minimum of 36 months of training must be spent in clinical neurosurgery, along with three months in clinical neurology and three months in neuroradiology. Depending on the program, operative experience and patient responsibility usually increase every year. Within the neurosurgical experience, residents are usually required to participate in at least one full year of research, either basic or clinical. Many different hospital environments are typically encountered during residency training, including county, private, academic, and VA facilities.

Upon completion of a neurological surgery residency, residents should be proficient in operative procedures involving tumors, the spine, pediatrics, and vascular neurosurgery. They should efficiently and effectively manage the clinical care of neurosurgical patients and be able to critically evaluate relevant neurosurgical research. It should be noted that the field of neurosurgery continues to evolve, with advances in radiographic imaging, gamma knife radiosurgery, and endovascular treatments now becoming the standard of care.

Neurological surgery is an extremely rewarding surgical specialty, providing opportunities to participate in critical clinical situations, to undertake advanced clinical or basic research, and to become involved in an ever-changing and challenging field. However, this specialty is notorious for remaining one of the most competitive fields in medicine despite its demanding schedules and high attrition rate. Balancing work and personal life is challenging for any field in medicine, but this is especially true in neurosurgery because of its demanding hours and stressful work. Residents in neurosurgery work the maximum hours allowed. Many programs have a 10% exception to the work hours rules, which permits 88 hours per week. This continues beyond junior years and extends through the chief resident experience.

> Some programs have exceptions to the 80-hour workweek and allow 88 hours per week.

The requirements for success in residency can be divided into three categories: clinical judgment, technical skills, and research capabilities. Preparing for success in each of these categories requires specific training and acquisition of particular skill sets. Clinical judgment is built through experience, which is initially obtained during subinternships and by neurosurgical knowledge. Technical skills are critical to any surgical subspecialty, and learning the basics smooths the transition to residency and accelerates the student's learning curve. Neurosurgery requires

# Quick Stats

## NEUROLOGICAL SURGERY

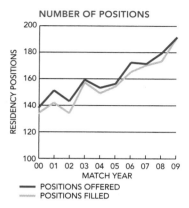

NUMBER OF POSITIONS

POSITIONS OFFERED
POSITIONS FILLED

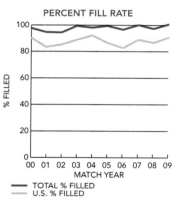

PERCENT FILL RATE

TOTAL % FILLED
U.S. % FILLED

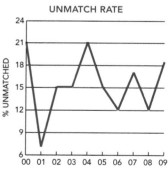

UNMATCH RATE

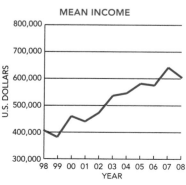

MEAN INCOME

manual dexterity and intense concentration when dealing with delicate parts of the nervous system. By the beginning of residency, students should be able to tie one- and two-handed knots, sew basic stitches effectively, and use simple neurosurgical tools such as the Cushing periosteal elevator. Finally, some experience with research techniques and exposure to scientific methodology allow new residents to hit the ground running with new or ongoing research projects. Furthermore, experience in managing projects provides an understanding of what is required to see a project to completion.

Neurosurgery residents are often described as hardworking, dedicated, tireless, passionate, and patient. Academic medical centers can be frustrating places in which to train, and residents are required to know an amazing amount of information about their patients and are ultimately responsible for their care. Good residents are able to balance these difficulties with the incredible responsibility of caring for critically sick patients.

Some programs offer fellowship training within or after the completion of a residency program. Generally, neurosurgery is broken down into six subspecialties: neurovascular, tumor, spine, functional, epilepsy, and pediatrics. Most academic programs have surgical cases divided evenly between cranial and spinal procedures. After residency, surgeons choose either academic or private practice. Academic surgeons work as a part of a larger medical center and split their practice between clinical work and research. In academia, surgeons typically subspecialize within neurosurgery and have one to two clinic days per week and one to two operative days per week. They spend the remainder of their time either pursuing basic science or laboratory research. This is in contrast to private-practice surgeons, who typically have three clinic days per week and two operative days per week. Their practice is usually 70–80% spine cases, with the remaining cranial caseload largely composed of tumors.

## APPLICATION TIPS

Positions in neurological surgery are now offered through the ERAS/NRMP main match. Given that neurological surgery is intensely competitive, applicants are expected to demonstrate a number of accomplishments prior to applying, such as a high USMLE Step 1 score (higher than the 80th percentile), election to AΩA, participation in research, and honors in clinical rotations (eg, general surgery). The strongest applicants will have completed one to three months of subinternships as well as some basic science or clinical research. One strategy to improve your chances is to participate in a subinternship at your institution of interest, especially if your home institution does not have a neurological surgery division or department of its own. One goal during an away subinternship is to obtain letters of recommendation from neurosurgeons in that program, including, but not limited to, the chairman and/or the residency program director. Programs look favorably on letters of recommendation from neurosurgeons, especially if they are from well-known institutions.

The optimal number of applications depends on your strength as a candidate, but it is recommended that applicants submit 30 to 40 applications and go to as many interviews as possible to increase their chances of matching. There are many factors to consider when selecting programs, including program strength, location, and your own interests within neurosurgery, as not every program is equally strong in all subareas of neurological surgery. One strategy for deciding which programs to approach is to ask neurological surgery residents at your home institution or at other institutions about the different programs. Another strategy is to attend one of the large annual neurosurgical meetings—for example, the American Association of Neurological Surgeons (AANS) or the Congress of Neurological Surgeons (CNS). These tactics can significantly improve your knowledge of what to look for in a program and strengthen your ability to distinguish among the different kinds and structures of neurological surgery programs.

## INTERVIEW TIPS

Most interviews last a single day, with a dinner either the night before or immediately following the interview day. Some programs reserve more than one day for interviews, but this is usually the case only in the larger programs. Most visits consist of similar activities, including grand rounds, campus/hospital tours, interviews, and meetings with residents. Individual interviews typically last 15 to 30 minutes. It is helpful to read about programs before interviewing, as most interviewers will ask if you have any questions about their program. Pertinent questions to discuss on your interview include available research opportunities, the number and variety of cases seen per year, and the amount of operative experience gained. Finally, it is always handy to have a photograph, a CV, and reprints of your publications with you during your interview should they be asked for.

### FOR MORE INFO . . .

**American Association of Neurological Surgeons**
5550 Meadowbrook Drive Rolling Meadows, IL 60008
(847) 378-0500
(888) 566-AANS
www.aans.org

**Congress of Neurological Surgeons**
www.cns.org

**American Board of Neurological Surgery (ABNS)**
6550 Fannin Street, Suite 2139
Houston, TX 77030
(713) 441-6015
www.abns.org

**TABLE 4-13**

**Top Five Most Frequently Encountered Conditions in Neurological Surgery**

1. Back pain/surgery
2. Brain tumors
3. Cervical pain/surgery
4. Trauma to nervous system
5. Vascular disease of nervous system

**TABLE 4-14**

**Selected Fellowship Training Opportunities in Neurological Surgery**

Cerebrovascular surgery: 1 year

Epilepsy surgery: 1 year

Interventional neuroradiology: 1 or 2 years

Neuro-oncology: 1 year

Neurosurgical critical care: 1 year

Pediatric neurological surgery: 1 or 2 years

Skull-base surgery: 1 year

Spine surgery: 1 year

Stereotactic and functional neurosurgery: 1 year

## NEUROLOGY

Neurology involves the investigation, diagnosis, and treatment of diseases related to the brain, spinal cord, peripheral nerves, muscles, and autonomic nervous system, as well as the relevant vasculature for each area. Neurologists treat patients of all ages and with a wide variety of disorders, from the common, such as headaches, cerebrovascular disease, seizure disorders, and neurodegenerative diseases, to the rare, such as movement disorders, neoplasms, and demyelinating diseases. Some

> As a neurologist, it is important to provide support for the patient as well as the patient's family or caretaker.

> Neurologists review their imaging scans, so a good understanding of neuroanatomy and neuroradiology is helpful.

## TABLE 4-15

### Top Five Most Frequently Encountered Conditions in Neurology

1. Headache
2. Epilepsy/seizures
3. Stroke
4. Dementia
5. Parkinson's disease

## TABLE 4-16

### Selected Fellowship Training Opportunities in Neurology

| | |
|---|---|
| Child neurology: 3 years | |
| Clinical neurophysiology: 1 year | |
| Critical care medicine: 1 or 2 years | |
| Neurodevelopmental disabilities: 4 years | |
| Pain management: 1 year | |
| Vascular neurology: 1 year | |

neurologists are also engaged in neurological rehabilitation. Many neurological problems are characterized by pain and can be chronic, debilitating, and often difficult to treat. A large portion of the practice of neurology is consultative, but the neurologist may also act as the primary physician. The specialty has the option of a combined certification board with psychiatry because of the close clinical relationship in treating cognitive and behavioral disorders.

Neurology requires a three-year residency program, preceded by an internship year in medicine, surgery, or transitional medicine. It generally works in the resident's favor to choose a medicine preliminary program, as such programs tend to be more relevant to later training in neurology. Look for preliminary program opportunities that might provide the flexibility to do neurosurgery electives, ophthalmology, or even neuroanatomy. Also keep in mind that the patient population and hospital setting may influence the quality and focus of training in certain areas (eg, trauma-related neurological diseases, HIV disease, or such chronic problems as stroke and dementia).

Neurology has greatly benefited from the recent explosion in technological research and pharmacology. Over the past few years, the specialty has grown and changed direction. It is now geared more toward treatment of previously intractable disorders. Practitioners in this field express hope and optimism that the future will bring even more successful interventions. However, there are still many conditions for which there is no treatment, and this can be a source of frustration and disappointment.

Exceptional residents in this field love working with their minds and have a strong preclinical knowledge base that is augmented by clinical foundations and diagnostic skill in medicine and psychiatry. On a personal level, the best physicians have a unique sensitivity to families and patients—neurological problems are often disabling, and patients and their families need encouragement and support. Since neurologists also spend a significant amount of time studying head CTs and MRIs, an interest in neuroradiology is also important. Neurologists are also invariably fascinated by the disease processes and the specialized neurologic exam, which has the power to be extremely diagnostic. Being able to perform a detailed neurological exam and elicit subtle deficiencies is one of the core competencies for neurology residents.

Most neurologists and residents feel that primary care physicians can take increasing responsibility for some chronic problems such as stroke, headaches, and uncomplicated seizures; however, more complex neurological problems require the care of a specialist. The management of acute stroke is now more sophisticated, with a high demand for neurologists to help in the emergency room setting. Neurology residency can be relatively busy with regular time on call and in the hospital. However, after completion of residency, attendings can choose the setting in which they wish to practice and the number of hours they wish to work. With a clinical practice, the typical lifestyle can be rather pleasant, with most private neurologists working normal daytime clinic hours. One of the drawbacks to this structure is the relatively low compensation for a specialty field. Alternatively, those working in a hospital may have more time on call. Job opportunities for neurologists seeking private or academic practices are readily available at present. In fact, some studies predict a critical shortage (up to 30%) in the supply of neurologists.

## APPLICATION TIPS

Positions for neurology residencies are filled through the main ERAS match. Senior neurology rotations should be completed early in the fourth year to ensure adequate time to request letters of recommendation. This is one field in which the reputation of the letter writer counts as much as the letter's substance. Generally, you should ask for letters from the best-known and most senior members of the neurology faculty, since their voices will resonate the loudest with the review committee. Away rotations at institutions of interest could also help, although opinion is divided on this issue.

To strengthen your application, you should include tangible proof of your commitment to the field of neurology, such as research experience, clinical volunteer experience, involvement in a neurology student interest group, or publications. Some programs will also look at the location of your internship institution and the type of internship to which you applied. In general, many programs prefer a medical internship located at either the same institution or a similarly prestigious one.

## INTERVIEW TIPS

Interviews range from individual sessions lasting about 30 to 45 minutes to group sessions conducted by a panel of faculty members. Each program has a different style, so be sure to ask about their format when you call to schedule your interview. Most of the time, the questions will be designed to gauge your dedication to and excitement about the field. In addition to the common interview fare (see Chapter 11), some interviewers will ask applicants to describe their research projects or to offer their opinions on ethical issues in neurological diagnosis and treatment. Some neurology programs have weaknesses in more recently developed specialty areas such as neuro-oncology, neurogenetics, and neuroimmunology. It is therefore important to determine the department's preparedness to teach these areas.

## FOR MORE INFO . . .

A student information packet can be obtained by calling or writing:

**American Academy of Neurology (AAN)**
1080 Montreal Avenue
St. Paul, MN 55116
(800) 879-1960
(651) 695-2717
www.aan.com

**American Board of Psychiatry and Neurology, Inc.**
2150 E. Lake Cook Road, Suite 900
Buffalo Grove, IL 60089
(847) 229-6500
www.abpn.com

## Quick Stats
### NEUROLOGY

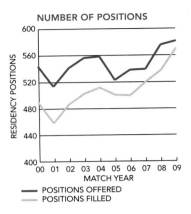

NUMBER OF POSITIONS

— POSITIONS OFFERED
— POSITIONS FILLED

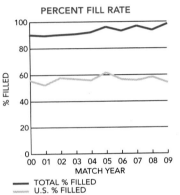

PERCENT FILL RATE

— TOTAL % FILLED
— U.S. % FILLED

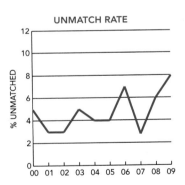

UNMATCH RATE

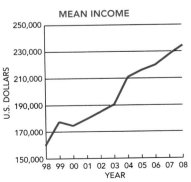

MEAN INCOME

## REFERENCES

Corboy JR, Boudreau E, Morgenlander JC, Rudnicki S, Coyle PK. Neurology residency training at the millennium. *Neurology* 58:1454–1460, 2002.

Ringel SP, Vickrey BG, Keran CM, Bieber J, Bradley WG. Training the future neurology workforce. *Neurology* 54(2):480–484, 2002.

## OBSTETRICS AND GYNECOLOGY

OB/GYN is a field limited only by the type of patients treated: female. From gynecologic evaluation to total obstetrical care, the obstetrician/gynecologist is essential to providing a continuum of women's health care. In addition, about half of all women utilize the OB/GYN as their sole source of health care. Therefore, the OB/GYN is in the unique position of providing both medical and surgical care to patients who may otherwise have no access to primary care. This field combines two specialties: obstetrics, which focuses on the care of women before, during, and after giving birth; and gynecology, which is a surgical specialty dealing with the diagnosis and treatment of diseases of the female reproductive system (vagina, ovaries, and uterus). Relationships with patients are often lifelong and last well beyond a woman's fertile period. There is also some exposure to male patients during the reproductive endocrinology and infertility portion of training, since andrology is an important aspect of infertility.

> Many patients rely on their OB/GYN as their only source of health care.

The length of residency training in OB/GYN is four years. The initial two years of training concentrate on general obstetrics, routine gynecology, outpatient care, gynecologic oncology, and basic surgical skills. The final two years involve increasing exposure to specialty areas. The upper-level resident must continuously hone teaching, management, and leadership skills. After finishing residency, a candidate must complete two years of practice before becoming board eligible. This would lead to a "generalist" practice in which the daily work would involve managing labor and delivery and treating gynecologic conditions both in the office and in the operating room. Additionally, there is a range of possible fellowships (see Table 4-18) that could lead to a practice that is primarily office based, as with reproductive endocrinology, or one that is primarily surgical, such as gynecologic oncology. OB/GYN residencies remain competitive. Even though fewer deliveries are being performed by OB/GYN physicians, the number of residency positions has remained stable.

> OB/GYN affords an exciting mix of clinical work and operating room experience.

As with many specialties, the best OB/GYN residents are both intelligent and efficient. For many, the skills needed to excel in OB/GYN begin during the fourth year of medical school while completing subinternships. This means taking ownership of your patients and demonstrating responsibility so that you can manage your patients independently. Self-starters can quickly complete the daily "check boxes" made for each patient's care. The other key aspect to excelling in this field is to learn how to present a patient in a clear, organized manner. Cogent presentations that are articulated clearly during morning rounds reflect well-conceived, organized plans. Therefore, medical students should try to emulate residents that present well. Presentations that ramble on minute details or that fail to provide

> Malpractice insurance costs in OB/GYN are becoming a national issue.

reasonable assessments reflect disorganized thought and ultimately "sloppy" care in the mind of the fellow or attending leading the team.

OB/GYN has benefited from impressive biomedical advances in recent years; enhanced maternal care and high-risk pregnancy management, in vitro fertilization, and increasing numbers of laparoscopic-assisted and in utero surgeries have lured candidates to the field. For the individual who appreciates interacting with patients in an outpatient setting but also enjoys high-tech procedural and surgical opportunities, OB/GYN may be the right choice. Practitioners in this field are also excited by taking care of the great variety of conditions that are unique to women and often feel unparalleled satisfaction in the delivery of a new life.

There are, however, some issues that make OB/GYN a challenging field. The high cost of malpractice coverage and the threat of litigation, for example, have become national problems. This may explain why career satisfaction is relatively low, with only 34.4% of practitioners reporting that they are very satisfied with the field. Those practicing only gynecology also report low job satisfaction, with only 27.3% reporting that they are very satisfied with their specialty. Residency program directors are aware of these concerns, and the vast majority of programs are incorporating some degree of formal medical-legal education into their residency curricula.

Additionally, there is competition for procedures due to the advanced training of nurse practitioners and nurse midwives who perform obstetrical services. Residents work long, stressful hours and are often sleep deprived, working at the 80-hour-per-week ACGME limit. Many residents suggest trying to maintain a peppy and positive attitude during this especially taxing period. However, not all of the rotations during residency are as busy—for example, clinic or ambulatory surgery rotations can provide more reasonable hours.

## APPLICATION TIPS

In a survey of OB/GYN residency program directors, the most important factors determining whether an applicant was invited for an interview were found to be grades, the MSPE, and USMLE scores. The program directors know that USMLE scores predict success on the OB/GYN boards. Some prestigious programs have further suggested that students try to complete away rotations at institutions that interest them, as a good impression on an away rotation improves the chances of being offered an interview. Strong evaluations in surgical rotations will similarly increase the applicant's strength. All application materials should be submitted as early as possible, usually by October.

## INTERVIEW TIPS

OB/GYN interviews are usually conducted in December and January. When you call to schedule, be aware that many programs have only a limited time period within which to interview large groups of applicants. Therefore, the earlier you submit your application, the more choices of dates you will have. Interview days may run long, lasting from 8 A.M. to 5 P.M., and generally consist of three to four interviews of 30 to 45 minutes each. Interviews may be individual or as a group

# Quick Stats

## OBSTETRICS AND GYNECOLOGY

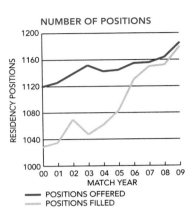

NUMBER OF POSITIONS

— POSITIONS OFFERED
— POSITIONS FILLED

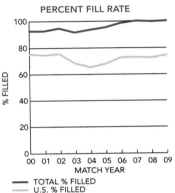

PERCENT FILL RATE

— TOTAL % FILLED
— U.S. % FILLED

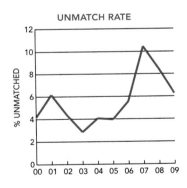

UNMATCH RATE

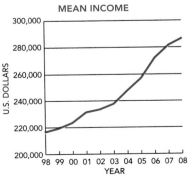

MEAN INCOME

## TABLE 4-17

**Top Five Most Frequently Encountered Conditions in OB/GYN**

1. Pregnancy/childbirth
2. Abnormal uterine bleeding
3. Menopausal concerns
4. Vaginitis
5. Pelvic pain

## TABLE 4-18

**Selected Fellowship Training Opportunities in OB/GYN**

Family planning: 3 years

Gynecology-oncology: 3 years

Maternal-fetal medicine: 3 years

Reproductive endocrinology: 3 years

Urogynecology: 3 years

depending on the program. When you interview, you should bear in mind that the "miracle of birth" is not a good enough reason for choosing this specialty. OB/GYN programs want to attract applicants who will become competent surgeons and have the capability to provide good primary care for women, so be prepared to present a case, discuss ethical issues related to the specialty, and explain why you want to be an OB/GYN.

You should be well versed in all important aspects of women's health and be aware of any major current ethical or policy issues that are relevant to the field. If you have done basic or clinical research, know your work inside out, as you will undoubtedly be questioned about it. For the most part, interviews are cordial and informal, offering the interviewer an opportunity to assess your personality.

## FOR MORE INFO . . .

Student information packets are available by calling or writing:

**American College of Obstetricians and Gynecologists (ACOG)**
409 12th Street, S.W.
P.O. Box 96920
Washington, D.C. 20090-6920
(202) 638-5577
www.acog.org

## REFERENCES

Bell JG, Kanellitsas I, Shaffer L. Selection of obstetrics and gynecology residents on the basis of medical school performance. *Am J Obstet Gynecol* 186(5):1091–1094, 2002.

Defoe DM, Power ML, Holzman GB, Carpentieri A, Schulkin J. Long hours and little sleep: Work schedules of residents in obstetrics and gynecology. *Obstet Gynecol* 97(6):1015–1018, 2001.

Leigh JP, Kravitz RL, Schembri M, Samuels SJ, Mobley S. Physician career satisfaction across specialties. *Arch Intern Med* 162:1577–1584, 2002.

Metheny WP, Ling FW, Holzman GB, Mitchum MJ. Answers to applicant selection from a directory of residency programs in obstetrics and gynecology. *Obstet Gynecol* 88(1):133–136, 1996.

Moreno-Hunt C, Gilbert WM. Current status of obstetrics and gynecology resident medical-legal education: A survey of program directors. *Obstet Gynecol* 106(6):1382–1384, 2005.

Taylor CA, Weinstein L, Mayhew HE. The process of resident selection: A view from the residency director's desk. *Obstet Gynecol* 85(2):299–303, 1995.

## OPHTHALMOLOGY

Understand the differences between ophthalmology and optometry and their political turf battles.

Ophthalmology is a medical, surgical, and rehabilitative specialty involved with the structure, function, diagnosis, and treatment of the visual system. This field extends beyond dysfunction of the globe and lens to include disorders of the extraocular muscles, eyelids, lacrimal system, cilia, orbit, and visual pathways. Ophthalmologists are also responsible for corrective vision services, including laser vision correction, glasses, and contact lenses.

Residencies in ophthalmology require one year of internship followed by three years of specialty training. Most residents choose to do a transitional year, but you can also do a preliminary medicine or surgical internship year. Some ophthalmology residencies also offer a customized internship year as a part of their program. Residents often rotate through both surgical and nonsurgical rotations, learning surgical techniques as well as the medical diagnosis and management of eye diseases. Board eligibility is achieved immediately after the completion of residency. Currently, there is no certification for subspecialties. Many fellowships are offered that range from one to two years and allow you to further hone your skills after completing residency. See Table 4-20 for a list of the fellowship opportunities following residency training in ophthalmology.

Ophthalmology has a good mix of surgical, clinical, inpatient, and outpatient work and offers continuity of care, as patients often are followed for many years. Thanks in large part to innovations in surgical and laser techniques, ophthalmology has recently taken off as a high-tech surgical and medical specialty with the ability to dramatically change a patient's quality of life. In addition, the field is heavily skill-based, from using magnifying lenses and a slit lamp for the basic ophthalmic exam to using an operating microscope and microsurgical instruments. Countless other devices used in everyday practice need to be mastered as well. Ophthalmologists also perform their own imaging procedures in the office, such as fluorescein angiograms, ultrasounds, and ocular coherence tomography scans.

Ophthalmologists typically work in an outpatient clinic with regular daytime hours, which enables a lifestyle conducive to outside interests and family life. Most ophthalmologists also take call responsibilities but these are minimal and rarely involve coming into the hospital for consults at night. The field is also attractive because it is expanding and will continue to be in high demand, since many of the conditions are highly prevalent in an aging population. Clinicians report that their patients are often very grateful, and the immediate appreciation that one receives is very rewarding. Most residents are happy during their residency and with their decision to pursue ophthalmology. Furthermore, the potential for humanitarian travel and international medical service is great, as the leading worldwide causes of blindness are generally preventable and treatable.

Despite all these attractions, challenges still remain for ophthalmologists. There is a high start-up cost for a new ophthalmology practice, as multiple pieces of basic, yet expensive equipment are needed for an office. As a result, most residency graduates join an established practice or an academic institution after completing residency. The relationship between ophthalmologists and optometrists is currently in flux. Many of the services provided by the two groups overlap, and there is ongoing debate regarding the boundaries between the two professions. Perhaps surprisingly, a recent survey reports relatively low career satisfaction among ophthalmologists, with 41.4% expressing a high level of satisfaction—a level below that of general surgery, orthopedic surgery, and urology.

Ophthalmology is a "hidden gem" that most students do not get exposed to during medical school. Therefore, medical students who are interested must take the initiative to schedule electives and advanced rotations in ophthalmology. As with any specialty, working hard and being responsible are generally the two most

# Quick Stats
## OPHTHALMOLOGY

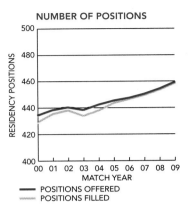

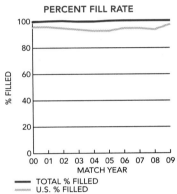

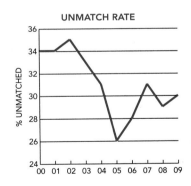

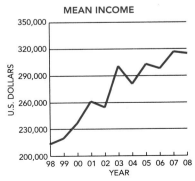

Most medical schools do not require a rotation in ophthalmology, so you will have to seek it out if you are interested.

Ophthalmology participates in the San Francisco Match, which has earlier deadlines than the NRMP Match.

## TABLE 4-19

**Top Five Most Frequently Encountered Conditions in Ophthalmology**

1. Glaucoma
2. Cataracts
3. Retinal disease
4. Refraction
5. Macular degeneration

## TABLE 4-20

**Selected Fellowship Training Opportunities in Ophthalmology**

Anterior segment surgery: 1 year

Cornea/external disease: 1 year

Glaucoma: 1 year

Neuro-ophthalmology: 1 year

Oculoplastics: 1 year

Ophthalmic pathology: 1 year

Pediatric ophthalmology: 1 year

Retina/vitreous: 2 year

Uveitis/immunology: 1 year

important elements to being a good resident. While work-hour limits are generally not an issue in ophthalmology, be prepared to spend a good deal of time studying and reading at home.

## APPLICATION TIPS

Ophthalmology remains one of the most competitive specialties. Positions in ophthalmology residencies are offered primarily through the Ophthalmology Matching Program run by the San Francisco Match. Applications should be submitted by late August, and ROLs by January. Match results are announced in time for applicants to learn their results before the deadline for the PGY-1 preliminary programs sponsored by the National Resident Matching Program (NRMP). Given the competition to enter the field, applicants should concentrate on doing well on the USMLE Step 1 as well as core clinical rotations and their senior ophthalmology rotation. Some programs use election to AΩA or Step 1 scores as a screening tool! Applicants should try to push the number of audition electives to the maximum allowed by their medical school—usually two or three. Supportive evaluations and recommendations from the senior ophthalmology faculty will boost your application.

Since this is another field in which most department heads know one another, connections can play an important part in getting you an interview invitation. In addition, any research experience, especially work resulting in publications or presentations, should be included in your CV. At present, most applicants are advised to submit about 20 to 35 applications in the hope of getting ten or more interviews. However, the right number for you will depend on the strength of your application, and some applicants apply to significantly more programs. Many advisors also suggest that you apply to a mix of strong and weak programs in order to increase your probability of matching.

## INTERVIEW TIPS

As with other surgical subspecialties, interviews for ophthalmology are more formal. Applicants often meet with the department head, one or two senior faculty members, and at least one resident. Most interviews last from 30 to 45 minutes, with many of the questions geared toward assessing the applicant's interest in the field, clinical and research background, and personality. If you have done research that you hope will give you an edge, be prepared to discuss your project in a polished manner. Some clinical questions may also be asked, depending on the interviewer. Given the competitiveness of the field, interviewers sometimes ask about your contingency plans in the event that you don't match in ophthalmology.

### FOR MORE INFO . . .

*Envision Ophthalmology: A Practical Guide to Ophthalmology as a Career Choice.* A free publication of the American Academy of Ophthalmology (AAO), this booklet includes general information about the application process as well as a practical discussion of factors to consider in selecting and assessing an ophthalmology program. To receive this excellent career guide, call or write:

American Academy of Ophthalmology
P.O. Box 7424
San Francisco, CA 94120-7424
(415) 561-8500
www.aao.org

American Board of Ophthalmology (ABO)
111 Presidential Boulevard, Suite 241
Bala Cynwyd, PA 19004-1075
(610) 664-1175
www.abop.org

Glaucoma Research Foundation (to inquire about research opportunities)
490 Post Street, Suite 1427
San Francisco, CA 94102
(415) 986-3162
(800) 826-6693
www.glaucoma.org

San Francisco Match Ophthalmology Matching Program
P.O. Box 7584
San Francisco, CA 94120-7584
(415) 447-0350
Fax: (415) 561-8535
E-mail: help@sfmatch.org
www.sfmatch.org

## REFERENCES

Andriole DA, Schechtman KB, Ryan K, Whelan A, Diemer K. How competitive is my surgical specialty? *Am J Surg* 84(1):1–5, 2002.

Leigh JP, Kravitz RL, Schembri M, Samuels SJ, Mobley S. Physician career satisfaction across specialties. *Arch Intern Med* 162(14):1577–1584, 2002.

## ORTHOPEDICS

Orthopedic surgeons are trained to evaluate the biomechanical function of the musculoskeletal system and provide treatment via medical, physical, or surgical methods. This field encompasses a broad range of conditions including trauma, sports injuries, degenerative diseases, congenital deformities, infections, and tumors of the hand, wrist, elbow, shoulder, spine, hip, knee, ankle, and foot. Orthopedic surgeons treat patients of all ages and are mostly focused on treating a patient's specific musculoskeletal complaint. Most recently, the field has made impressive strides in advancing surgical techniques and equipment. In fact, total hip arthroplasty was named the operation of the century by the journal *Lancet* for its ability to help people crippled by arthritis.

Orthopedic residencies require at least five years of training. The first year of residency is typically spent largely in general surgery rotations, and the last four years are spent in orthopedic surgery services. A postresidency practice period is required before you become board eligible, and various subspecialty training is available (see Table 4-22). After completing a fellowship, a specialist usually either joins an academic center or a private practice, and can expect to take call.

> The number of women going into orthopedics has been increasing over the past decade. However, it remains a heavily male-dominated field, with more than 21,500 male physicians and close to 1000 female physicians practicing in the United States in 2008.

> Even though some cases can be physically demanding, you do not have to have the build of a linebacker to be a successful orthopedic surgeon!

> High board scores, AΩA, many honors, and research experience are the keys to success.

## TABLE 4-21

**Top Five Most Frequently Encountered Conditions in Orthopedics**

1. Arthritis (any joint)
2. Fractures
3. Sprains/strains
4. Back pain
5. Carpal tunnel syndrome

## TABLE 4-22

**Selected Fellowship Training Opportunities in Orthopedics**

Adult reconstructive orthopedics: 1 year

Foot and ankle orthopedics: 1 year

Hand surgery: 1 year

Musculoskeletal oncology: 1 year

Orthopedics sports medicine: 1 year

Orthopedic surgery of the spine: 1 year

Orthopedic trauma: 1 year

Pediatric orthopedics: 1 year

---

One in seven U.S. seniors went unmatched in orthopedic surgery. Consider applying in a second field, such as general surgery, if you want to reduce your chances of going unmatched.

---

Orthopedic surgery continues to be a rewarding and gratifying field. Specialists have the opportunity to combine surgical techniques and orthopedic hardware (eg, microsurgery and joint prostheses) with work in physical rehabilitation for the treatment of acute and chronic orthopedic problems. In addition, earnings for orthopedic surgeons continue to be well above average. However, increasing professional liability insurance premiums and overhead costs are reducing overall compensation. On the whole, 47.1% of orthopedic surgeons evaluate their career as very satisfactory, which represents a relatively high percentage among medical specialties.

Being a good resident in orthopedics requires a dedication to learning and clinical care. The resident must be well organized and able to multitask. It helps to have a thick skin and to be quick with the right answer. Having good spatial reasoning capabilities and hand-eye coordination is imperative. Interested applicants are advised to work hard while on the orthopedics rotation—never try to leave early or leave things unfinished. The more cases you do as a medical student, the more comfortable you will be when you start residency. The best students show interest in learning and ask a lot of questions. As with other specialties, the most successful residents are those who are efficient, thorough, and hard working.

The orthopedic surgery physician faces many challenges. Long hours both in the clinic and OR are just the beginning; a successful orthopedic surgeon will be busy and average greater than 60 hours per week with patient care. As a resident, count on being one of the busier residents in the hospital and working close to the maximum number of hours allowed (80 per week). Another potential drawback is that many orthopedic patients have issues with pain and can be dependent on pain medications, which can be difficult to manage. Additionally, orthopedic surgeons are typically involved in legal discussions involving assessments of disability secondary to accidents.

## APPLICATION TIPS

Orthopedics is a challenging specialty and is among the most competitive surgical specialties. As a result, it is imperative to excel in all aspects of medical school. Doing well during your first two years is important, but excelling on the USMLE Step 1 is paramount. Unfortunately, most programs use it as a standard to compare students. It is not necessary to realize that you are an "orthopod" from the day you start medical school, but you should know that you want to enter orthopedics by the middle of your third year of medical school in order to plan your subinternships. Most students do one subinternship at their home institution and at least one, if not two, subinternships away. Subinternships allow you to intimately evaluate other programs and also allow you to show those programs what kind of candidate you will be.

Excelling in your orthopedic rotations is obviously important, but you should do well in all your rotations, especially surgery. Research during medical school is important, but not absolutely essential. Letters of recommendation are an important part of the application, and the best way to get these is to make yourself known to the attendings by being engaged and asking appropriate questions during cases in the OR.

Bernstein et al. summarized the process and criteria that orthopedic surgery residency program directors have used for selection of residents. Academic credentials, including class rank and USMLE scores, are heavily weighted. The prestige of AΩA election is now widely recognized as well; 54% of all successful candidates are members of AΩA. Also well established and documented in the Bernstein study is the enormous importance of performing well during an audition elective, or "orthopedic clerkship," at the program director's institution.

The interview process in orthopedics is directed toward "getting to know" the applicant and is probably not useful in distinguishing one outstanding applicant from another. However, 5% of programs tested manual skills, and 18% used clinical scenarios as part of the interview process. While the assumption is often made that research is a necessity to match in orthopedics, this is not supported by the literature. Also important to note is a recent study by Dale et al., which found that some candidates "falsified research citations on their applications to orthopedic programs." Falsification or overstatement of your achievements is not only unethical, but is extremely dangerous and could cause you to lose your chance at a residency program altogether.

## INTERVIEW TIPS

Interviews in orthopedic surgery are difficult to obtain, so if you are offered one, it means that you've proven yourself academically. As stated previously, the Bernstein review suggests that 18% of program directors use clinical scenarios, so be prepared, at a minimum, to present an interesting or memorable case. If you have done research, be particularly careful to accurately describe your findings and their significance. Interviews are usually conducted from mid-November to early February.

## FOR MORE INFO . . .

For a brochure on careers in orthopedic surgery, call or write:

**American Academy of Orthopedic Surgeons (AAOS)**
6300 North River Road
Rosemont, IL 60018-4262
(847) 823-7186
(800) 346-AAOS
**www.aaos.org**

## REFERENCES

Bernstein AD, Jazrawi LM, DellaValle CJ, Zuckerman JD. Orthopedic resident selection criteria. *J Bone Joint Surg Am* 84:2090–2096, 2002.

Dale JA, Schmitt CM, Crosby LA. Misrepresentation of research criteria by orthopedic residency applicants. *J Bone Joint Surg Am* 81:1679–1681, 1999.

Leigh JP, Kravitz RL, Schembri M, Samuels SJ, Mobley S. Physician career satisfaction across specialties. *Arch Intern Med* 162:1577–1584, 2002.

Learmonth ID, Young C, Rorabeck C. The operation of the century: Total hip replacement. *Lancet* 370:1508–1519, 2007.

# Quick Stats
## ORTHOPEDICS

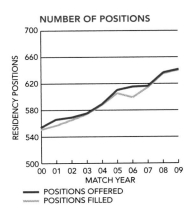

NUMBER OF POSITIONS

— POSITIONS OFFERED
— POSITIONS FILLED

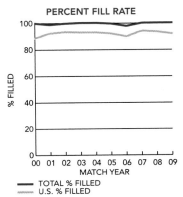

PERCENT FILL RATE

— TOTAL % FILLED
— U.S. % FILLED

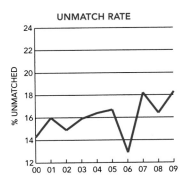

UNMATCH RATE

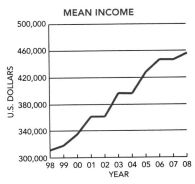

MEAN INCOME

## OTOLARYNGOLOGY

Otolaryngology, also known as ear, nose, and throat (ENT), is a relatively small field that sees an extremely diverse patient population and performs a vast array of clinical and surgical procedures. However, its size belies the demand for these busy, specialized surgeons. Otolaryngologists enjoy some of the best aspects of both surgery and clinical medicine. Although the primary care specialties might take over allergy treatment, as well as simple procedures such as tympanotomy, ENT physicians continue to play key roles in academics, head and neck oncology, pediatric otolaryngology, laryngology, rhinology, and the growing fields of facial plastics, otologic implants, and allergy.

Otolaryngology is an exciting field that combines the best of both surgical and medical roles. In general, most medical students are attracted to the field through a surgical rotation because ENT is a surgical subspeciality. As a result, interest in surgery and spending time in the OR are important considerations. Of equal importance, interest in clinical medicine is critical because otolaryngologists spend more than half of their time outside of the OR, conducting medical management of patients prior to counseling them regarding surgical options. Medical students considering the field should not be discouraged by the competitiveness of the application process.

If you are really passionate about becoming an otolaryngologist but do not have the strongest application, do not exclude applying. There are many opportunities either during or after medical school to pursue a research project in otolaryngology, do an away rotation, attend academic conferences, and strengthen your application.

The attractions of otolaryngology are many, including the opportunity to help patients with disorders that affect quality of life, the diversity and complexity of head and neck pathophysiology, and the physicians in the field, who are generally considered to be congenial, approachable, and well-rounded. Otolaryngologists have a wide variety of career options since it is such a diverse field. They see patients of all age groups, have the option to pursue either mainly a clinical or surgical career in either an academic or private setting, and can also perform research. As a result, training is rigorous, with the goal of providing exposure to all aspects of the field. However, with the diversity of pathophysiology, it may be difficult to become proficient in some particular areas, such as plastic and reconstructive surgery, without pursuing fellowship training.

> Otolaryngologists can tailor their practice to be more clinical or more surgical.

In order to excel in the field of otolaryngology, it is important to be well-rounded in medical school and learn not only the fundamentals of surgery but also those of medicine, pediatrics, radiology, and critical care medicine. Otolaryngology is a broad subspeciality and is comprised of both surgical and clinical responsibilities. In addition, the field is constantly evolving, with the advent of new technology and breakthroughs in research. Therefore, it is important to continue reading and to develop the philosophy early in medical school that learning never ends—it really only takes off when starting residency.

To excel as a resident, many attendings have said that a good resident usually fulfills the three "A's" of success: affability, availability, and ability. Attendings are relying on you to take good care of their patients. A good resident is a team player who is conscientious, detail oriented, hardworking, and eager to learn. Although there is not much time outside the hospital, it is important to keep learning and continue to read at least an hour or so every day to become knowledgeable and competent in the field. You are constantly learning on the job, but concepts need to be solidified through constant reading and discussion. In addition, standardized testing does not end in medical school; it continues throughout residency! Performance on the annual "in-service exam" is critical and is used to determine your preparation to eventually take the board examination, which consists of oral and written portions.

The daily life of an otolaryngologist is varied, depending on whether an academic or private career is pursued. Some otolaryngology attendings are able to combine both worlds. Academic otolaryngologists, or "surgeon scientists," see more complex cases and incorporate research into their careers. Most academic otolaryngologists are fellowship trained in a particular area and specialize in that field. An important part of academic life is teaching residents and medical students. Otolaryngologists who pursue private practice also see a wide variety of patients with head and neck diseases. They usually practice in a community setting within a group of other otolaryngologists and tend to refer more complex cases to academic centers. Many private otolaryngologists are also fellowship trained and can choose to focus on that field or can see a diverse group of patients, depending on their interests. An attractive aspect of the field is the flexibility to make your career what you want it to be.

Life after residency is good no matter what! There is a great demand for otolaryngologists. In general, half of otolaryngology residents pursue fellowship, while the other half start working in private practice.

As of the 2006 Match, all otolaryngology programs switched from the early Match to the regular Match and participate with both ERAS and the NRMP. Most ENT programs are five-year programs and include a one-year internship that combines general surgery rotations with rotations such as emergency medicine, anesthesia, neurosurgery, and critical care medicine. A few of the more prestigious, heavily academic programs offer positions with another year or two for research, usually between the general surgery and ENT years.

## APPLICATION TIPS

The keys to success in this highly competitive field are much the same as those in many of the other competitive specialties. Strong board scores are almost a prerequisite to a successful application. Students scoring below the 80th percentile on the USMLE Step 1 exam should seriously consider applying in another field in addition to ENT as a contingency. One recent study found that ENT matching success strongly correlates with high medical school GPAs (if available), high board scores, high class rank (if available), honors in both general surgery and medicine, and AΩA selection. Some of the very competitive ENT programs suggest that applicants do an audition rotation at their hospital to increase their likelihood of being invited for an interview.

In general, it's a good idea to do externships if you are aiming for specific programs where your application is less competitive than you'd like. Because there are only 100 or so programs in ENT and no more than a few spots available per

# Quick Stats

## OTOLARYNGOLOGY

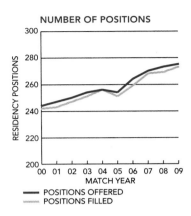

NUMBER OF POSITIONS

—— POSITIONS OFFERED
—— POSITIONS FILLED

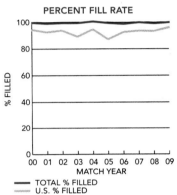

PERCENT FILL RATE

—— TOTAL % FILLED
—— U.S. % FILLED

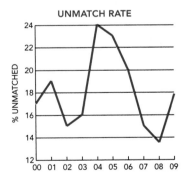

UNMATCH RATE

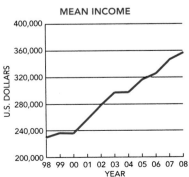

MEAN INCOME

program, you are also operating at a serious disadvantage if you are restricted to applying in a particular geographic region.

Deadlines for applications will vary by program, with most being in October, but it is beneficial to submit your completed ERAS application as early as possible. You are allowed to submit up to four letters of recommendation via ERAS. The most balanced approach is to submit two to three letters from ENT faculty and one from a clinical attending from another major clerkship (eg, medicine, surgery). If you did ENT research, your research adviser can be one of your letter writers. If you did research outside of ENT, try to get two to three letters written by ENTs, with the third or fourth letter from your research adviser. Otolaryngology is a small community of physicians, and for the most part everyone knows everyone else. As a result, it is helpful to obtain letters from chairs of otolaryngology programs at which you have rotated.

## INTERVIEW TIPS

The ENT interview season runs from mid-October into early February, with most interviews taking place in December and January. If you're offered an interview at one program, it would not hurt to call other programs you have approached in that geographic region to ask if they are willing to grant you an interview while you are in the area. Most ENT programs, however, have only two to three interview dates per season, so clustering interviews is often very difficult. Be ready to crisscross the country to get all the interviews you need, and prepare to spend anywhere from $3000 to $5000 on this process, from buying suits to paying travel expenses. The conventional wisdom is that going to eight interviews is a good indication that you'll match; most applicants go to between 12 and 15 interviews.

An applicant will typically sit for six to eight interviews during the visit, each lasting 15 to 30 minutes—although it is not unheard of to have up to 13 half-hour interviews in one day! Interviews are generally held with one to two faculty members; panel interviews are relatively rare. This schedule usually includes an interview with the department chair, who in some cases is also the program director. During the interview, emphasize your strengths and interests that are most compatible with the philosophy of the particular program. It is also a good idea to highlight your academic and research interests when you are interviewed by the department chair, even if the program is more clinically oriented. You should also feel free to drop names, assuming that the interview is going well and that you are well liked by the people whose names you drop. ENT is a small field in which anyone who's anyone knows everyone.

Some interviews may include a practical session in which you are asked to suture, tie, carve soap, produce differential diagnoses, or identify radiologic landmarks. These types of interviews are becoming exceedingly rare, however. Generally, the main point of these exercises is not to test your knowledge base but rather to see how you think under and deal with pressure. The best information on a particular program's interview style can be garnered from people who have already interviewed with that program; if you share your interview experiences, most other applicants will give you the skinny on places they have been. The best way to prepare for the unknown is to keep a case presentation ready for discussion. This

> If asked to demonstrate practical skills at an interview, remain calm, cool, and collected.

is fair game and may be requested several times during the course of the interview season, even during the most benign interview sessions.

## FOR MORE INFO . . .

**Baylor University** has a great Web site with links to most other otolaryngology programs:
www.bcm.tmc.edu/oto/others.html

**American Academy of Otolaryngology—Head and Neck Surgery (AAO-HNS)**
One Prince Street
Alexandria, VA 22314
(703) 836-4444
www.entnet.net

**American Academy of Facial Plastic and Reconstructive Surgery**
310 South Henry Street
Alexandria, VA 22314
(703) 299-9291
(800) 332-FACE
www.facial-plastic-surgery.org

**Otomatch,** a Web site for medical students applying in otolaryngology, with a discussion board, interview dates calendar, and other match related information:
www.otomatch.com

**American Board of Otolaryngology (ABOto)**
3050 Post Oak Boulevard, Suite 1700
Houston, TX 77056
(713) 850-0399
www.aboto.org

**Association for Research in Otolaryngology**
www.aro.org

## REFERENCES

Calhoun KH, Hokanson JA, Bailey BJ. Predictors of residency performance: A follow-up study. *Otolaryngol Head Neck Surg* 116(6 Pt 1):647–651, 1997.

Kay DJ, Lucente FE. Otolaryngology residents' objectives in entering the workforce. *Laryngoscope* 112(10):1766–1768, 2002.

## TABLE 4-23

**Top Five Most Frequently Encountered Conditions in Otolaryngology**

1. Sinusitis/sinus disease
2. Otitis media
3. Hearing loss
4. Head and neck cancers/tumors
5. Allergies

## TABLE 4-24

**Selected Fellowship Training Opportunities in Otolaryngology**

| |
|---|
| Neurotology: 2 years |
| Pediatric otolaryngology: 1 or 2 years |
| Plastic surgery of the head and neck: 1 year |
| Laryngology: 1 year |
| Rhinology: 1 year |
| Sleep medicine: 1 year |

## PATHOLOGY

A consulting specialist, the pathologist has long been known as the "doctor's doctor." One of the most traditional fields in medicine, pathology is the study of the mechanisms and manifestations of disease at the tissue, cell, and, increasingly, the molecular level. It is a specialty that allows the physician to spend much of his working hours thinking about disease pathogenesis and discussing the ramifications of the diagnosis on the treatment and outcome of the patients. Pathology is especially well suited for those who want to combine lab-based research with clinical practice.

In many illnesses and diseases, the gold standard of diagnosis still relies on the work of a pathologist. The manner in which pathology is practiced has evolved dramatically from both a scientific and an economic perspective. The recent ex-

# Quick Stats

## PATHOLOGY

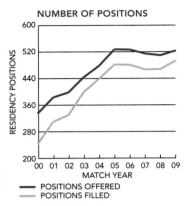

NUMBER OF POSITIONS

RESIDENCY POSITIONS

MATCH YEAR

— POSITIONS OFFERED
— POSITIONS FILLED

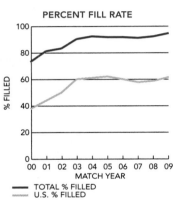

PERCENT FILL RATE

% FILLED

MATCH YEAR

— TOTAL % FILLED
— U.S. % FILLED

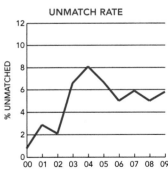

UNMATCH RATE

% UNMATCHED

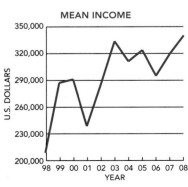

MEAN INCOME

U.S. DOLLARS

YEAR

plosion in biomedical technology, especially in the area of genetics, has had a profound effect on the field. Furthermore, many practices are hiring subspecialized pathologists, especially in large urban centers. More residents are therefore delaying graduation from their training programs, choosing instead to acquire more distinctive fellowship skills to make themselves more desirable to potential employers. Rumors of a steeply declining job market for pathologists across the board have not materialized, however.

Becoming board certified in either anatomic pathology (AP) or clinical pathology (CP) requires a minimum of three years. Most applicants enter through the combined AP/CP track, which is a total of four years. There is no transitional or preliminary year. If you are certified in only one specialty, you might be limited to working in large hospitals that can afford to employ separate specialists. This option may be ideal for those who have a combined MD/PhD degree or are quite certain that they want to stay in academic pathology with a significant research component to their work. It may also be the best pathway for those who already know what subspecialty they want to pursue. (For example, neuropathologists often do only AP training, and directors of blood banks need only CP training.)

Anatomic pathology residency training comprises core rotations required for board certification, including surgical pathology, cytopathology, autopsy, and subspecialty rotations particular to the institution's set curriculum. Clinical pathology, also called laboratory medicine, encompasses blood banking and transfusion medicine, hematopathology, clinical chemistry, microbiology, immunology, and laboratory management.

Anatomic pathology is very attractive to those who learn visually and have good spatial reasoning and pattern recognition skills. Clinical pathology is great for those who are excited about the possibilities and limits of diagnostic tests and are interested in bringing new tests to bear on medical dilemmas. Those with an interest in basic science or translational research may be particularly suited to working on the molecular tools that are advancing the frontiers in both AP and CP. There are a lot of opportunities to teach in this field, not just to residents and medical students, but also to other physicians. As for lifestyle, pathology offers better hours than most other specialties, and overnight calls are generally home calls with relatively few instances of being called in to the hospital.

It is important to consider the obvious distance between pathologists and patients before applying to pathology. Even in subspecialties where you may see patients routinely, like blood bank/transfusion medicine, you have to be comfortable with not ever being the primary care provider for your patients. With regard to daily challenges, hours that residents spend "grossing," or cutting specimens for slide preparation, vary a lot by institution. This is something to look into and consider before making your rank list.

## APPLICATION TIPS

The importance of doing a rotation in pathology cannot be overemphasized. You simply won't get a good grasp of this field without having experienced it firsthand. This is not something you can extrapolate from your experience in histology lab. Also important to consider is doing some of your elective time in laboratory medicine (CP), because this will help you figure out if you want to do a combined AP/CP program or do only CP.

Because training programs in pathology have different emphases, it is important for you to find a program that matches your career goals. This is especially true for combined clinical and anatomic pathology programs, which may be strong in only one department. Ask for help from a senior pathologist you have met with on a rotation or through research to help you choose the right programs to apply to. It's a relatively small field, so most pathologists have a good understanding of the strengths and weaknesses of different programs. A strong evaluation in the senior elective, accompanied by solid letters of recommendation (with at least one from a pathologist), is essential in this process. So is a well-considered and well-written personal statement. Some applicants feel unduly pressured to demonstrate research interests, especially when interviewing at top-tier academic programs. However, even those programs take a number of residents each year who do not have a research background, so this should not be a deterrent.

## INTERVIEW TIPS

As with any field, most interviewers will be curious to know why you are interested in their specialty, so be prepared to answer questions about your particular interests, research background, and any plans you might have for your future career. Interviews often last roughly 30 minutes, with four to ten interviews a day depending on whether you are applying to an AP only, CP only, or combined program. Even with the rise in applicants, most programs try to keep the numbers of interviewees per interview day down to a handful so that it feels more personal. A few programs hold large-scale interviews (on the order of 30 applicants) and have applicants rotate through the interviewers like musical chairs. Expect to answer some questions about your postresidency plans, such as conducting research, receiving extra training, or going straight into practice.

Carefully assess programs for the breadth and depth of their training, resident satisfaction, research opportunities, flexibility, and staff support. It is advisable to know, before you interview, whether you prefer to learn by subspecialty signout (eg, learning GI pathology separately from breast pathology) or general signout. Some programs have the residents rotate on a three-day basis with "grossing" on day 1, previewing on day 2, and signing out with the attending on day 3. Others have the residents do all three activities in one day, every day. It is hard to know what you prefer if you haven't done an elective in pathology, which is all the more reason to do so.

## FOR MORE INFO . . .

*Student Information Packet.* This free packet includes several articles and a slick brochure about career opportunities in pathology. The College of American Pathologists (CAP) also produces a promotional video that it lends out at no cost. To receive an information packet or borrow the video, call or write:

**College of American Pathologists**
325 Waukegan Road
Northfield, IL 60093
(800) 323-4040
www.cap.org

---

> Having a good visual memory is a plus in pathology.

## TABLE 4-25

**Top Five Most Frequently Encountered Conditions in Pathology**

1. Cancer
2. Biopsies
3. Benign neoplasms
4. Inflammatory diseases
5. Pap smears/GYN screening

## TABLE 4-26

**Selected Fellowship Training Opportunities in Pathology**

| |
|---|
| Blood banking/transfusion med: 1 year |
| Chemical pathology: 1 year |
| Cytopathology: 1 year |
| Forensic pathology: 1 year |
| Hematology (pathology): 1 year |
| Immunopathology: 1 or 2 years |
| Medical microbiology: 1 year |
| Neuropathology: 2 years |
| Pediatric pathology: 1 year |

# Quick Stats

## PEDIATRICS

### NUMBER OF POSITIONS

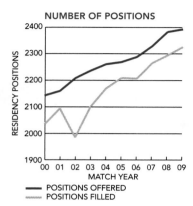

— POSITIONS OFFERED
— POSITIONS FILLED

### PERCENT FILL RATE

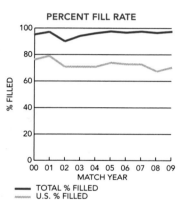

— TOTAL % FILLED
— U.S. % FILLED

### UNMATCH RATE

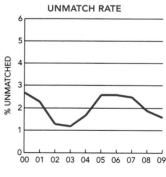

### MEAN INCOME

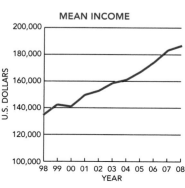

**American Society for Clinical Pathology (ASCP)**
2100 West Harrison Street
Chicago, IL 60612-3798
(312) 738-1336
(800) 621-4142
www.ascp.org

## REFERENCES

Alexander CB. Trends in pathology graduate medical education. *Hum Pathol* 32(7):671–676, 2001.

Bryant J. Underemployment: Another aspect of the oversupply in pathology. *Hum Pathol* 30(9):1118–1119, 1999.

Kent JA. A tale of two systems: Pathology resident recruitment in and out of the National Resident Matching Program. *Hum Pathol* 32(7):677–679, 2001.

## PEDIATRICS

Pediatricians care for children from birth to young adulthood and are often able to develop meaningful long-term relationships with their patients as they grow up. They also interact significantly with the parents or guardians to educate them and to help direct the patient's continued health and growth. Depending on the work environment, pediatricians can see many healthy patients in well-child visits, which focus on normal development and disease prevention. Alternatively, they can work in hospitals or intensive care units and manage children with serious medical problems.

In some practices the routine procedures and well-child care in the outpatient setting is performed by nurse practitioners, physician assistants, and family practitioners. This means that pediatricians, if they wish, can focus on the care of the more seriously ill children. General pediatrics tends to be more and more office based and is increasingly oriented toward group practice. Career satisfaction tends to be higher than in other primary care fields.

Residencies in pediatrics require three years of training. About 30–40% of graduates do additional subspecialty training, sometimes after years of primary care practice. Similar to internal medicine, pediatric programs are also divided into categorical and primary care programs. The categorical programs are geared more toward inpatient care, with ample opportunity to explore subspecialty options, while primary care focuses on general pediatrics. Pursuing a primary care track will not close the door on future subspecialty training.

Pediatrics programs can be roughly classified according to their setting: children's versus non–children's hospitals. Children's hospitals have more pediatrics specialists available and in general offer more comprehensive training and education. In a children's hospital, everything is geared toward kids, from the intubating equipment in the ER to the wallpaper in the CT units. Children's hospitals also tend to be located in large cities and have more of a tertiary care focus. Good children's hospitals have affiliations with adult centers for obtaining delivery room experience.

By contrast, residencies in non–children's hospitals provide more interaction with faculty and house staff from other primary care specialties that involve children, such as family practice, OB/GYN, and internal medicine. These programs can be further categorized into community, university, and county/municipal settings. These are discussed in more detail in Chapter 6.

## APPLICATION TIPS

In the coming years, there will be excellent opportunities for both U.S. graduates and IMGs seeking positions in pediatrics. Since the quality of programs varies and some smaller programs may have difficulty providing residents the opportunity to see an adequate range of disorders, it is the applicant who must carefully decide where to apply. It goes without saying that your personal statement and CV should emphasize any involvement you might have with children, community or public health care, and volunteer activities. As in the other primary care specialties, the type of individual you are and your long-term goals will provide fodder for question-and-answer sessions.

## INTERVIEW TIPS

Most interviews for pediatrics programs are scheduled from late November through January. The interview day typically runs from 8 A.M. to 3 P.M. Expect two to four interview sessions, each 20 to 45 minutes in length. Interviews in this specialty are generally low key and nonconfrontational. In addition to having the qualities typically desired in all house officers, you must package yourself as an individual who interacts well with parents and children. Good interpersonal skills are a must. Remember that most of your interviewers are parents themselves and want to know that you are the kind of person to whom they could entrust the care of their children.

## FOR MORE INFO . . .

*Pediatrics Information Packet.* In addition to giving a general profile of the specialty, this packet includes fact sheets detailing current socioeconomic statistics on pediatrics practice. To receive this information for free, call or write:

**American Academy of Pediatrics (AAP)**
141 Northwest Point Boulevard
Elk Grove Village, IL 60007
(847) 434-4000
www.aap.org

*Selecting a Pediatric Residency: An Employment Guide.* This is a comprehensive, step-by-step guide to selecting, applying to, and interviewing at pediatrics residency programs. It also discusses family and marriage considerations, employment issues such as contract and salary guidelines, and certification licensing requirements. It is available to medical students for $5 plus shipping costs. To order, call or write:

**AAP Publications Department**
P.O. Box 747
Elk Grove Village, IL 60009-0927
(888) 227-1770

> While physician income tends to be lower than in many other fields, job satisfaction is higher!

### TABLE 4-27
**Top Five Most Frequently Encountered Conditions in Pediatrics**

1. Upper respiratory tract infections
2. Allergies and asthma
3. Behavioral problems
4. Otitis media
5. Gastrointestinal disorders

### TABLE 4-28
**Selected Fellowship Training Opportunities in Pediatrics**

Adolescent medicine: 3 years

Allergy and immunology: 2 years

Cardiology: 3 years

Child neurology: 3 years

Child and adolescent psychiatry: 2 years

Critical care medicine: 3 years

Endocrinology: 3 years

Gastroenterology: 3 years

Hematology and oncology: 3 years

Infectious diseases: 3 years

Medical genetics: 2–4 years

Neonatal/perinatal medicine: 3 years

Nephrology: 3 years

Pediatric emergency medicine: 3 years

Pulmonary disease: 3 years

Rheumatology: 3 years

## Quick Stats

### PHYSICAL MEDICINE AND REHABILITATION

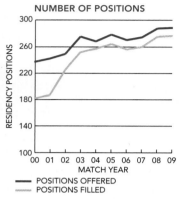

NUMBER OF POSITIONS

— POSITIONS OFFERED
— POSITIONS FILLED

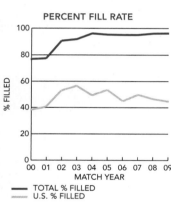

PERCENT FILL RATE

— TOTAL % FILLED
— U.S. % FILLED

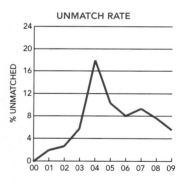

UNMATCH RATE

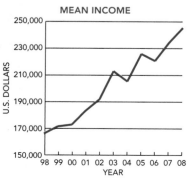

MEAN INCOME

## REFERENCES

Bradford BJ. Pediatric career choices. *Pediatrics* 110:647–648, 2002.

Pan RJ, Cull WL, Brotherton SE. Pediatric residents' career intentions: Data from the leading edge of the pediatric workforce. *Pediatrics* 109:182–188, 2002.

Shelov SP, Burg FD. The pediatric residency match: A worrisome horizon. *Ambul Pediatr* 2:417–418, 2002.

## PHYSICAL MEDICINE AND REHABILITATION

Physical medicine and rehabilitation (PM&R), also known as physiatry or rehabilitation medicine, is a relatively new and exciting field concerned with the treatment of musculoskeletal diseases, focusing on reducing pain and improving function. Physiatrists see patients with a broad range of acute and chronic pain and musculoskeletal problems. Patients include those with more common problems such as back and neck pain, pinched nerves, and fibromyalgia, as well as patients who have had major catastrophic events. Some examples include traumatic brain injuries, strokes, or orthopedic injuries. They also treat patients with neurologic disorders such as multiple sclerosis, polio, and amyotrophic lateral sclerosis (ALS).

Physiatrists can treat patients individually or as consultants, and frequently are the ones to coordinate the services of an interdisciplinary rehabilitation team. They are able to form and maintain relationships with their patients and see a wide variety of patient problems. They enjoy a comfortable lifestyle, often with minimal or no night calls. These attributes have led to PM&R residency becoming more popular and satisfying as a specialty. Some physiatrists may have broad practices, but the newer trend is to specialize in single areas such as pediatric rehabilitation, sports medicine, geriatric medicine, EMG and nerve conduction studies, and brain injury rehabilitation.

Residency training consists of one year in a transitional or preliminary program, followed by three years in a PM&R residency. Some institutions offer a four-year program that includes the internship, while others combine their programs with internal medicine and pediatrics.

PM&R is growing in popularity because it offers the physician the chance to practice holistic medicine, emphasizes building a relationship with the patient, and is associated with a very comfortable lifestyle. In addition, the use of techniques such as fluoroscopy is making the field more exciting, particularly in the areas of sports medicine and interventional pain management.

## APPLICATION TIPS

PM&R residency programs are imbalanced in the sense that the top programs are extremely competitive, while the rest of the programs are progressively less competitive. This disparity offers U.S. graduates and IMGs many opportunities to match in good to very good programs. Programs vary greatly in terms of the relative amount of inpatient rehabilitation training, musculoskeletal medicine, EMG training, and outpatient rehabilitation medicine that is offered. Some programs also incorporate a year of electives and research opportunities. Applicants should investigate these options closely and try to match them with their own preferences. It is a good idea to perform an elective rotation at your program(s) of choice before making a final decision.

## INTERVIEW TIPS

The applicant should show some understanding of the field to demonstrate a strong interest. At the top-rated programs, research experience and electives can make the difference. Expect three to four interviews of 15 to 30 minutes each. Interviewers generally take a relaxed approach and are usually very interested in the applicant's reason for choosing PM&R. Opportunities for research and specialized electives vary greatly among programs, and the interview is a good opportunity to obtain more specific information.

## REFERENCES

Braddom RL, Crawford J, DeLisa JA, Heilman D. Analysis of current practices in recruitment of residents for physical medicine and rehabilitation. *Am J Phys Med Rehabil* 77(4):317–325, 1998.

De Lisa JA, Jain SS, Campagnolo D, McCutcheon PH. Selecting a physical medicine and rehabilitation residency. *Am J Phys Rehabil* 71(2):72–76, 1992.

Millis SR, Campagnolo DI, Kirshblum S, Elovic E, Jain SS, DeLisa JA. Improving resident research in physical medicine and rehabilitation: Impact of a structured training program. *J Spinal Cord Med* 27(5): 428–433, 2004.

Smith J, Krabak BJ, Malanga GA, Moutvic MA. Musculoskeletal education in physical medicine and rehabilitation residency programs. *Am J Phys Med Rehabil* 83(10):785–790, 2004.

> Most medical students are not exposed to PM&R. So if you are interested, seek out a physician to shadow or do an elective.

## TABLE 4-29
### Top Five Most Frequently Encountered Conditions in PM&R

1. Back pain/injury/surgery
2. Stroke
3. Neck pain/injury/surgery
4. Spinal cord injury
5. Arthritis

## TABLE 4-30
### Selected Fellowship Training Opportunities in PM&R

| |
|---|
| Pain management medicine: 1 year |
| Spinal cord injury medicine: 1 year |

## PLASTIC SURGERY

Plastic surgeons are masters of reconstruction. They deal with restoring function and form to disfigured regions of the body whether the defect is caused by trauma, burns, cancer, developmental abnormalities, chronic wounds, or other disease processes. This typically means that plastic surgeons operate beyond just the skin to also include the underlying musculoskeletal system, breasts and body wall, craniofacial structures, extremities, external genitalia, and hands. No other surgeon operates on more regions of the body, which means this field requires an extraordinary anatomical knowledge base.

In general, there are two paths to becoming a plastic surgeon. The first is to match directly from medical school. This is through the regular (NRMP) Match, and the residency is most often a six-year track, though a few programs are seven years in length. There are both integrated and combined programs via this direct match pathway. An integrated program means you are considered a plastic surgery resident from day one. You are under the directorship of the plastic surgery program, and your rotations are guided by the plastic surgery program director. In the combined program, the first three years of residency are in general surgery with the general surgery program director guiding your education. After satisfactory

> Plastic surgery is one of the most competitive fields! Apply to many programs and consider applying in a second field such as general surgery.

# Quick Stats

## PLASTIC SURGERY

### NUMBER OF POSITIONS

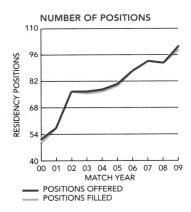

POSITIONS OFFERED
POSITIONS FILLED

### PERCENT FILL RATE

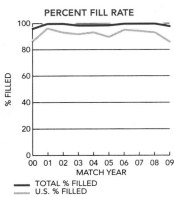

TOTAL % FILLED
U.S. % FILLED

### UNMATCH RATE

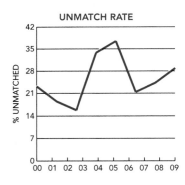

### MEAN INCOME

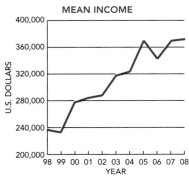

completion of these three years, you automatically transition into plastic surgery residency at the same institution.

The alternative to matching into plastic surgery straight out of medical school is to do a plastic surgery fellowship after at least three years in general surgery or completion of residency in otolaryngology, orthopedics, urology, or neurosurgery. This match is administered by the Plastic Surgery Matching Program (PSMP), which is a component of the San Francisco Matching Program.

Plastic surgery is a relatively new field. It incorporates many skills and techniques from general surgery, ophthalmology, otolaryngology, orthopedics, and oral and maxillofacial surgery. What sets plastic surgeons apart is that they are specifically trained in tissue transfer and microsurgery as it pertains to the use of grafts, flaps, and reimplants. Aesthetic surgery is also a principal component of the plastic surgeon's practice. The ability to enhance beauty comes from the skill and understanding acquired through reconstruction. Plastic surgeons frequently cite the variety of patients and problems as one of the strengths to the field, along with the instant gratification of changing someone's life for the better. In addition, plastic surgery affords the opportunity to participate in both domestic and international philanthropic work.

A plastic surgery residency is a significant commitment and clinicians suggest that those interested in the field attain a good understanding of the field and its demands before applying. Talking to residents, faculty advisors, and practicing plastic surgeons can help those interested to make an informed decision. Sub-internships are also important in this process. The most successful residents value working hard as part of a team, problem solving, and having good interpersonal skills. Beyond this, operative judgment, creativity, technical expertise, attention to detail, a good aesthetic sense, and ethical behavior are especially important. Life as a plastic surgery resident is a busy one. There are plenty of OR cases, clinics, and emergency room consults to keep an entire service of residents busy. A typical day can easily be 12 hours, with a call schedule that can vary from every third to fourth night.

Life after residency is what you make of it. There are plenty of opportunities in both the academic and private sectors, with a vast majority of plastic surgeons working in private practice. Most cosmetic surgery is performed in these private practices, while major reconstructions are typically done in academic practices. This diversity enables the plastic surgeon to find a practice that particularly suits his or her interests and lifestyle preferences. Keeping up with all the information and surgical expertise can be a big challenge. Very long microsurgical cases (greater that 15 hours) and an oversaturation of plastic surgeons in desirable metropolitan areas can also be drawbacks for some.

## APPLICATION TIPS

Plastic surgery is one of the most competitive specialties due to the small number of residency positions and high number of students who apply. Therefore, all aspects of the application are important. Many programs use AΩA status, high USMLE Step 1 board scores, honors in clinical rotations, research experience, and a glowing chair's letter as selection criteria. The letters of recommendation from well-regarded plastic surgeons carry significant weight since plastic surgery is a small field in which most practitioners know each other well, especially at academic institutions. Therefore, it is beneficial to maximize the number of away subinternships and meet as many faculty as possible in the hopes of attaining letters of recommendation. Most applicants apply to at least 30 programs nationally and also rank general surgery programs as a backup.

## INTERVIEW TIPS

As with any highly competitive field, make sure you are well prepared for the interview. If you have been offered an interview, it means your application was strong enough that the program considers you a potential resident. Usually only 10% of applicants are offered an interview. Make sure that your interview does not compromise your chances. Hold several practice interviews and think through your answers to the common interview questions described in Chapter 11. You should have a good explanation for everything mentioned in your application, and leave your interviewers with the impression that you are intelligent, professional, and enthusiastic. Of course, come prepared with questions to ask the faculty and residents to express how interested you are in each program.

The interview is typically a two-day commitment with an informal dinner the night preceding the interviews so that applicants can meet the residents and faculty. Interviews will vary by institution but expect four to nine interviews lasting from 15 to 20 minutes each. Most interviews will be directed by one to three faculty members. It is not unheard of to be asked clinical questions during the interview, but this is increasingly rare. Be prepared for some "pressure sessions" in which you are asked rapid-fire questions that are intentionally antagonistic.

All plastic surgery program directors have a strict policy of no contact following the conclusion of the interview. Therefore, thank-you notes are forbidden as well as any contact between the applicant and members of the faculty. The only exception is logistical questions directed toward the program administrator.

## FOR MORE INFO . . .

**American Society of Plastic Surgeons**
444 E. Algonquin Rd.
Arlington Heights, IL 60005
847-228-9900
www.plasticsurgery.org

## TABLE 4-31

**Top Five Most Frequently Encountered Conditions in Plastic Surgery**

1. Cosmetic (all types)
2. Skin cancer
3. Breast reconstruction
4. Breast reduction surgery
5. Hand surgery

## TABLE 4-32

**Selected Fellowship Training Opportunities in Plastic Surgery**

| |
|---|
| Aesthetics: 1 year |
| Burn surgery: 1 year |
| Craniofacial surgery: 1 year |
| Hand surgery: 1 year |
| Pediatric plastic surgery: 1 year |

## PSYCHIATRY

Psychiatrists specialize in diagnosis and treatment of mental, emotional, and addictive disorders. Advances in the understanding of the neurobiology of mental illness and its complex interactions with social and environmental factors, as well as recent innovations in diagnostic, therapeutic, and imaging techniques have been catalysts for a growing interest in psychiatry among medical students. A recent national study in career satisfaction within specialties showed significant career

> Personal attributes, especially good interpersonal and communication skills, are highly valued in applicants.

# Quick Stats

## PSYCHIATRY

### NUMBER OF POSITIONS

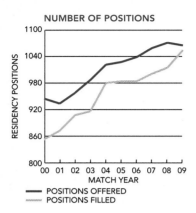

### PERCENT FILL RATE

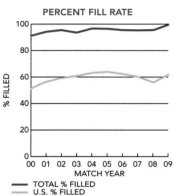

### UNMATCH RATE

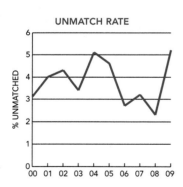

### MEAN INCOME

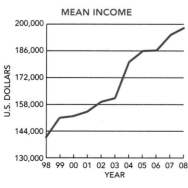

satisfaction in psychiatry, particularly in child and adolescent psychiatry. This satisfaction is in part due to factors such as manageable working hours and controllable lifestyle. Psychiatry offers the opportunity to work in a range of different settings such as inpatient, outpatient, research facilities, and private practice, and call responsibilities are relatively light compared to other specialties.

Residencies in psychiatry generally require a preliminary year, preferably in medicine, followed by three years of training in psychiatry. Most programs have a three- to nine-month rotation in medicine and neurology within the first postgraduate year, followed by three years of rotations of variable length of inpatient, outpatient, and psychiatric subspecialties. The fourth year has some elective time, but some programs incorporate training in neurology or geriatrics during this year.

Depending on the orientation of the program, training may place an emphasis on either psychotherapy or on the biological aspects of mental illness. For this reason, it is important to determine whether the orientation of a particular program matches your expectations and area of interest. Alternatively, you can evaluate whether the program offers good exposure to different areas in psychiatry, giving you the option to later decide your area of interest. The residency should, however, provide you a broad range of patients and exposure to different settings such as outpatient, inpatient, and psychiatric hospitals. As with any specialty, try to gauge the satisfaction among current residents in the programs you visit.

Psychiatry offers a range of subspecialties such as child, forensic, geriatric, addiction, and psychosomatic psychiatry. There is a growing need for psychiatrists in most subspecialties currently throughout the United States, especially in child and geriatric psychiatry.

## APPLICATION TIPS

A combination of good academic credentials, good recommendation letters, and personal attributes—especially good interpersonal and communication skills— are highly valued in applicants. Strong undergraduate backgrounds in behavioral sciences or experience working or volunteering in mental health demonstrates significant interest in psychiatry. Some residency programs value prior research experience.

## INTERVIEW TIPS

Expect to have three to five interviews with different attendings and at times with chief residents. Questions tend to probe the applicant's desire to enter psychiatry, communication skills, and the ability to interact with other people. Interviews also seek to corroborate the information found in the applications, particularly the personal statement.

## FOR MORE INFO . . .

*Directory of Psychiatric Residency Training Programs.* Although this directory is not updated as often as AMA-FREIDA, it has a more logical, user-friendly format. Information unique to the directory includes contact names and numbers for student electives, house staff contact names, and diagrams of a typical resident rotation schedule. The directory also offers general advice about residency applications. It is available at your psychiatry department or can be ordered for $25 with a student discount from:

**American Psychiatric Publishing, Inc.**
1000 Wilson Blvd., Suite 1825
Arlington, VA 22209
(800) 368-5777
www.appi.org

**American Psychiatric Association (APA)**
1000 Wilson Blvd., Suite 1825
Arlington, VA 22209-3901
(888) 35-PSYCH
(703) 907-7300
www.psych.org

**American Academy of Child and Adolescent Psychiatry (AACAP)**
3615 Wisconsin Avenue, N.W.
Washington, D.C. 20016
(202) 966-7300
www.aacap.org

## REFERENCES

Leigh JP, Tancredi DJ, Kravitz RL. Physician career satisfaction within specialties. *BMC Health Serv Res* 9:166, 2009.

Leigh JP, Kravitz RL, Schembri M, Samuels SJ, Mobley S. Physician career satisfaction across specialties. *Arch Intern Med* 162(14):1577–1584, 2002.

Lehrmann JA, Walaszek A. Assessing the quality of residency applicants in psychiatry. *Acad Psychiatr* 32:3, 2008.

Moran M. Medical school grads' interest in psychiatry holds steady. *Psychiatr News* 42(8):1, 2007.

Yudowsky R, Elliott R, Schwartz A. Two perspectives on the indicators of quality in psychiatry residencies: Program directors and residents. *Acad Med* 77(1):57–64, 2002.

*National Resident Matching Program, Results and Data: 2009 Main Residency Match.* National Resident Matching Program, Washington, D.C., 2009.

### TABLE 4-33
**Top Five Most Frequently Encountered Conditions in Psychiatry**

1. Anxiety disorders
2. Depressive disorders
3. Bipolar disorder
4. Substance abuse disorders
5. Schizophrenia

### TABLE 4-34
**Selected Fellowship Training Opportunities in Psychiatry**

Addiction psychiatry: 1 year

Child and adolescent psychiatry: 2 years

Forensic psychiatry: 1 year

Geriatric psychiatry: 1 year

Hospice and palliative medicine: 1 year

Pain management: 1 year

Psychosomatic medicine: 1 year

Sleep medicine: 1 year

## RADIOLOGY

Diagnostic radiology incorporates a variety of radiologic methodologies and techniques to diagnose problems and guide therapies. The field has grown tremendously over the last decade, thanks primarily to advances in image acquisition and image viewing technology. Having good visual orientation and spatial reasoning is critical. A radiology resident must continuously translate two-dimensional images into three-dimensional anatomy. Detail orientation is also necessary to consistently read every portion of every film. This will distinguish a superior resident from one who relies on a "gestalt" impression and misses something in the corner of a film. Being a radiologist requires focus because of the stationary and repetitive nature of the work.

It is also beneficial to be sociable and have a good sense of humor. In contrast to other specialties where the resident and attending may only interact for a few hours during rounds, a radiology resident is in the same room as the attending all day and, for a good portion of that time, directly interacts with that attending while reviewing cases. The ability to maintain stimulating and entertaining conversation makes the day more enjoyable for everyone and is an indispensable skill for a resident.

# Quick Stats

## RADIOLOGY

### NUMBER OF POSITIONS

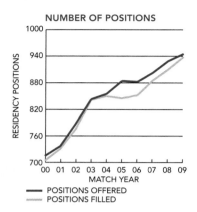

- ■ POSITIONS OFFERED
- ■ POSITIONS FILLED

### PERCENT FILL RATE

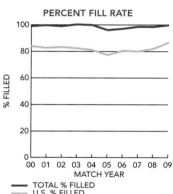

- ■ TOTAL % FILLED
- ■ U.S. % FILLED

### UNMATCH RATE

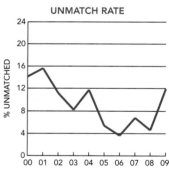

### MEAN INCOME

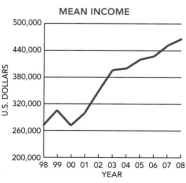

If you appreciate the rewards gained from the interaction with patients, radiology can be challenging because of the minimal patient contact. Radiologists do not have their own patients. Even in interventional radiology, the interaction with the patient is brief and mostly introductory as he or she has been referred from another physician who has already done the primary workup. Radiologists act as consultants to their fellow clinicians in a manner where efficiency is prioritized.

Training in radiology generally requires one preliminary year followed by four years of diagnostic radiology. The preliminary year can be satisfied through completion of a transitional, surgical, or preliminary medicine year. The transitional year internship is probably the most popular choice among radiology residents because of the variety of experience it affords and the amount of exposure to specialized areas of medicine that have field-specific terminology and concepts. The style of radiology training depends on the institution, but all institutions will cover the major imaging modalities, including nuclear medicine, and training in interventional radiology.

A typical workweek in residency is about 60 hours. Postresidency fellowships (one to two years) are offered in a wide variety of organ-based specialties. Fellowships can either lead to a Certificate of Added Qualification (CAQ), such as neuroradiology, pediatric radiology, interventional radiology, and nuclear medicine, or can simply be a focused training without a formally recognized additional certification, such as musculoskeletal radiology, mammography, and body MRI.

Radiologists for the most part continue to enjoy a good lifestyle, relatively high income, flexible work hours, and a good amount of vacation time. Practitioners in other fields, such as cardiology, gastroenterology, and urology, are performing many imaging-guided procedures that compete with the interventional radiology workload. Nevertheless, radiologists are in high demand in many areas of the country. They can practice in either the academic or private setting. Academic positions often pay significantly less but have much lighter workloads. Academic sections often read fewer studies; the attending moves through them more slowly because they are simultaneously teaching, and there is less paperwork since residents do most, if not all, of the dictations. Private practice can be taxing due to the drive to read more studies in order to maximize reimbursement for the practice. However, the higher pay attracts a number of physicians to that arena.

The best preparation for radiology residency is to focus on the motivation behind ordering diagnostic studies for patients. Understanding how differential diagnoses are generated and tested will prepare you conceptually for the types of questions you will have to answer as a radiologist. Also, become familiar with the vernacular of different specialties, names and concepts behind the slew of medical instruments (eg, catheters and drains), and common procedures that patients undergo. This requirement is why a transitional year is a popular choice among applicants.

## APPLICATION TIPS

Strong evaluations in the senior clinical rotations, especially radiology, support the successful application. High board scores and excellent letters of recommendation by senior radiology faculty members are next in importance. Research experience or a technical background prior to entering medical school is also viewed favorably. As with other competitive specialties, early completion of application material is important. You will need to be well organized if you are to coordinate applications for both internship and residency positions. Students are usually advised to apply to at least 20 to 30 programs in order to obtain a comfortable 10 to 15 interviews. However, the best number of programs to apply to varies widely. For applicants whose academic record or board scores are not as competitive, it is not unusual to apply to 50 or more programs.

## INTERVIEW TIPS

Because of the small number of spots available, residency programs in radiology tend to offer interviews only to strong applicants in whom they are seriously interested. A candidate's visit typically includes two to five interviews, each 15 to 30 minutes in length. Interviews for radiology often tend to be relaxed, placing major emphasis on the applicant's reason for entering the field and interviewing at the particular institution. You might also be invited to attend a clinical case conference, but almost no one expects you to be able to read an x-ray on the spot. Quantifying a "good eye" in radiology is even harder than evaluating manual dexterity for a surgical field, so programs don't even try. During the interview sessions, it may be particularly important to assess resident working conditions and satisfaction, which vary significantly among programs.

## FOR MORE INFO . . .

**Career Information Packet.** This packet includes a brochure describing the field of radiology as well as several articles describing job prospects, average earnings, and practice characteristics. This information can be obtained free of charge by calling or writing:

**American College of Radiology (ACR)**
1891 Preston White Drive
Reston, VA 20191-4397
(703) 648-8900
(800) ACR-LINE
www.acr.org

## REFERENCES

Anzilotti K, Kamin DS, Sunshine JH, Forman HP. Relative attractiveness of diagnostic radiology: assessment with data from the National Residency Match Program and comparison with the strength of the job market. *Radiology* 221(1):87–91, 2001.

Pretorius ES, Hrung J. Factors that affect National Resident Matching Program rankings of medical students applying for radiology residency. *Acad Radiol* 9(1):75–80, 2002.

> Many residents do a transitional year in order to gain broad exposure to both medical and surgical fields.

> In competitive fields, ask several mentors how many programs to apply to.

### TABLE 4-35

**Top Five Most Frequently Encountered Conditions in Radiology**

1. Trauma
2. Cancer/malignancy
3. Central nervous system disease
4. Respiratory diseases
5. Breast disease and mammography

### TABLE 4-36

**Selected Fellowship Training Opportunities in Radiology**

Abdominal radiology: 1 year

Cardiothoracic radiology: 1 year

Interventional neuroradiology: 1 year

Musculoskeletal radiology: 1 year

Neuroradiology: 1 or 2 years

Nuclear radiology: 1 year

Pediatric radiology: 1 year

Vascular and interventional radiology: 1 year

## RADIATION ONCOLOGY

Radiation oncologists are an essential part of the multidisciplinary management team for cancer patients, collaborating closely with other physicians. Radiation oncology uses ionizing radiation in the treatment of patients with cancer and

# Quick Stats

## RADIATION ONCOLOGY

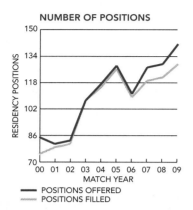

NUMBER OF POSITIONS

- — POSITIONS OFFERED
- — POSITIONS FILLED

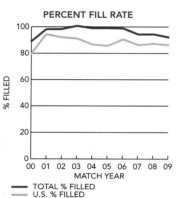

PERCENT FILL RATE

- — TOTAL % FILLED
- — U.S. % FILLED

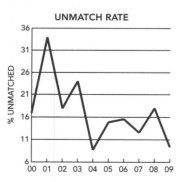

UNMATCH RATE

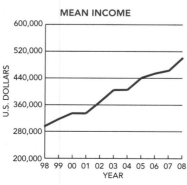

MEAN INCOME

other diseases. Some of the treatment modalities include external beam radiation, brachytherapy, combined chemotherapy, and radiotherapy. They treat tumors at a wide variety of sites in patients of all ages. The field is attractive to some because of its relatively easy lifestyle and minimal call duties. As a result, it is becoming increasingly competitive.

Radiation oncologists enjoy treating a diverse population and working with colleagues in surgical and medical oncology. The field requires an excellent command of the literature and provides lifelong intellectual challenge. Radiation oncology also combines the localized treatment approach of surgery with the intellectual challenges of medicine. This field can be both mentally and psychologically challenging. The mental challenge comes from the wealth of literature and information that must be mastered for each and every disease site. The psychological challenge comes from the significant portion of patients who are receiving palliative care, with some actively dying. However, providing longitudinal care gives an opportunity for meaningful and rewarding relationships with patients.

A one-year internship either in internal medicine, family practice, pediatrics, OB/GYN, or surgery, or a transitional year is required for this specialty, followed by four years of residency in radiation oncology. A typical resident workweek is about 65 to 70 hours. The majority of radiation oncology is outpatient work. Your week consists of clinic time, simulations, and procedures. The clinic time is broken down into new visits, follow-up visits, and on-treatment visits. You will usually attend multidisciplinary tumor boards and classes in radiobiology and physics. The residency also requires a large amount of outside reading. Treating nearly every type of cancer, radiation oncologists must master every disease site on the same level as the surgeon and medical oncologist who specialize in treating that site.

The majority of residents choose to go into practice directly following residency, though there are many opportunities for further clinical or research training. Whether an academic or community practice path is chosen, work hours can be well balanced with life outside the hospital or clinic.

## APPLICATION TIPS

Given the increasing competitiveness of radiation oncology and the small number of positions available at each institution, applicants should do their best to have a strong application so as to increase their chances of matching. Strong letters of recommendation from internal medicine specialists, oncologists, and radiation oncologists are important, as are excellent board scores and clerkship grades. In addition, because it is a research-heavy field, extensive experience with and a demonstrated commitment to clinical or laboratory research is extremely important. Ideally, the research should be within the field of radiation oncology. However, any research experience will be a big plus.

## INTERVIEW TIPS

Interviews are usually conducted one-on-one with an attending. Expect three to four interviews lasting approximately 30 minutes each. Students should express interest in caring for cancer patients and in the basic science on which the field is based. Lifestyle is usually a clear advantage in this field of medicine but should not be the major factor governing its selection. Opportunities for academic medicine and research pursuits may be limited in some programs. In the course of your discussions with residents, ask about the quality of the basic science teaching, and make sure there are adequate staff to teach these principles of the discipline.

> Research experience is a huge plus. Be sure to highlight it in your application.

## FOR MORE INFO . . .

**American College of Radiation Oncology (ACRO)**
4350 East West Highway, Suite 401
Bethesda, MD 20814
(301) 718-6515
www.acro.org

**American Society for Therapeutic Radiology and Oncology (ASTRO)**
12500 Fair Lakes Circle, Suite 375
Fairfax, VA 22033-3882
(800) 962-7876
(703) 502-1550
www.astro.org

## REFERENCES

Bushee GR, Sunshine JH, Schepps B. The status of radiation oncology training programs and their graduates in 1999. *Int J Radiat Oncol Biol Phys* 49(1):133–1138, 2001.

Radiation Oncology Resident Training Working Group. Radiation oncology training in the United States: Report from the Radiation Oncology Resident Training Working Group organized by the Society of Chairman of Academic Radiation Oncology Programs (SCAROP). *Int J Radiat Oncol Biol Phys* 45(1):153–161, 1999.

Zeman EM, Dynlacht JR, Rosenstein BS, Dewhirst MW. Toward a national consensus: Teaching radiobiology to radiation oncology residents. *Int J Radiat Oncol Biol Phys* 54(3):861–872, 2002.

**TABLE 4-37**

**Top Five Most Frequently Encountered Conditions in Radiation Oncology**

1. Lung cancer
2. Breast cancer
3. Prostate cancer
4. Metastatic cancer to the bone
5. Colorectal cancer

**TABLE 4-38**

**Selected Fellowship Training Opportunities in Radiation Oncology (typically 1 year)**

Brachytherapy

Proton therapy

Pediatric radiation oncology

Lymphoma

## TRANSITIONAL-YEAR PROGRAM

A transitional year is a one-year internship that involves broad training and time for a number of electives. It fulfills the internship requirement for residencies in fields such as anesthesiology, radiology, radiation oncology, and dermatology. For those on a quest for a flexible internship, transitional-year programs (TYPs) continue to be a popular choice. In contrast to the preliminary medicine or preliminary surgery years, transitional internships allow for exposure to many other fields, such as OB/GYN, EM, orthopedics, pediatrics, and anesthesia, as well as traditional medicine and surgery. The length of each rotation and the type of work involved are usually flexible and can be tailored to each individual's needs and interests. Some programs will have certain required core rotations that must be satisfied. The best TYPs are found at institutions that have strong departments in all the fields in which you would rotate (particularly in medicine, pediatrics, and surgery). The variety of experience in TYPs is ideal for anyone entering a residency such as radiology, in which a wide base of knowledge is desirable.

Other students take a TYP because they're undecided on a specialty, but this can prove to be a difficult undertaking. By the time your year starts, the application process is already upon you. In addition, finding time for interviews during the year

# Quick Stats

## TRANSITIONAL-YEAR PROGRAM

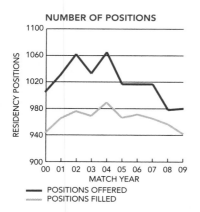

NUMBER OF POSITIONS

— POSITIONS OFFERED
--- POSITIONS FILLED

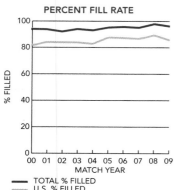

PERCENT FILL RATE

— TOTAL % FILLED
--- U.S. % FILLED

> The Urology Match is run by the American Urological Association (AUA), not the NRMP.

> Urology is gaining popularity among female medical students and residents.

can be challenging. So make sure you reach an understanding with the program director/chief resident regarding the time you will need to apply and interview. If you can't take sufficient time off, it may be preferable to take a year off for research or an MPH degree.

## APPLICATION TIPS

As with most internship programs, the competitiveness of the TYP depends on the reputation of the institution and on the flexibility of the program. Applicants should have strong clinical evaluations, good letters of recommendation, and convincing reasons for seeking a transitional internship. Board scores tend to be less important except at highly prestigious institutions. Early submission of application material is important. Despite the February date posted by many programs, the recommended deadline is early November.

## INTERVIEW TIPS

Interviews are casual and are even optional for some programs. The applicant will usually be scheduled for two or three sessions lasting 30 minutes each. Questions attempt to ascertain the candidate's ability to fit in with the program, desire for a transitional residency, and long-term plans. Interviews for TYPs should center on how the immediate needs of the program and long-term goals of the applicant can be mutually beneficial.

## FOR MORE INFO . . .

*Transitional Year Program Directory.* More popularly known as the "Purple Book," this annually updated directory is available at your student affairs office. You can order your own copy by calling or writing:

**Association for Hospital Medical Education Council of Transitional Year Program Directors**
419 Beulah Road
Pittsburgh, PA 15235
(412) 244-9302
(866) 617-4780
www.ahme.org

## UROLOGY

There are many reasons that people pursue careers in urology and many aspects of urology that you should evaluate when considering applying in urology. One attraction is the wide range of surgeries and procedures. The field provides a balance between surgery and office-based care in which you have the opportunity to perform complicated cystectomies for cancer, ureteroscopy for stone disease, or quicker vasectomies and cystoscopies in the office setting. A second aspect is the continuity of care. There is an opportunity to have an ongoing relationship with patients as you follow them years before or after surgery and counsel them about their diseases, which may range from cancer to voiding dysfunction.

While urology is a surgical field, the lifestyle can be more manageable than many other surgical fields. The training is rigorous. However, since urologists remain in short supply and there are few urologic emergencies, once you finish training there remains good job availability, reasonable hours, and competitive financial compensation compared to many other fields. While it is not necessary to complete a fellowship to find a job, there are many options and opportunities for those interested in further training. Some urologic fellowships include oncology, infertility, female urology, pediatric urology, trauma and reconstruction, and endourologic/laparoscoic/robotic surgery. Robotic and laparoscopic surgery has become a major component of many urologic surgeries and represents a growing and innovative aspect of this field. Although urology remains a male-dominated field, women represent a small but growing minority of residents in training.

Residency training in urology is typically five years in length. The first one or two years of training are in general surgery, followed by at least three to four years in a urology training program. The urology residency match is carried out under the auspices of the American Urological Association (AUA). Some urology programs also use the Electronic Residency Application Service (ERAS).

Many medical school programs do not include urology as a required third-year rotation, and therefore you may not have exposure to the field before the early application deadline. If you might be interested in urology, try to set up an elective as soon as possible. It is encouraged to participate in subinternship rotations at both your home and outside institutions prior to applying.

## APPLICATION TIPS

Urology applications go through an early match managed by the AUA. It is recommended that students submit their applications as soon as possible. Although the deadline for applications is usually November or December, applications should be mailed by October. Factors that will make your application stronger include AΩA status, high USMLE scores, a high GPA, particularly with respect to medicine and surgery clerkship grades, and a recommendation from the chief of urology. Research or special experience in urology provides a competitive advantage. The AUA reports that in 2009 the average number of applications per individual was 43 and the average number of interviews was nine.

## INTERVIEW TIPS

Interviews may be conducted on a group or individual basis and are usually informal and relaxed. There are usually two to three interviews lasting 30 to 45 minutes each. Interviewers attempt to ascertain your personality and whether it is compatible with the program. Applicants should be prepared to describe how they acquired their interest in urology. Expect direct questions about your interest in the clinical and/or research aspects of the program to which you are applying.

# Quick Stats
## UROLOGY

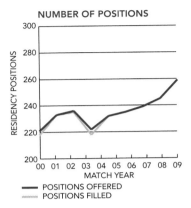

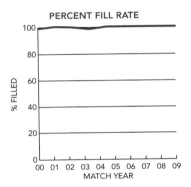

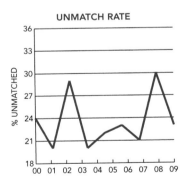

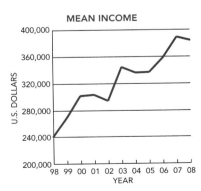

> If you are interested in urology, try to schedule your rotations and subinternships as early as possible.

## TABLE 4-39

**Top Five Most Frequently Encountered Conditions in Urology**

1. Benign prostate disease
2. Prostate cancer
3. Kidney stones
4. Urinary tract infections
5. Sexual dysfunction

## TABLE 4-40

**Selected Fellowship Training Opportunities in Urology**

| |
|---|
| Endourologic laparoscopic fellowship: 1 or 2 years |
| Female urology: 1 or 2 years |
| Male reproductive health: 1 or 2 years |
| Pediatric urology: 1 year |
| Urologic oncology: 1 or 2 years |

## FOR MORE INFO . . .

**American Urological Association Residency Matching Program**
2425 West Loop South, Suite 333
Houston, TX 77027-4207
(800) 282-7077, ext. 86
(713) 622-2700, ext. 86
Vacancy hotline: (800) 282-7077, ext. 88
**www.auanet.org**

**Listing of Accredited Urology Programs, Accreditation Council for Graduate Medical Education**
515 North State Street, Suite 2000
Chicago, IL 60610
(312) 755-5000
**www.acgme.org**

**American Board of Urology**
2216 Ivy Road, Suite 210
Charlottesville, VA 22903
(434) 979-0059
**www.abu.org**

**UrologyMatch,** a forum and informational Web site for medical students applying to urology programs:
**www.urologymatch.com**

## REFERENCES

Andriole DA, Schechtman KB, Ryan K, Whelan A, Diemer K. How competitive is my surgical specialty? *Am J Surg* 184(1):1–5, 2002.

Kerfoot BP, Mitchell ME, Novick AC. Grappling with the evaluation of clinical competencies: A view from the Residency Review Committee for Urology. *Urology* 60(2):223–224, 2002.

Teichman JM, Anderson KD, Dorough MM, Stein CR, Optenberg SA, Thompson IM. The urology residency matching program in practice. *J Urol* 163(6):1878–1887, 2000.

## FELLOWSHIP TRAINING

When considering which residency to choose, it is worth thinking several steps ahead, to possible fellowship training and your ultimate career goals. Most residencies have several fellowships in which further training can be pursued, some of which lead to additional certification. Selected fellowships in some of the more popular fields are described here, along with practical tips on how to boost your chances of getting a spot in a competitive fellowship.

## SELECTED MEDICAL SPECIALTIES

### TABLE 4-41
Match and Income Data for Selected Medical Fellowships Involved in NRMP, 2009

| Fellowship | U.S. Graduate Applicants | Total Applicants | Positions Offered | Programs | % Filled by U.S. Grads | Total % Filled | Median Physician Income 2008 |
|---|---|---|---|---|---|---|---|
| Allergy and Immunology | 128 | 174 | 115 | 70 | 77.4 | 93.9 | $258,459 |
| Cardiology | 496 | 1159 | 712 | 166 | 59.1 | 98.6 | $427,068 |
| Clinical Oncology | 78 | 191 | 44 | 12 | 45.5 | 90.9 | $264,329 |
| Endocrinology | 130 | 325 | 223 | 110 | 44.4 | 87.4 | $197,832 |
| Gastroenterology | 309 | 608 | 339 | 153 | 64.6 | 96.8 | $449,014 |
| Hematology and Oncology | 277 | 706 | 426 | 119 | 51.2 | 96.9 | $373,037 |
| Infectious Disease | 162 | 331 | 303 | 127 | 50.2 | 88.1 | $221,149 |
| Nephrology | 149 | 578 | 367 | 142 | 36 | 94.8 | $283,226 |
| Pulmonary Medicine | 2 | 86 | 20 | 10 | 5 | 100 | $292,596 |
| Pulmonary and Critical Care | 228 | 607 | 397 | 122 | 49.6 | 97.5 | $316,463 |
| Rheumatology | 104 | 243 | 181 | 99 | 48.6 | 92.8 | $218,697 |

*National Resident Matching Program, Results and Data: Specialties Matching Service 2009 Appointment Year.* National Resident Matching Program, Washington, D.C., 2009. (www.nrmp.org/data/resultsanddatasms2009.pdf).

*Physician Compensation and Production Survey 2009.* Medical Group Management Association, Englewood, CO, 2009.

## ALLERGY AND IMMUNOLOGY

Allergy and immunology (AI) is a specialty focused on the evaluation, physical and laboratory diagnosis, and management of disorders involving the immune system. This field goes beyond asthma and autoimmune diseases to include diverse situations such as adverse immunologic reactions and organ transplantation. These specialists typically are involved in discovering patient-specific allergens and then advising how to best alleviate the symptoms. The allergist-immunologist's role is expected to expand as our understanding of the immune system broadens.

AI is one of the few medicine subspecialties without significant call. The lifestyle is not much different than that of a dermatologist. Most of the work is in an ambulatory clinic setting with occasional hospital consults. A typical clinic day may go from 8 A.M. to 5 P.M. You will cover sick call after normal office hours, and this duty can be shared if there are other allergists or nurse practitioners in the practice. Allergists often take a day off during the week to run errands or to catch up on paperwork. Some young allergists may work weekends while they are building their practice. The average workweek is 40 to 50 hours. Most of the work is cognitive, with few procedures that the allergist needs to personally perform. Because the specialty has a conjoint board, you will see both pediatric and adult populations. If you are an academic allergist, you will do more inpatient consults and have the ability to focus on either children or adults, depending where your faculty appointment is.

There are two paths into a two-year AI fellowship: completion of a residency in either medicine or pediatrics. This is the only subspecialty that has a conjoint board [ie, it has two parent boards: the American Board of Internal Medicine (ABIM) and the American Board of Pediatrics (ABP)]. Applicants applying to AI are typically interested in the clinical, academic, and research aspects of this specialty.

There are many attractions to the field of AI. The work is gratifying, as most of the disease entities are manageable and improve over time with current treatment options. The pay is good, and the work hours are very reasonable with little inpatient involvement, which is attractive to many people. From the academic side, there is a huge demand for academicians right out of fellowship. There are good opportunities to conduct research on both the clinical and basic science sides of AI. Translational immunology research often involves other fields, including oncology, nephrology, pulmonology, and gastroenterology. There are ample teaching and research opportunities for private practitioners near academic medical centers or through industry clinical trials. Academic allergists are paid a half to a third less than their counterparts in private practice.

There are, however, still challenges in AI. Depending on your practice setting, you may be restricted to mostly "bread and butter" asthma and rhinosinusitis cases and will not see the clinical diversity that you may have been accustomed to during fellowship training. There may be local "turf" issues with some specialties, such as ENT for allergic rhinitis and pulmonologists for asthma. Allergists earn part of their income though immunotherapy (ie, allergy shots) for allergic asthma and rhinitis. There is a concern that the allergist's income may be affected in the future if immunotherapy is superseded by other preferred therapeutic options.

## APPLICATION TIPS

Applicants tend to be above-average residents with a strong interest in clinical immunology and how it can be applied in disease diagnosis and management. To be competitive for an AI fellowship, you need strong clinical letters and some research experience in the area, preferably with an accepted abstract or a review paper as evidence of your intellectual capability and interest. If you are interested in it, you should consider doing multiple AI electives, performing clinical or basic

> You can do an AI fellowship following residency in either internal medicine or pediatrics.

## TABLE 4-42

### Top Five Most Frequently Encountered Conditions in Allergy and Immunology

1. Allergic rhinitis/conjunctivitis
2. Asthma
3. Urticaria/angioedema
4. Sinusitis
5. Dermatitis

AI research, and attending a national meeting. Fellows who do well have a strong interest in developing ongoing patient relationships and enjoy the cognitive challenge of disease management.

## FOR MORE INFO . . .

**The American Academy of Allergy, Asthma and Immunology**
www.aaaai.org

**The American College of Allergy, Asthma and Immunology**
www.acaai.org

## CARDIOLOGY

Cardiology is an extremely popular and competitive field. It is a subspecialty of internal medicine that is concerned with the diagnosis, prevention, and treatment of diseases of the heart and cardiovascular system. Cardiologists can become involved in a wide range of activities depending on their interests. They can choose to work in outpatient or inpatient settings, perform cardiac imaging, or, with further training, perform interventional procedures. In the hospital, cardiologists frequently work on consult services, advising various services on how best to manage their patients' cardiovascular disease while in the hospital. This is typically a busy role because many elderly adults have heart disease. They also function as interventionalists in the catheterization lab by placing stents under fluoroscopic guidance, and perform electrophysiology ablations that are used to treat atrial fibrillation and ventricular tachycardia. These can be very rewarding specialties where you can witness your interventions improve the prognosis of critically ill patients. There was a time when cardiothoracic surgeons were viewed as the saviors of patients with myocardial infarction, but that paradigm is slowly shifting as cardiologists are able to treat those patients both medically and through procedural interventions.

Another key element in the cardiologist's skill set involves noninvasive imaging such as echocardiography, nuclear cardiology (ie, stress testing), CT angiography, and cardiac MRIs. Cardiac care units are run by cardiologists, who are treating the most critically ill patients and those awaiting transplantation. Cardiologists may also see patients in a typical continuity clinic setting and help to manage outpatient medication needs.

Following medical school and a three-year residency in general internal medicine, a cardiology fellowship requires an additional three years of training. Typically, residents apply during their second year of residency; however, it is still possible to obtain a position during the third year of residency. There is also a "fast-track" program, which consists of applying during one's intern year. This is usually more competitive and oriented for candidates who have an MD/PhD or significant research experience. This option also necessitates that the applicant only apply to his or her home program.

Success in a fellowship is based on various factors, but two that will make you stand out are your willingness and undying commitment to take the best care of the patient and a drive for self-directed learning. Those interested in cardiology

> Cardiology is popular and competitive. Get involved in cardiology research as a resident if you can.

**TABLE 4-43**

Top Five Most Frequently Encountered Conditions in Cardiology

1. Coronary artery disease/angina
2. Congestive heart failure
3. Hypertension
4. Arrhythmias
5. Hyperlipidemias

should demonstrate a consistent zeal to learn, honesty, and an understanding of their own limits. Since medicine is a team endeavor, you must have patience and a willingness to help when interacting with colleagues, coworkers, and nurses. Additionally, it is helpful to be familiar with the scientific method, since the ability to perform research during your fellowship will make for a well-rounded fellowship experience.

One challenging aspect of cardiology is the enormous growth in the field that makes it difficult to keep current. Like many areas of medicine, it can also be a struggle to successfully manage both your professional and private life, since patient care can become all encompassing. Significant opportunities are available for both basic and clinical research in cardiology, and in academic institutions there is increasing pressure to perform research; however, there is often little time and incentive to perform it.

## APPLICATION TIPS

Remember that cardiology is a very competitive fellowship, with more than 500 applications for five to six spots at each specific program. Most commonly, programs interview about ten applicants for one position. Therefore, a top-tier residency program and a strong background in research will a go a long way in securing an interview.

After the three years of general cardiology fellowship, physicians are eligible to sit for the general cardiology boards. However, for those interested in subspecialization, additional training is available in any of the following areas: electrophysiology (additional one to two years), interventional (one year), noninvasive imaging (one year), and advanced heart failure/transplant (one year).

### FOR MORE INFO . . .

**American College of Cardiology**
www.acc.org

**American Heart Association**
www.americanheart.org

**American College of Chest Physicians**
www.chestnet.org

**American College of Physicians**
www.acponline.org/index.html

## ENDOCRINOLOGY

Endocrinology is a subspecialty of internal medicine that deals with the diagnosis and management of disorders of the endocrine system, as well as diabetes and metabolic disorders. Now that obesity is fast becoming one of the most common patient conditions, diabetes and metabolic syndrome are the typical conditions that an endocrinologist encounters. Thyroid disorders and cancer, abnormalities in bone metabolism, and pituitary disorders are other common conditions.

Endocrinology is about feedback loops and the eternal problem of cause and effect. It is an ongoing quest for the basis of diseases and conditions, rooted in principles of physiology and the application of this knowledge to the management of patients. Therefore, a strong grasp of physiology, as well an innate thirst to answer the questions "Why?" and "Now what?" are required. Natural curiosity and the willingness to ponder over complex feedback loops and their effect on various conditions and disease states are essential in a future endocrinologist. The best endocrinologists are those who have a good grasp of the pathophysiologic principles of endocrinology, as well as a strong foundation in internal medicine.

As a fellow, excellent history taking and physical exam skills, meticulousness, thirst for learning, and humility are important characteristics to possess. A focused, but detailed, history is needed, with attention to certain symptoms that are particular to hormonal abnormalities. One must also be adept at performing a physical exam and have a good eye for picking up small details and nuances. Physical exam findings in endocrinologic conditions more often than not are very subtle, such as atrophy of the thenar eminence in uncontrolled diabetes, proximal muscle weakness in Cushing's syndrome, or subtle visual field cuts in a patient with pituitary adenoma. Organizational skills are also a necessity. There are often numerous tests, results, and rechecks that must be followed.

> A good understanding of physiology and an attention to detail are important in endocrinology.

There are four paths that most endocrinologists take after fellowship. The first and most common is private practice. These physicians are usually affiliated with a nearby hospital where they have privileges to see their patients who are admitted. They are also called upon for consults for inpatients. The second pathway is the academic life in a university setting. These endocrinologists see outpatients in the clinic, as well as hospital inpatients. However, they have the added responsibility of serving as medical school faculty or in a residency/fellowship program in the university-based hospital. The third option is research, ranging from bench research to clinical research. A final pathway is any combination of these three options.

The hours and lifestyle of endocrinologists are definite attractions of the field. Since most patients are outpatients, the hours are the typical clinic hours. On-call fellows take calls at home after hours and on weekends. Most matters can be dealt with over the phone. There are only extremely rare emergencies that require the endocrinologist's presence in the middle of the night. Because this field deals with chronic diseases, endocrinologists develop a long-term relationship with their patients, which is both rewarding and fulfilling. However, endocrinology is not known for its financial rewards. A large percentage of the income is from clinic visits and inpatient consults. Procedures, which are typically billed at higher rates, are rare in endocrinology. The only procedures performed by endocrinologists are thyroid ultrasounds and fine-needle aspirations.

**TABLE 4-44**

**Top Five Most Frequently Encountered Conditions in Endocrinology**

1. Thyroid disease
2. Diabetes mellitus
3. Hypertension
4. Hyperlipidemia
5. Osteoporosis

## APPLICATION TIPS

Entrance into an endocrinology fellowship requires completion of a residency in internal medicine. Research experience is looked on favorably, and as in any subspecialty, publications are a big plus. Because endocrinology relies on a strong foundation in internal medicine, a record of competence and a high standard of patient care are important.

**FOR MORE INFO . . .**

The American Association of Clinical Endocrinologists
www.aace.com

The American College of Endocrinologists
www.aace.com/college

## GASTROENTEROLOGY

Gastroenterology is a specialty of internal medicine concerned with the diagnosis, management, and treatment of disorders of the digestive tract from mouth to anus. This includes but is not limited to diseases of the esophagus, stomach, small and large intestine, pancreas, liver, and gallbladder. With the increasing prevalence of endoscopy, gastroenterology is becoming a more procedure-intense specialty.

Gastroenterology is an exciting subspecialty, in part because it is one of the few medical subspecialties that involve diseases intrinsic to multiple organs, each of which have unique physiology and pathophysiology. In addition, gastroenterologists can train to specialize in multiple types of procedures, such as diagnostic esophagogastroduodenoscopy (EGD), diagnostic colonoscopy, endoscopic treatment of upper and lower GI bleeding, endoscopic retrograde cholangiopancreatography (ERCP), endoscopic ultrasound, liver biopsy, endoluminal stenting, esophageal dysplasia ablation, esophageal stricture dilatation, and percutaneous endoscopic gastrostomy tube placement. Therefore, the field requires mastery of both intellectual knowledge and procedural knowledge, which provides a diverse experience when caring for patients.

> Many people are attracted to gastroenterology because it provides the opportunity to perform procedures.

The challenges of the field parallel the attractions of the field. Because gastroenterology encompasses disease of multiple organs, it is challenging and perhaps impossible to have expertise in all aspects of gastroenterology. Gastroenterologists will often subspecialize in a certain aspect of gastroenterology (eg, inflammatory bowel disease, general hepatology, motility disorders, pancreaticobiliary diseases) to acquire and maintain expertise within a specific niche.

There are several keys to success in internal medicine residency and gastroenterology fellowship. Organizational skills and the ability to prioritize are paramount. As an intern and resident, there are an overwhelming number of daily tasks. These include examining patients; evaluating and analyzing labs, imaging studies, and data; discussing cases with colleagues and consultants; counseling patients and families; and entering patient care orders. One must develop the ability to determine the order in which tasks must be executed and ensure that all of them are completed in a timely manner. Communication skills with both patients and colleagues are also a priority. One must be able to succinctly, accurately, professionally, and empathetically communicate with others. In addition, perseverance, composure under pressure, intellectual curiosity, and patience are key.

In a gastroenterology fellowship, hours are limited by Accreditation Council for Graduate Medical Education (ACGME) requirements that are similar to those of residency. However, since fellowship call is taken as "home call," the work-hour regulations are modified such that the total number of hours worked per week must be less than 80 hours, inclusive of the hours spent in the hospital when taking call.

The training required to be board eligible for gastroenterology includes four years of medical school, three years of internal medicine or primary care residency, and three years of gastroenterology fellowship. A fourth year of gastroenterology fellowship to obtain further training is optional. The two fourth-year fellowships are either in advanced endoscopy (ERCP and/or endoscopic ultrasound) or transplant hepatology.

## APPLICATION TIPS

As with any subspecialty, a strong background in internal medicine is crucial. If you are interested in gastroenterology, try to complete rotations in it as a resident to get a feel for whether you enjoy the procedural aspect, as well as any particular part of the field that interests you most (eg, hepatology or inflammatory bowel disorders). Research in the field is always a plus.

### FOR MORE INFO . . .

**American College of Gastroenterology**
www.acg.gi.org

**American Gastroenterological Association**
www.gastro.org

**American Society for Gastrointestinal Endoscopy**
www.asge.org

**TABLE 4-45**

**Top Five Most Frequently Encountered Conditions in Gastroenterology**

1. Gastroesophageal reflux disease
2. Irritable bowel syndrome
3. Colon cancer screening
4. Hepatitis
5. Inflammatory bowel disease

## HEMATOLOGY AND ONCOLOGY

Hematology/oncology (heme/onc) is a specialty of internal medicine or pediatrics that has a dual focus on benign hematologic conditions as well as hematologic malignancies and solid tumors. Heme/onc physicians diagnose, follow up, treat, and offer palliative care to the wide range of patients with these conditions. Oncologists also play a major role in health care policy by establishing the principles of cancer screening for populations. Oncologists serve as the primary coordinators of care for patients with cancer, but frequently interact as a team with radiologists, pathologists, surgeons, and clinical researchers. Heme/onc also has a strong research component, with practitioners frequently involved in laboratory projects. It is not uncommon for MD/PhDs to choose this specialty, because it provides an invigorating academic environment in which clinical medicine and basic science research can flourish and allow a seamless transition from bench to bedside.

Depending on the practice, the average clinical provider spends about two to three days/week in clinic and attends on service approximately 12 weeks/year. Outpatient management of patients varies from a single initial consultation and follow-up with primary care providers to frequent clinic visits for administration of chemotherapy, blood product support, or intravenous therapy. Inpatient coverage usually includes overnight call responsibilities, that is, taking calls from the house staff on the wards and in the emergency rooms. Inpatient responsibilities include management of the resident staff in caring for patients admitted for any number of reasons: initial cancer diagnosis, chemotherapy, fever and neutropenia, sepsis, blood product support, vaso-occlusive pain crisis, acute chest syndrome, splenic sequestration, stroke, deep vein thrombosis, pulmonary embolism, and other bleeding diatheses.

The care of children and adults with cancer and blood disorders can be challenging in terms of the emotional connection that physicians feel for their patients over the months or years of treating them. The logistics of getting the necessary support services in place for these patients can also be difficult. There are limited home care nursing, pharmacy, and hospice services, which can cause physicians to become frustrated when they are not able to deliver the best quality of care.

The most talented fellows demonstrate confidence, humility, and an overall determination to learn all aspects of the field. A heme/onc fellowship is three years in length and requires the completion of a residency in internal medicine or pediatrics. The first year of fellowship is much like residency, although with greater responsibility. The clinical fellowship year is extremely intense and is spent managing the immediate needs of the entire inpatient and outpatient service by guiding and mentoring of the clinical staff. Thereafter, the focus shifts to a dedicated research effort. Completion of a scientifically meaningful project is a requirement of all fellowships. There are opportunities to pursue either clinical or basic science research projects, depending on your interests. During these two to three years, you will gain experience reading and reviewing academic literature, preparing your own research findings for publication, and learning how to draft applications to fund-granting agencies. Again, depending on your interests, you may choose to seek out opportunities to continue your research or to join the faculty of an academic practice as clinical staff.

> It is possible to specialize in hematology or oncology alone, but the combined heme/onc track is most common.

## TABLE 4-46

### Top Five Most Frequently Encountered Conditions in Heme/Onc

1. Myeloid cancers
2. Anemia
3. Lung cancer
4. Colon cancer
5. Breast cancer

## APPLICATION TIPS

Applications are sent through ERAS, and applicants participate in the subspecialty's NRMP Match. Since heme/onc is a field that values research, it is helpful to have experience in research during residency, especially on a topic related to heme/onc. There are also fellowships offered in hematology or oncology alone. However, the combined heme/onc fellowship is more common and allows for greater flexibility and diversity in future practice.

## FOR MORE INFO . . .

**American Society of Hematology**
www.hematology.org

**American Society of Clinical Oncology**
www.asco.org/portal/site/ascov2

**American Society of Pediatric Hematology/Oncology**
www.aspho.org

## INFECTIOUS DISEASE

Pathogens are ubiquitous and infect patients of all sorts—those who are generally healthy and those who are chronically ill. Therefore, infectious disease (ID) specialists are critical at all levels from outpatient to intensive care. Their broad expertise is necessary for optimal patient care, research, directing public health efforts, and developing new antimicrobial agents. It is particularly useful training for those with an interest in global health. Consequently, training in ID attracts highly motivated individuals with varying interests who all desire to solve important problems.

Traditionally, an adult ID fellowship is undertaken after three years of training in an internal medicine residency, while pediatric ID fellowships follow residency training in pediatrics. Since ID specialists do not focus on any particular organ or system, they must have a broad knowledge of internal medicine and hence are among the finest clinicians. A wise internal medicine program director once said, "What you do not learn during residency, you will not learn during fellowship." This foundation is built upon one's dedication to outstanding patient care during internal medicine residency: taking a careful history; finely honing physical exam skills; constantly reading; and personally reviewing radiology films, blood smears, and biopsy results. Prior to matriculation, some residents and students will have had exposure to tropical medicine or some type of basic, translational, or clinical research. This is not a prerequisite for fellowship but may help guide one's future career. Some residents choose to "fast track" into an adult ID fellowship after two years of residency training. Fellowship training can occur in large university settings where research is an essential component, or in community settings where the emphasis is on direct patient care, and the fellowship is typically three or two years, respectively.

Given the demand for ID physicians in hospitals, there is hardly a typical day. Consistently, however, the hours are long, problems are challenging, and the work is always intellectually and personally satisfying. As an ID fellow, time can also be spent performing basic, translational, or clinical research or being directly involved in patient care. The scheduling depends on the institution (eg, some require all clinical training in the first year followed by protected research time in the subsequent years while others intersperse clinical care blocks with research blocks for the duration of the fellowship).

The majority of patient care is delivered in the inpatient setting with a smaller component in an outpatient clinic (general infectious diseases or the longitudinal HIV/AIDS clinic). In the inpatient setting, ID physicians can serve as the primary team for patients or act as consultants to medical and nonmedical services. When caring for inpatients, fellows evaluate data in the microbiology lab daily and review films and slides in the radiology and pathology departments, respectively. Call is taken from home with the schedule varying by institution. It is common to answer clinical questions over the phone, and it is not uncommon to go into the hospital to tend to a sick patient. Finally, depending on institutional support, tropical

> ID is a field of problem solving that requires close attention to detail.

medicine electives may be arranged. Again, the days are not typical, but the field is very rewarding at multiple levels.

A genuine interest in solving problems and keen eye for detail separate ID specialists from many other physicians. This involves a dedicated amount of time, so patience is necessary. One must be a lifelong learner and be able to communicate effectively with the microbiology lab, patient, primary team, and other consultants. Furthermore, ID specialists must understand and respond to the needs and specific practices of other medical and surgical disciplines. In addition to the complex clinical care outlined, the diversity of career opportunities is also one of the attractions.

While a difficult exercise, as a medical student, you should ask yourself, "Where do I see myself in five or ten years?" Once you identify your interests, you should seek out appropriate individuals who are currently in that area of mutual interest and "pick their brain" with questions such as: What are pros and cons of the position? How did the individual get to where they are now? If they could go back in time, what would they change? Finally, aside from traditional medical student rotations on an inpatient ID consultative service or outpatient clinic, consider doing a tropical medicine rotation, spending time in a microbiology or virology lab, or rotating with the department of public health. Again, the need for ID physicians is broad, so you can make your career what you want it to be!

## APPLICATION TIPS

As in any specialty, successful trainees will be most productive at a place where their research interests and organizational culture are similar to those of the institution. After identifying your own interests, scan recent literature and the Web. Is there a particular investigator or study group from an institution that consistently publishes on a topic you are interested in? Currently funded research projects are accessible online through Web sites such as www.clinicaltrials.gov or http://projectreporter.nih.gov. Finally, talk to your mentors and program director about your interests and goals, as they can give you crucial insights about ID programs. In preparing your application, follow all directions posted, provide ample time to collect the letters of recommendation, and try to have a focused, clear, and concise personal statement.

By the time you are interviewing for an ID fellowship, you will already be familiar with the interviewing process from your internal medicine interviews. Beyond traditional questions about your experiences gained during internal medicine residency, your career goals, and why you are interested in ID, interviewers may focus on your prior scholarly activity (publications, presentations, or posters) and how your future research and clinical interests match those of the institution. Some institutions will require you to identify a potential mentor or research project while applying. If you are interested in ultimately making your mark in ID in global health, it is important to take advantage of any clinical and/or research opportunities that are available during your residency (and even in medical school). Fellowship directors want to see evidence of your commitment to and passion for global health.

## TABLE 4-47

**Top Five Most Frequently Encountered Conditions in Infectious Disease**

1. HIV/AIDS
2. Pneumonia
3. Osteomyelitis
4. Sepsis
5. Fever

## FOR MORE INFO . . .

**The Infectious Diseases Society of America** has a wealth of information for prospective students, residents, and current fellows. Go to **www.idsociety.org**, then click on the "Education and Training Tab" located at the top of the page.

# NEPHROLOGY

Nephrology is a branch of internal medicine that deals with the kidney in health and disease. It offers great variety in patient care. The patients seen by a nephrologist may range from the relatively healthy to those in the intensive care unit. Nephrologists are frequently consulted for help in the care of patients with electrolyte disorders, acid-base disorders, and severe hypertension. Renal replacement therapy for patients suffering from kidney failure represents a large component of the field and includes providing acute and chronic dialysis as well as care for patients after kidney transplantation. Transplantation introduces added complexity in its intersection with the field of immunology.

Entrance to an adult nephrology fellowship requires completion of an internal medicine residency, while entrance to a pediatric nephrology fellowship requires completion of a residency in pediatrics. Fellows become board eligible after two years of training. Most training programs are two years in length. However, some combined research and clinical pathway programs require three years. A few university hospitals offer an additional one-year fellowship to subspecialize in transplant nephrology. Depending on the fellowship program, most renal fellowships are extremely busy with long working hours. The fellow frequently has to come in at night to provide urgent dialysis in patients suffering from multiorgan failure in the intensive care unit.

Compared to cardiology and gastroenterology, nephrologists do not perform a large number of procedures except for placing catheters for dialysis access and performing kidney biopsies. Interventional radiologists, depending on the hospital and private practices, are also performing some of these procedures. Private nephrologists often have a large patient population, with many dialysis patients.

Nephrology has a very strong basis in physiology, and many diseases, such as electrolyte disorders, cardiogenic shock, and sepsis, require a deep understanding of the underlying pathophysiology, rather than memorization of a list of facts. In addition, nephrology requires a solid grounding in internal medicine in order to deal with consults on patients with a wide variety of concomitant conditions or illnesses. Nephrologists have the opportunity to have short encounters with patients that greatly impact their care as consultants, and can also develop long-term relationships with their end-stage renal disease (ESRD) or transplant patients. However, the care of patients with ESRD who require chronic dialysis can be very challenging. This patient population overall has a short life expectancy and requires frequent hospitalization.

Nephrology continues to be a field that has close ties to physiology departments and can involve basic science research. If physiology fascinates you and

> Nephrology requires a deep understanding of the physiology and pathophysiology of the kidney.

## TABLE 4-48

**Top Five Most Frequently Encountered Conditions in Nephrology**

1. Chronic renal failure and transplantation
2. Hypertension
3. Diabetes mellitus
4. Acute renal failure
5. Electrolyte imbalances

you like caring for patients with complex disorders, then nephrology is a field you should strongly consider.

## APPLICATION TIPS

Training programs vary largely depending on the interests of the faculty. Programs may focus on basic science research, clinical research, or in training individuals who will go directly into clinical practice. None of these programs will exclusively take fellows that match their department's general orientation, but will certainly favor applicants with similar interests.

Once you begin interviews, be sure you are well prepared. Anticipate the questions that will be asked: Why have you chosen this specialty? What fascinates you about nephrology? Are you interested in basic science or clinical research? Where do you see yourself in ten years? What have you done so far in the field (eg, case reports, research experience, attended meeting, references who are nephrologists who supervised you during your residency)? Read about the faculty and the research they perform so that you can discuss it with them.

## FOR MORE INFO . . .

**American Society of Nephrology**
www.asn-online.org

## RHEUMATOLOGY

Rheumatologists rely on detective-like skills as they evaluate patients who have had extensive workups but whose diagnosis remains elusive. They diagnose and treat patients with systemic autoimmune diseases such as rheumatoid arthritis, systemic lupus erythematosus, and scleroderma, many of which are rare and have fascinating presentations. Rheumatologists also medically manage more common arthritic conditions such as osteoarthritis and gout. The advent of several new biological agents has begun a new era in the management of autoimmune diseases. An inquisitive mind, patience, and compassion are all traits that will serve a rheumatologist well.

Entry to an adult rheumatology fellowship requires completion of a three-year internal medicine residency. To acquire eligibility for the board certification examination in rheumatology, two years of fellowship training are required. Although most programs are two years in length, some of the more academic programs are three years, where the first year is predominantly clinical, and the second and third years are usually research based. Get to know the programs before applying so that you know whether they are geared toward those interested in academics or are more clinically based. The number of fellows recruited each year varies from one to four. In programs recruiting only one fellow per year, as a first-year fellow you will be on the consult service for the majority of the year. Many academic programs offer opportunities to obtain MPH or PhD degrees. There are also a dozen or so combined rheumatology and allergy programs.

After a fellowship, there are three common pathways that are pursued. One is academic rheumatology, which involves either clinical or basic science research. The second is clinical practice, and the third is industry positions. The hours are lighter compared to other specialties, but accordingly the compensation remains at the low end of the spectrum for the internal medicine subspecialties.

Rheumatology is a field in which you can develop a close relationship with your patient, sometimes acting as their primary care provider. Managing chronic persistent pain becomes both a science and an art. Because many of the conditions are rare and can have diverse presentations, there is the thrill of going after the diagnosis. Procedures such as joint injections, which give immediate relief, can be very rewarding and add a practical dimension. It is a very intellectual specialty, and a firm grasp of immunology is important in understanding the pathogenesis of autoimmune diseases and their treatments.

Rheumatologists have to be able to deal with uncertainty and help their patients to do the same. Despite many investigations, the diagnosis may not always be clear. Rheumatologists are often working alongside other specialists and allied medical professions to manage complicated patients. Therefore, effective and frequent communication is necessary and may be time consuming. A fellow can expect to spend equally as much time (or more) with follow-ups and paperwork as with the actual patient in a clinical setting.

> Rheumatologists frequently see patients who have puzzling arrays of symptoms, and must figure out the diagnosis.

## APPLICATION TIPS

Applications are sent through ERAS, and should be submitted by early December (18 months before the fellowship start date). The majority of programs participate in the internal medicine subspecialties NRMP match, and results are announced in mid-June.

Rheumatology exposure during residency can vary, so it is important to arrange an elective early and preferably in a hospital with a fellowship program. Letters of recommendation from senior rheumatology faculty who demonstrate that they have worked closely with you will make for a stronger application. Fellowship programs in big cities, in the Northeast, and on the West Coast tend to be more competitive. Relevant research and publications are not a requirement, but program directors look more favorably at candidates who have them.

Interview season usually runs from mid-January to mid-May. As rheumatology departments are small, and most of the faculty want to meet applicants, be prepared for several (sometimes up to 12) interviews in one day. Almost every interviewer wants to know where you see yourself in ten years to gauge if you are headed for research or a clinical career. Make sure you are aware of the research interests of the department. The opinions of current fellows in a program are invaluable. Ask them about their experiences on the consult service, the teaching experience of the faculty, how well the clinics are run, and if they are able to see a wide cross-section of rheumatologic diseases. It is an advantage if you have an idea of the career path you would like to pursue after fellowship when applying.

### TABLE 4-49

**Top Five Most Frequently Encountered Conditions in Rheumatology**

1. Rhematoid arthritis
2. Osteoarthrits
3. Systemic lupus erythematosus
4. Fibromyalgia
5. Osteoporosis

## FOR MORE INFO . . .

American College of Rheumatology
www.rheumatology.org

## SELECTED SURGICAL SPECIALTIES

### TABLE 4-50

**Match and Income Data for Selected Surgical Fellowships Involved in NRMP, 2009**

| Fellowship | U.S. Grad Applicants | Total Applicants | Positions Offered | Programs | % Filled by U.S. Grads | Total % Filled | Median Physician Income 2008 |
|---|---|---|---|---|---|---|---|
| Abdominal Transplant Surgery | 25 | 86 | 78 | 61 | 32.1 | 70.5 | $390,000 |
| Colon and Rectal Surgery | 81 | 113 | 78 | 43 | 82.1 | 97.4 | $363,000 |
| Pediatric Surgery | 42 | 61 | 40 | 40 | 75 | 100 | $444,195 |
| Surgical Critical Care | 73 | 95 | 143 | 75 | 47.6 | 59.4 | $259,856 |
| Thoracic Surgery | 76 | 101 | 118 | 86 | 60.2 | 79.7 | $438,724 |
| Vascular Surgery | 76 | 101 | 118 | 86 | 60.2 | 79.7 | $385,609 |

### REFERENCES

*National Resident Matching Program, Results and Data: Specialties Matching Service 2009 Appointment Year*. National Resident Matching Program, Washington, D.C., 2009. (www.nrmp.org/data/resultsanddatasms2009.pdf).

*Physician Compensation and Production Survey 2009*. Medical Group Management Association, Englewood, CO, 2009.

## ABDOMINAL TRANSPLANT SURGERY

Abdominal transplant surgery is a surgical subspecialty that requires a broad knowledge of surgery and medicine. Abdominal transplant surgeons treat patients with end-stage hepatic, renal, intestinal, and pancreatic diseases. They also manage the immunosuppresive treatments for patients following transplantation. As a result, transplant surgeons maintain a lifelong relationship with their patients.

Organ transplantation is an exciting but very challenging field. Attractions of the field include the complexity of cases and the long-term relationship with the patients. Also, for individuals who enjoy immunology, transplantation is a career option. Transplant surgeons are often trained in multiorgan transplantation, though many later choose to focus on either kidney/pancreas transplantation or liver/intestinal transplantation. Some surgeons perform a variety of operations consisting of transplants, liver resections, and dialysis access. Other transplant surgeons may continue to perform a wide variety of general surgery procedures as well.

The field of organ transplantation is very rewarding but demanding. Because of the unpredictability of when a transplant donor will be available, the hours involved in transplantation can be difficult and variable. The hours after fellowship are slightly better but not vastly improved. However, seeing a patient who had

> Transplant surgeons must perform the operations when an organ becomes available, whether that is between 9 A.M. and 5 P.M. or in the middle of the night.

been in fulminant hepatic failure walk out of the hospital after a liver transplant is truly amazing. Some transplant surgeons may seek to have a more predictable schedule and can have careers in hepatobiliary or general surgery.

Entry into a transplant surgery fellowship requires completion of a general surgery residency. Most fellowships are two years in length, although some centers offer a third year that focuses on specialized areas such as intestinal transplantation or pediatric liver transplantation. The number of fellows recruited to each program per year varies from one to four. Most programs are structured around four rotations: renal transplantation, donor service, pancreas transplantation, and liver transplantation. After a transplant fellowship, most surgeons pursue a career in academics. Positions are usually clinically based with opportunities to be involved in basic science research.

## APPLICATION TIPS

Instructions for applying to transplant surgery fellowships are found on the Web sites of most programs. The American Society of Transplant Surgeons (ASTS) has a list of accredited transplant surgery fellowships, as well as the focus of each program (ie, renal, pancreas, liver, or intestinal transplantation). The ASTS Web site (www.ASTS.org) also has a listing of important dates for the abdominal transplant surgery match. Most applicants apply in the fourth year of surgery residency.

Each program generally requires a personal statement, CV, and three letters of recommendation. Letters of recommendation from any surgical faculty member are accepted, but many programs favor letters from other transplant surgeons who have worked with you and can attest to your potential in transplantation. Although there are approximately 70 active transplant fellowship positions each year, nearly 30% go unfilled. Fellowship programs that are multiorgan focused tend to be more competitive. Relevant research in immunology or transplantation is not a requirement, but program directors view candidates with research more favorably.

Interviews are conducted from February to May, the NRMP rank list for programs is due by the beginning of June, and the Match results are available late in June. Since transplant fellows are an integral part of the transplant program, many of the faculty and transplant coordinators will want to meet applicants on interview day. The discussion with the transplant fellows at every program where you interview is important. Ask them about their operative experience. This is especially important in liver transplants. Also, ask each fellow about his or her experience with the job search and where previous fellows have gone for faculty positions. Currently, the market for transplant surgeons is a major concern, and some programs may have fellows who cannot find job positions. The top five most frequently encountered conditions are not included here, as they were not available for abdominal transplant surgery.

## ▌ FOR MORE INFO . . .

**American Society for Transplant Surgery**
www.ASTS.org

## CARDIOTHORACIC SURGERY

Cardiothoracic surgery is the surgical specialty focused on diseases of the thorax, which typically include disorders of the heart and great vessels along with the lungs, conducting airways, and the esophagus. While the surgical interventions of these diseases remain the focus of this profession, there is an increasing push from within the community for cardiothoracic surgeons to be involved in noninvasive diagnostic procedures. This is an area that is currently in flux, and the future remains undecided.

As with the other surgical specialties, cardiothoracic surgery blends an interest in anatomy, pathology, and physiology. Beyond that, cardiothoracic surgery is especially challenging technically and employs a varied skill set for a broad spectrum of procedures. Most of all, operating on the heart and putting a patient on "pump" are privileged experiences that hold intrinsic value for those who are enthusiastic about the field. For general thoracic surgery, operations for early-stage lung and esophageal cancers provide good cure rates, and the outcomes can be very rewarding.

It is no secret that the number of coronary artery bypass graft (CABG) surgeries has decreased with the growing use of stents. As a result, fewer jobs currently exist, the surgical patients are sicker, and reimbursements are lower. There has been a subsequent decline in applicants for training, though more than half of currently practicing surgeons are expected to retire in the next 12 years. Consequently, there will be a shortage of cardiothoracic surgeons by the year 2020, even if all CABG cases are eliminated.

Cardiothoracic surgeons have had to reinvent themselves amidst the drop in CABG cases, and this has fueled exciting technological advances in minimally invasive surgery, ablative procedures for atrial fibrillation, endovascular treatment of aortic disease, percutaneous valve replacement, and off-pump coronary revascularization. Regardless, the training in cardiothoracic surgery rightly focuses on the acquisition of basic skills, such as performing a good vascular anastomosis, putting a patient on bypass, managing an acute aortic dissection, and working up a lung mass. Success in these endeavors should guide one's evaluation of a residency program for training.

There are now multiple routes of training available to become a cardiothoracic surgeon. The most common path is to enter a two- or three-year specialty training in cardiothoracic surgery after completion of a general surgery residency. Candidates apply during their fourth year of residency as part of a match. While they are eligible to sit for the boards in general surgery, this is no longer required for American Board of Thoracic Surgery (ABTS) certification. Residents are now also required to choose a concentration: "cardiothoracic," which places an emphasis on cardiac and vascular surgery; or "general thoracic," which focuses on the lungs and airway, foregut, chest wall, diaphragm, and tumors of the mediastinum. Each track determines the number of cases required for graduation, but both lead to full ABTS certification.

Recently, two alternatives to the traditional pathway have emerged: "integrated" and "fast-track." The integrated pathway is a six-year program that starts right after medical school. Depending on the program, the first two years involve varying amounts of time in general surgery, vascular surgery, cardiology, interventional radiology, and trauma surgery. This is followed by four years of standard cardiothoracic training at the same institution. The fast-track pathway is seven years and starts off with traditional training in general surgery. One applies after the second year for a fast-track position at the same institution. There is an early emphasis on cardiothoracic training by the fourth year. Only a handful of integrated and fast-track programs currently exist, and the results of this training method are not yet known. However, the ABTS has proposed that the integrated approach become the sole pathway for certification by 2020.

The ideal type of training model has been a matter of debate, and the best fit may vary according to the individual. While medical students with strong aspirations for the field may benefit from the integrated pathway, many people will need more time and experience before making the commitment, so starting with general surgery would be more appropriate. If one's interest eventually leads to general thoracic surgery, then longer training in general surgery may also be desirable. The fast-track model might be a suitable intermediate between the other two pathways. Of course, the traditional model has time-proven results, and future colleagues and employers have a lot of faith in that system.

Those interested in subspecialty training have many options. For example, to train in congenital cardiac surgery, you must first complete a cardiothoracic residency through any of the three pathways, which provides fundamental exposure to the field. Thereafter, you must undergo a 12-month ACGME-approved fellowship leading to ABTS certification. Other fields available for additional training include minimally invasive surgery, cardiac transplantation, aortic and endovascular surgery, and congenital heart surgery. This training may take the form of an ACGME-approved fellowship, as in congenital heart surgery, or less formal "super-fellowships" that may last six months to two years.

Both adult cardiac and thoracic patients tend to have multiple comorbidities, and postoperative management can often be challenging. With the need to fit in the requisite clinical and operative experience, average hours during residency easily approach 80 hours per week. Depending on a variety of factors, average hours for an attending generally range from 60 to 80 hours per week.

For those who choose an academic milieu, one usually focuses on either cardiovascular or general thoracic surgery. In private practice, there is more of a blend. In either case, the first year out is widely regarded as the time when technical maturity becomes more solidified.

## APPLICATION TIPS

Those wishing to apply in this field should develop a good foundation in critical care, as it informs much of the decision making in cardiothoracic surgery. Also, the chief year in general surgery is a prime opportunity to mature technically and clinically. Finally, good surgical mentors can be invaluable. Important characteristics of a cardiothoracic fellow are integrity, efficiency, and a willingness to work as hard as an intern, even after being chief resident in general surgery. A passion for the field also helps to overcome many obstacles.

> There are now three paths to CT surgery: an "integrated" path, a "fast-track" path, and the traditional two to three years of training following general surgery residency.

### TABLE 4-51

**Top Five Most Frequently Encountered Conditions in Cardiothoracic Surgery**

1. Lung cancer
2. Noncardiac vascular disease
3. Coronary artery disease
4. Valvular heart disease
5. Congenital heart disease

## REFERENCES

Grover A, Gorman K, Dall TM, Jonas R, Lytle B, Shemin R, Wood D, Kron I. Shortage of cardiothoracic surgeons is likely by 2020. *Circulation* 12:488–494, 2009.

## FOR MORE INFO . . .

**American Academy of Thoracic Surgeons**
www.aats.org
This Web site has good sections for both medical students and residents interested in the field.

**American Board of Thoracic Surgeons**
www.abts.org

## COLON AND RECTAL SURGERY

Colon and rectal surgery is a surgical subspecialty that focuses on the diagnosis and management of benign and malignant diseases of the colon, rectum, and anus. Diseases encountered by the colorectal surgeon include, but are not limited to, colorectal cancer, inflammatory bowel disease, diverticulitis, and pelvic floor and anorectal disorders. A unique aspect of colorectal surgery is the ability of surgeons to both diagnose and manage their patients. They perform endoscopic (sigmoidoscopy, colonoscopy), physiologic (manometry, electromyographic studies, etc.), and radiologic (defecography, endorectal or endoanal ultrasound) studies to diagnose the disorder, and then manage the problem as indicated by their workup. A successful colorectal surgeon will have an inquiring mind that can meet the challenges of elusive diagnoses or poorly understood diseases, and a steady hand that can perform lifesaving surgeries or push the boundaries of advanced laparoscopy.

Entry into a colorectal surgery residency requires the completion of a five-year general surgery residency at an ACGME-accredited institution. Board certification requires the completion of a one-year fellowship in an ACGME accredited program in colon and rectal surgery, followed by written and oral examinations administered by the American Board of Colon and Rectal Surgery. The number of residents recruited each year varies from one to five, depending on the program. Some of the programs are more suited for training surgeons aspiring for private practice careers, while others are better suited for academic careers. Most people choose either an academic career that can include clinical or basic science research, or private practice. The clinical practice in both is similar except that academic colon and rectal surgery tends to involve less endoscopy due to the availability of gastroenterologists in academic centers. An important consideration after training is to assess participation in general surgery cases and the call that goes along with it. At some of the smaller practices, colorectal surgeons participate in general surgery call pools, while the larger practices tend to have a purely colorectal surgery practice.

Colorectal surgeons perform a wide variety of both outpatient and inpatient procedures, ranging from endoscopies to complex laparoscopic cases. Abdominal cases include laparoscopic or open partial colectomies, low anterior resections, abdominoperineal resections, proctocolectomies, rectopexies, pelvic exonerations, stricturoplasties, small bowel resections, intestinal bypasses, and others. Anorectal cases include hemorrhoidectomies, fistulotomies, sphincterotomies, sphincteroplasties, anorectal flaps, prolapse repairs, transanal excisions, and others. The multitude and variety of procedures ensures the colorectal surgeon is always challenged and occupied.

Residents completing general surgery are attracted to colon and rectal surgery for several reasons. A large part of the training in the senior years in general surgery is in abdominal surgery, and more specifically in intestinal surgery—this engenders a natural transition to colon and rectal surgery. The latest advancements in general surgical training have been in minimally invasive surgery, and these emerging technologies have revolutionized colorectal surgery. Furthermore, some advanced technologies like natural orifice surgery that are being explored in certain surgical specialties have existed as established procedures for several years in colorectal surgery (eg, transanal endoscopic microsurgery). Also, unlike most other surgical fields that focus on either benign or malignant disease, colorectal surgery training offers expertise in both. The disorders managed by a colorectal surgeon can range from benign disorders that can be truly disabling (eg, hemorrhoids and incontinence) to some of the malignancies that have the best outcomes in oncology. This ability to cure disabling or malignant disorders successfully assures patient satisfaction, thereby directly augmenting the surgeon's satisfaction.

After the grueling years of general surgery training with long hours and endless calls, colorectal surgery call is benign, with few emergencies that need long operations at midnight. Finally, colon and rectal surgery is the board-certified specialty requiring the shortest duration of training after surgical residency. It is a technologically advanced field with a comfortable lifestyle and a high job satisfaction. These factors keep colon and rectal surgery a desirable and competitive fellowship.

> Colorectal surgeons can decide whether to perform mostly shorter, outpatient procedures, or to do complex, major surgeries.

## APPLICATION TIPS

Residency applications are through ERAS, and are submitted starting in late July (11 months before the residency start date). All programs participate in the NRMP match, and by late November, results are announced. In 2008, there were 126 applicants and 43 programs, making this a highly competitive surgical specialty, where excellent recommendation letters from program directors and chairmen are of paramount importance. The colon and rectal surgeons are a small, well-knit community, so it is beneficial to meet the program directors at the national meeting that takes place in May or at regional meetings, and to request recommendation letters from colorectal surgery faculty at your institution. Research and publications in colon and rectal disorders are not mandatory, but are definitively viewed favorably, especially if a spot in a program geared toward an academic career is desired.

Interview season usually runs from August to early November (even a few days before the rank-order list submission deadline). Contact the programs that you are seriously interested in after the ERAS submission to inquire about interview dates so that you can block away some time for your favorite programs before making engagements with less desirable programs. Most programs will have you meet with

## TABLE 4-52

**Top Five Most Frequently Encountered Conditions in Colon and Rectal Surgery**

1. Colon cancer
2. Anorectal problems
3. Hemorrhoids
4. Inflammatory bowel disease
5. Gallbladder disease

each of the faculty, so be prepared for anywhere from 2 or 3 interviews to as many as 12 or 15 in one day. Make sure to inquire about the case volumes (endoscopic, abdominal, and anorectal), the exposure to various disorders, presence of a chief resident on the service (as this can hinder your operative experience), and the placement of fellows in past years. If you are interested in an academic career, inquire about the research interests of the faculty, while understanding the caveat that this is a one-year clinical training program that may not leave a lot of room for extensive research. Also find out about anesthesiology, pathology, and radiology teaching, as you will be tested on these materials in the course of your certification exams. Most importantly, talk to the current colorectal fellows. Their input about the program is invaluable to assess if a program is the right place for you to spend the last year of your training.

## FOR MORE INFO . . .

**American Board of Colon and Rectal Surgery**
www.abcrs.org

## TRAUMA SURGERY AND SURGICAL CRITICAL CARE

Trauma surgery and surgical critical care is a fellowship that can be pursued following general surgery residency. While the two fields are usually combined in both training and practice, physicians can focus on one or the other separately if desired. Physicians in this specialty care for previously healthy trauma victims as well as those with multiple comorbidities undergoing elective or emergent operations. As a result, they have the opportunity to treat a wide array of disease processes.

Trauma surgeons and surgical intensivists care for some of the most complex patients. Patients who require operations or become injured can have any known disease process as a comorbidity. Caring for these patients requires a deep understanding of the basic physiology of all organ systems and the impact of each system on the others. The manipulation of these relationships requires some of the broadest training of all medical specialties. It also allows for collaboration and comanagement with providers from nearly every other medical specialty and subspecialty.

Trauma surgeons begin providing care in the emergency department for critically injured patients. They perform a wide variety of procedures, ranging from routine establishment of intravenous access to median sternotomy and repair of cardiac lacerations. There are few, if any, other fields in surgery that operate on as wide a range of anatomic locations. And while the trauma surgeon's care may start in the emergency department, it continues to the operating room, intensive care unit, regular hospital ward, and the outpatient clinic. Some of the problems trauma surgeons must contend with include pneumothorax, hemothorax, bony fractures, airway compromise, solid organ injury, traumatic brain injuries, major vascular injury, acute blood loss anemia, hypothermia, and bowel injuries.

Surgical intensivists are frequently consulted to assist or direct the management of postsurgical patients who require mechanical ventilation, vasoactive medications, large-volume resuscitation, and blood component therapy. Frequently, these patients also have electrolyte disturbances, acid-base disorders, sepsis, ileus, coronary artery disease, acute coronary syndrome, pulmonary emboli, acute lung injury/adult respiratory distress syndrome (ARDS), or malnutrition. Different combinations of these conditions and others often occur in the same patient and offer a challenge to the intensivist, who must prioritize their treatment.

Three challenges of the field are prioritizing competing disease processes, making rapid diagnostic and therapeutic decisions, and dealing with end-of-life issues. Treatment of one injury may exacerbate another of the patient's underlying comorbidities. The outcome of a critical patient may hinge on the swift recognition and intervention of a remediable problem. End-of-life discussions with both patients and families are an unfortunate but necessary part of the care of the critically ill patient. Sensitivity and compassion are indispensable assets during these conversations.

The fellowship is one to two years, depending on the program. Two-year programs typically offer more opportunity for operative time and research. There are some accredited programs that focus on critical care only. Following fellowship training, most trauma surgeons practice at large hospitals in group practices. Frequently, these are in large cities at academic hospitals, though opportunities do exist for private practice and community settings. Surgical intensivists work in intensive care units in hospitals of all sizes. Both trauma and surgical critical care can be combined with a general surgery practice. There is a growing demand for physicians trained to deal with the multiply injured and critically ill.

## APPLICATION TIPS

Some training programs are slanted either toward trauma or critical care. This is often largely based on the location and the interests of the faculty. The volume and type of trauma (blunt vs. penetrating) may give some insight as to which way the program is skewed. Choose a program that fits your interests, complements your strengths, and fills any weaknesses in your general surgery training. You may be asked which aspect of the field, trauma or critical care, you prefer. As with most fellowships, research is looked upon favorably but is not a requirement. Having a definite research interest is helpful but not essential. Know why you want to go into trauma and critical care.

When evaluating a potential program, there are some important questions you should ask to get a feel for the training you would receive there. For example: What is the typical ICU census and length of stay? What is the acuity of the typical ICU patient? (How sick is a typical patient?) Is there opportunity to work in nonsurgical or trauma ICUs? What is the mix of blunt versus penetrating trauma? What is the volume of trauma evaluations, admissions, and operations? How often do the fellows operate? (Ask to see a typical operative case log.) What types of cases are the fellows doing? You should also ask about where former fellows are practicing, which is a good gauge of the quality of the program.

> In some settings, surgeons can decide whether to focus on trauma surgery or critical care, but frequently they perform both.

### TABLE 4-53
**Top Five Most Frequently Encountered Conditions in Surgical Critical Care**

1. Sepsis
2. Shock
3. Respiratory failure
4. Acute renal failure
5. Acid-base disorders

### TABLE 4-54
**Top Five Most Frequently Encountered Conditions in Trauma Surgery**

1. Solid organ injury
2. Pneumothorax/hemothorax
3. Traumatic brain injury
4. Bowel injury
5. Major vascular injury

## VASCULAR SURGERY

Vascular surgery is one of the most rapidly evolving fields in surgery. In addition to being a pillar of traditional open surgical training, the field of vascular surgery has rapidly embraced endovascular technology. This burgeoning technology offers patients "minimally invasive" treatment modalities. The increase in endovascular procedures, the introduction of new grafts and devices, and the launching of five-year training programs marked the beginning of a new era for vascular surgeons.

There are several ways to become a vascular surgeon. The traditional way is to complete a five-year general surgery residency and then apply to a two-year fellowship program in vascular surgery. This is still the most common track at present, through which most vascular surgeons in the United States are trained, and graduates are eligible for board certification in both vascular and general surgery. A less common, alternate track that some general surgery residents take is early specialization. Certain residency programs allow residents to begin a two-year fellowship in vascular surgery training during what would be their chief year in general surgery, with the end result that they spend four years in general surgery, followed by two in vascular surgery. Graduates of these programs are also board eligible in both general and vascular surgery.

In 2007 the first integrated vascular surgery programs formed that accepted residents straight out of medical school to train them as vascular surgeons, and do not require prior certification in general surgery. In 2007 there were only four positions of this type available in the United States. This pathway has grown considerably since then, with 21 programs in the United States offering integrated positions, compared with 100 offering vascular surgery fellowship positions. The number of integrated positions available is expected to increase in coming years. Integrated programs can be five or six years in length, and may follow a "3 + 3" model or a "0 + 5" model. In the 3 + 3 model, residents spend the first three years of residency in general surgery rotations, followed by three years of training in vascular surgery. In the 0 + 5 model, two years of general surgery rotations are performed, but they are integrated throughout the first four years of residency, and the rest of the training is in vascular surgery. Graduates of integrated programs are board eligible in vascular surgery only.

Vascular surgery is the specialty that deals with diseases related to the arteries, veins, and lymphatics. Vascular surgeons are trained as specialists who understand the pathophysiology and natural history of disease processes related to these systems, and can offer medical, endovascular, or open surgical treatment suited to each individual patient. One major pathology seen in the field is blockages in arterial blood flow. These develop most commonly from atherosclerosis, but also from autoimmune diseases, congenital conditions, and trauma. Arterial flow is reestablished to organs through endarterectomy or open bypass procedures using endogenous veins or prosthetic grafts. Blockages in an artery can also be treated less invasively in some cases, using percutaneous balloon angioplasty and stenting under radiological guidance through a single groin puncture. Blockages in lower extremities lead to claudication, rest pain, ulceration, and ultimately to limb loss. In the carotid arteries, blockage leads to strokes and transient ischemic attacks. When the blockages form in the visceral arteries, they can cause mesenteric ischemia.

Arteries can also become aneurysmal or dilated and are at risk for rupture or thrombosis. Abdominal aortic aneurysms are relatively common and can be treated with open or endovascular repair. All of these situations can require the expertise of a vascular sugeron for definitive treatment. Patients with vascular disorders are typically elderly and frequently have significant comorbidities. This renders the decision-making process challenging based on a patient's wishes, level of activity, medical problems, and anatomy. In addition, it means many of the patients have high risk for negative outcomes during surgery and require complex intraoperative and postoperative care.

Technological advances in vascular surgery over the past decade have increased the interest of vascular surgeons in venous disease. Varicose veins are now treated with laser or radiofrequency ablation as outpatient, office-based procedures requiring small puncture sites. Deep venous thrombosis causing severe swelling of the lower extremity can be opened with catheters and lytic agents to prevent long-term sequelae and post-thrombotic syndrome. Vascular surgery is also one of the specialties that helps care for patients with end-stage renal disease who are on dialysis, by creating arteriovenous fistulae or grafts to allow venous access. Thus, the modern vascular surgeon must be well trained and highly capable in both traditional, open surgical as well as endovascular techniques in order to perform a broad spectrum of procedures with variable complexity and anatomy.

## APPLICATION TIPS

In order to apply for integrated residency positions in vascular surgery, you should have completed a subinternship in the field as a medical student and be able to articulate your reasons for wanting to become a vascular surgeon. Spots in integrated programs are highly competitive, so it is normal to apply to general surgery programs as well, with the intention of completing a vascular surgery fellowship following residency. As with any competitive field, high board scores and honors in your surgical rotations are important. If you are applying after completing a general surgery residency, then be sure to highlight any research you have performed in the field of vascular surgery during your residency.

## FOR MORE INFO . . .

**The Society of Vascular Surgery (SVS)** Web site has a comprehensive Web page on training options:
www.vascularweb.org/Residents_and_Students/Vascular_Training_Options.html

A resource to help interested students find a mentor to guide them is also available at:
www.vascularweb.org/index.html

**TABLE 4-55**

**Top Five Most Frequently Encountered Conditions in Vascular Surgery**

1. Peripheral vascular disease
2. Abdominal aortic aneurysms
3. Carotid disease
4. Venous disease or insufficiency
5. Dialysis access

# International Medical Graduates and the Match Process

## INTRODUCTION

An international medical graduate (IMG) can be broadly defined as anyone who has graduated from a medical school outside the United States, Canada, or Puerto Rico. IMGs have been divided into U.S. citizen IMGs and non-U.S. citizen IMGs. The group as a whole represents roughly one-quarter of both U.S. residents and U.S. practicing physicians. The provision of medical care and the filling of residency programs in the United States have always relied heavily on applications from IMGs, who continue to play an important role in providing health care for Americans in both urban and rural areas. The number of residency spots offered in the United States exceeds the number of graduates from U.S. medical schools by roughly 30%. These spots must be filled, and residency programs often look to IMGs for this purpose (see Table 5-1).

> IMGs continue to play an important role in providing health care for Americans.

In 2006, about 217,700 IMGs received medical degrees from more than 200 countries. This represented about 24% of the 915,500 physicians currently practicing in the United States. There are differences and similarities in the demographics of IMGs as a whole in comparison to U.S. medical graduates. For example, more than half of all IMGs train in primary care, as compared to only one-third of U.S. graduates. Internal medicine has been the most popular primary specialty with IMGs, followed by family medicine, pediatrics, surgery–preliminary, psychiatry, and neurology. The IMG population has increased by more than 100,000 physicians since the 1970s, predominantly in these previously mentioned specialties. In terms of total physician counts in the United States, IMGs accounted for approximately 21% of the total in the 1980s and currently represent the aforementioned 24.5% of the total physician count. The states with the highest concentrations of IMGs are New Jersey and New York, where nearly 40% of physicians are IMGs. Illinois and Florida also have a large number of IMGs, who account for approximately 30% of all physicians. A recent study on initial practice locations for IMGs found that they were more likely to be located in the same state where they received their graduate medical education (GME) training and less likely to choose a market with more stringent licensure requirements. Furthermore, this study showed that IMG physicians were more likely to locate in markets with established higher proportions of IMG physicians, suggesting that networks among established IMGs played a role.

A study in *JAMA* described some changes that have taken place in the demographics of IMGs in the United States. Specifically, this study found that between

## TABLE 5-1

### IMGs in the Match

| Applicants | 2006 | 2007 | 2008 | 2009 |
|---|---|---|---|---|
| U.S.-citizen IMGs | 2435 | 2694 | 2969 | 3390 |
| % U.S. citizens accepted | 50 | 50 | 52 | 48 |
| Non-U.S.-citizen IMGs | 6442 | 6992 | 7335 | 7484 |
| % non-U.S. citizens accepted | 49 | 46 | 42 | 42 |

1995 and 2001, the number of IMGs initiating the accreditation process in the United States was reduced by 46%. This change was thought to have resulted from the declining number of residency positions available in the United States. However, even with this precipitous drop in the number of IMGs seeking certification, the authors concluded that the applicant pool continues to supply an ample number of capable individuals to fill U.S. residency positions.

Another study looking at board specialty certification among U.S. graduates and IMGs found that IMGs generally have lower board-certification rates than do U.S. graduates. A subgroup analysis showed that the non-U.S.-citizen IMGs had better certification rates than did U.S.-citizen IMGs. In addition, after the devastating terrorist attacks on September 11, 2001, the process of immigrating and obtaining visas has become more challenging. Taken together, these findings make it evident that IMGs who are applying to train in the United States must be armed not only with the medical skills and knowledge needed to be good doctors but also with a detailed understanding of the numerous steps required to gain residency and accreditation. These complicated steps are addressed in this chapter and elsewhere in this book.

> IMGs must be prepared with medical skills and knowledge, as well as a detailed understanding of the residency process.

As compared to U.S. graduates, the IMG has to go through a longer residency application process, which is followed by an interview process that may seem less friendly to IMGs. Indeed, some studies have shown that when comparing IMGs and U.S. medical graduates with similar skills and abilities, U.S. medical graduates were favored in the recruitment process for several reasons, including the pressure to rank U.S. graduates higher so as to avoid a reduced complement of U.S. medical graduates in the program. Despite this inequity, the overall process is streamlined to ensure that there is little difference in quality among residents, whether they graduated from medical school in the United States or abroad.

## THE GENERAL APPROACH

The financial, emotional, and time commitments required throughout the application and Match process are certainly important factors for any applicant. IMGs face the added challenges of traveling from abroad, applying for visas, obtaining security clearances, and settling down in a new country. However, this objective is not impossible to realize as long as you are organized, use a stepwise approach, and keep your eyes on the prize: Match Day. A strong commitment and a resilient spirit are two of the most important ingredients for success during the matching process.

If you want to pursue postgraduate training in the United States, start planning while you are still in medical school. Usually, the best time is during the third or fourth year, when elective rotations are completed. The goal is to match the typical credentials of the U.S. medical graduate applicant. Most seniors in U.S. medical programs will have done electives in specialties corresponding to their desired residency. Some will also rotate at institutions where they will apply for residency positions. Hence, IMGs should try to do an elective at a U.S. institution in their specialty of choice, and this process must start early in the clinical years.

> Your goal is to match or exceed the typical credentials of the U.S. medical graduate applicant.

An elective performed in the United States has many advantages:

- Obtaining firsthand experience of U.S. clinical settings. It is extremely difficult to obtain clinical exposure in the United States once you are finished with medical school for medical/legal and insurance reasons.

- Creating a favorable impression with U.S. faculty and identifying potential future writers for letters of recommendation.

- Taking advantage of improved accessibility to some institutions where IMGs are more accepted as medical students.

- Improving the potential for interview offers at institutions where IMGs have previously performed electives.

- Applying for a visa to participate in elective rotations may make it easier to obtain one for residency, as some of the prerequisites may be the same.

Obviously, doing an elective in the United States creates extra expenses that need to be budgeted for, such as airline tickets, visa costs, expenses for food and accommodations, and in-country travel.

Even though there are many benefits to doing an elective in the United States as a medical student, it is by no means a requirement for success in the Match. Indeed, most IMGs have not done electives prior to arriving in the United States. For each IMG, the first step toward establishing a medical career in the United States is resolving the question: "When should I go to the United States?" If you are not able to participate in an elective in the United States during medical school, then you would still need to visit the United States in order to take the USMLE Step 2 CS, and then again during the interview process. All who wish to be accredited by the U.S. board in their specialty of choice must do all their training, from PGY-1 (internship year) onward, in the United States.

It is important to get in touch with the Educational Commission for Foreign Medical Graduates (ECFMG) for the application materials. Their Web site (www. ecfmg.org) has information on the application and a time line of events with application deadlines for United States Medical Licensing Examination (USMLE) Steps. (Information on these exams is provided later in this chapter.)

After making the choice to train in the United States, it is important to gather information on individual programs in your desired specialty throughout the United States. You may be able to get more information via specific program coordinators or through official program Web sites. An important source of information is current doctors or residents in training. For example, Web-based forums, such as www.studentdoctor.net or www.imgforum.com, may give you better insight into individual programs. It is important to keep in mind, however, that these web-based forums are not sources of official information and may represent the opinion of the person writing the post. Communication with individual programs may also reveal lists of residency program alumni who do not mind being contacted.

The next big step is to prepare for the USMLE exams. It is usually best to take these exams during or immediately after medical school, when the knowledge is freshest in your mind. Whereas high scores on the USMLE do not necessarily grant the IMG a place in residency, such scores can help to improve the chances of getting good interviews, thus opening more doors in the Match process. Most of the USMLE exams can be taken in your home country (more information can be

---

> Doing an elective in the United States has numerous advantages.

> Deciding when to go to the United States for medical training is the first key question you must answer.

> IMGs have outperformed U.S. medical graduates on internal medicine in-training exams.

found on the ECFMG Web site). Currently, the Step 2 Clinical Skills (CS) exam is administered at selected centers in the United States only. Once you have completed the exams, you can apply for the residency of your choice via the Match.

One of the most troubling questions for IMGs is whether their USMLE score will be good enough to secure interviews in the United States. The section that follows has strategies to enhance your chances as an IMG. However, even IMGs with near-perfect scores have matched at less desirable residency locations, while those with average scores have matched well due to research experience, publications, U.S. elective experience, or strong letters of recommendation. The bottom line is that while USMLE scores may serve as a numeric cut-off for screening applicants, many other factors determine one's success during the matching process.

It is possible to do a residency in your home country and then come to the United States for specialty training. If you wish to be licensed by the U.S.-based board in your specialty, however, you must begin and finish postgraduate (residency) training in the United States. Once you have decided that you wish to enter the U.S. Match, it will be worth your while to consider the specialty in which you are going to apply. As mentioned above, many IMGs apply to primary care residencies because it is widely perceived that IMGs have a higher success rate in this field. In fact, the numbers do support this approach. Recently, one in four family medicine residents was an IMG, whereas only 2% of ophthalmology residents were IMGs. Although these numbers clearly do not prevent IMGs from applying in other fields, they do offer an indication of where IMGs have historically achieved the most success (see Chapter 4 for details on your specialty). At the same time, the notion that IMGs perform at the bottom of every field is not substantiated by current data. For example, a recent article from the *Annals of Internal Medicine* observed that IMGs have outperformed U.S. medical graduates on internal medicine in-training exams.

Once you have chosen the field in which you wish to match, you will find that the process of applying to the programs is much like that for U.S. medical graduates. The necessary components are listed in Table 5-2.

## THE USMLE

The USMLE Steps 1, 2 Clinical Skills (CS), and 2 Clinical Knowledge (CK) are a set of medical exams that are designed to evaluate your readiness to enter a U.S. residency program. Directors of residency programs in the United States often have a difficult time comparing U.S. medical graduate applicants because of the different grading schemes, requirements, and levels of competition found at various U.S. medical schools. Not surprisingly, many program directors also find that comparing IMGs to U.S. medical graduates or to one another is extremely challenging. The USMLE Steps provide at least one objective criterion against which to make such comparisons (see Table 5-3 for pass rates for first-time test takers). It is therefore essential that any IMG who is considering residency in the United States excel on all three Steps, and particularly on Step 1. Refer to *First Aid for the USMLE Step 1*, *First Aid for the USMLE Step 2 CS*, and *First Aid for the USMLE Step 2 CK* for additional information and advice on this subject. Here are some key facts about the USMLE:

**TABLE 5-2**

**Steps in Your Application to Various Programs**

1. Have your school verify that you have completed the two years of basic science training.

2. Apply for and pass the United States Medical Licensing Examination (USMLE) Step 1.

3. Apply for and pass the USMLE Step 2 Clinical Knowledge (CK).

4. Graduate from medical school and obtain your degree.

5. Send a copy of your medical degree to the Educational Commission for Foreign Medical Graduates (ECFMGs).

6. Obtain a current ECFMG certificate.

7. Pass the USMLE Step 2 Clinical Skills (CS) within 1 year of graduating from your medical school.

8. Send for an Electronic Residency Application Service (ERAS) application.

9. Register as an "independent applicant" with the National Resident Matching Program (NRMP).

10. Research and choose programs to apply to electronically through ERAS.

11. Obtain interview invitations and interview.

12. Rank programs through the NRMP.

13. Review visa options from various programs and begin your visa paperwork.

14. Review licensing requirements in each state in which you applied, and consider beginning licensing paperwork in your preferred state.

## TABLE 5-3

**2009 Pass Rates for First-Time USMLE Test Takers**

|          | U.S. Students (%) | IMGs (%) |
|----------|-------------------|----------|
| Step 1   | 94                | 73       |
| Step 2 CK | 97               | 83       |

Don't feel singled out by the CS exam. The U.S. medical students have to take it, too!

Testing performance is an important determinant of success in the Match for IMGs. Be prepared.

## TABLE 5-4

**USMLE Step 2 CS Pass Rates\* for First-Time Test Takers**

| U.S. students | 97% |
|---------------|-----|
| IMGs          | 73% |

*From 2008–2009.

- The USMLE Steps 1 and 2 CK are now administered exclusively by computer and are given on a continuous basis throughout the world.
- The test is administered to IMGs by the ECFMG rather than by the National Board of Medical Examiners (NBME).
- In order to register for the USMLE Step 1, you must first have taken the basic sciences coursework at your medical school.
- Registration for the USMLE Step 2 Clinical Knowledge (CK) and Clinical Skills (CS) exams also requires that you be within one year of graduation from your medical school.
- To be certified by ECFMG, international medical graduates must, among other requirements, pass a medical science examination. Obtaining a passing score on both Steps 1 and 2 CK currently fulfills this requirement for certification. You can take Step 1 or Step 2 CK in either order, provided you meet the eligibility requirements for these exams.
- Step 2 CS replaced the Clinical Skills Assessment (CSA), formerly administered by the ECFMG. The CS exam is offered throughout the year in five locations: Atlanta, Chicago, Houston, Los Angeles, and Philadelphia. The purpose of this test is for students to demonstrate the ability to collect and analyze data and to communicate well with patients. (See Table 5-4 for CS results.)
- Registration for the USMLE Step 3 is possible only after you have completed between one and three years of residency or if you are a physician not participating in the Match.
- You will need to pass Step 3 if you intend to apply for an H-1B visa (see below). In addition, there are time restrictions regarding how many years after taking Step 1 you are still eligible to take Step 3. Typically, this is seven years. However, you should confirm with the USMLE Web site for exact time limits as they apply to your situation.

The definitive source of information on USMLE exams is the *USMLE Bulletin of Information*, which can found on the USMLE Web site (www.usmle.org).

## THE ECFMG CERTIFICATE

If you are an IMG, the ECFMG will serve as the rough equivalent of your dean's office in the matching process. ECFMG certification can be a tedious process, but it is essential if you are to be considered by U.S. residencies. Indeed, according to U.S. legal statutes, IMGs who do not have an ECFMG certificate are "invisible" to U.S. residency programs. In addition to passing the required exams, applicants for ECFMG certification must meet certain medical education credential requirements. All IMGs must have had at least four credit years (academic years for which credit has been given toward completion of the medical curriculum) in attendance at a medical school that is listed in the International Medical Education Directory (IMED) on the ECFMG Web site. The physician's graduation year must be included in the medical school's IMED listing.

Additionally, ECFMG requires copies of your medical education credentials, which are verified by the appropriate officials at your medical school. If you have already graduated from medical school when you submit your application to ECFMG, you must include copies of your medical diploma and a recent photograph with your application. If you are still a student, you must send the copies of your diploma and your photograph as soon as you graduate. You must also provide an English translation if the document you provide is not in English. When ECFMG sends your medical diploma to your medical school for verification, ECFMG will request the medical school to include your final medical school transcript when the school returns the verification of your medical diploma to ECFMG. ECFMG will notify you in writing when it sends your credentials for verification and when it receives verification of your credentials from your medical school.

> Be sure to stay on top of the credentialing process.

## THE MATCH

See Chapter 1 for general information about the Match.

The National Resident Matching Program (NRMP) Web site (www.nrmp. org) has an "Applicant User Guide," which contains specific information for IMGs. IMGs need to fulfill all requirements by September in order to have complete certification prior to submission of the Rank Order Lists (ROL) in mid-January. If you have not passed the USMLE by September, you may not be able to enroll in the NRMP. You may, however, apply for residency positions outside of the Match.

While U.S. medical graduates apply to 8 to 12 programs if applying in less competitive specialities and 15 to 20 if applying in more competitive specialities, IMGs should submit applications to a minimum of 20 to 30 programs if applying in less competitive specialties, and 30 to 40 programs if applying in more competitive specialties, consisting of both teaching and community hospitals. Applications should be sent in as early as possible. While you are waiting, you can begin to research your visa options and even get started on some of the paperwork for medical licensure in the state(s) where you hope to match. On Match Day, if all has gone well, you will know where you are going and can begin to work on your visa.

> Apply to a wide range of programs to cover your bases.

## ERAS

The Electronic Residency Application Service, or ERAS, has almost universally replaced the paper applications of old, transmitting residency applications and credentials via the Internet. It is important to note that some programs and specialties including pediatric neurology, neurotology, and ophthalmology still require paper applications. In addition, certain specialties have an "early match" date, and so all deadlines are earlier (see Chapter 4 for detailed information about each specialty). ERAS is available to all U.S. medical graduates as well as those outside the United States and Canada through ECFMG. More information on the ERAS and early match applications can be found in Chapter 7.

IMGs are advised to apply to a broad range of programs, as the climate for acceptance can fluctuate from year to year. IMGs should also note that their personal statements will be closely scrutinized for their use and mastery of the English language. Therefore, pay close attention to your personal statement and have it read by a native English speaker. When it comes to proofreading your personal statement, remember that more reviewers looking for mistakes will help you avoid more errors. Please see Table 5-5 for what to leave out of a personal statement.

### TABLE 5-5

**What *Not* to Include in a Personal Statement**

- Discussion of U.S. politics or U.S. foreign policy.

- Discussion of your monetary goals.

- Discussion of religious beliefs.

- Any work that is not your own. Do NOT copy your statement from Web sites that claim "perfect" personal statements. This will guarantee that you do not obtain a position in the United States if you are caught.

- Discussion of extremely controversial topics such as abortion, euthanasia, the death penalty, and gay rights.

## INTERVIEWS

> The interview is a good time to get a feeling for how IMG-friendly a program is.

If all has gone well thus far, you will be invited to interview at a subset of the programs to which you applied. You will interview along with U.S. medical graduates on predetermined days and should follow the advice presented in Chapter 11 of this book. There are, however, some additional points that should be mentioned.

- You should get a feel for each program's overall approach to IMGs on the day of your interview. Are there many IMGs at the program, or have there been at least a few in the past?

- Other IMGs are excellent resources from whom you can glean valuable information about immigration issues as well as an idea of the level of support the program provides to IMGs.

Keep in mind that a positive experience with an IMG from your medical school in the past may open doors for you in that program.

In addition to the interview tips presented in Chapter 11, consider the following advice:

- Describe your school in the most positive of terms. U.S. program directors and interviewers are not necessarily biased against foreign medical schools, but they are wary of unknown entities.

> IMGs who prepare well continue to match at competitive programs every year.

- If you portray your school in a positive light, it is more likely to be perceived that way.

- It may be prudent to save questions about visas for other residents and program administrators, as program directors may not know this information.

- Keep the discussion on medicine and training, since these are universal goals of residents, applicants, and program directors.

- The goal of your interview should be to convince your interviewer that due to your shared interest in medicine, you both have more in common than he or she may think, even if you are the only IMG the program has ever interviewed.

## MAXIMIZING YOUR CHANCES

> U.S. research experience will put the IMG ahead of the pack.

As an IMG you may face disadvantages when applying to programs at top-tier institutions, such as teaching hospitals affiliated with renowned universities and research centers. In some cases, IMGs will not even be considered for an interview simply because there are too many qualified U.S. graduates from the university's own medical school and other U.S. schools. However, that is not the end of the road for the IMG, because there is a subset of IMGs who continue to match every year at competitive institutions. The following are some ways to maximize your chances as an IMG.

## DOING MEDICAL RESEARCH

Explore all possible options, beginning with research positions, fellowships, and even research assistantships.

- Ironically, most of the big research universities and hospitals usually have multiple opportunities for research-based positions that are simply unfilled.

- These positions may not pay that well or may be unfilled because there are no U.S. medical graduates willing to take up a one- to two-year research fellowship.

- In addition, these very programs also almost always have a research director's office or dean for research. This office can provide the IMG with a very useful list of potential job openings, often with visa support for the right candidate.

> It helps if the IMG has had interaction with the program director, faculty, and residents.

The ideal research position is within the department in which the candidates wishes to do a residency. For example, surgical residencies are very competitive; however, over the last few years some IMGs have matched in orthopedics, plastics, neurosurgery, and general surgery. They may have started as research fellows, completed one to three years of research, and proved themselves as viable applicants. The goal is to get some recognition through research. Once your name is recognizable via presentations, papers, and publications, program directors might be more willing to rank you favorably.

Contrary to popular belief, large research-based university centers actually are more open to IMGs since they want to have an international feel—but the IMG has to be known to the program director, faculty, and residents. Working at a well-known research institution increases your chances of being called for interviews by other teaching hospitals. This experience will also give you the opportunity to generate letters of recommendation from U.S. teaching faculty.

Some positions that are open at university hospitals may not be salaried for the first year but provide a stipend for future years. While this may seem unattractive, IMGs who have taken this approach have had good results. Program directors may think highly of applicants who prove their mettle through determination in the face of hardship. In addition, it demonstrates an applicant's ability to work on research projects both independently and as part of a team.

## OBTAINING AN ADVANCED DEGREE

Getting advanced degrees in the United States can be a major boost toward getting interviews at desirable programs. The IMG will stand out because of the additional skills, research, and maturity acquired during the program for an MPH or MS degree—attributes that teaching/university programs find attractive. While working toward the advanced degree, it also does no harm for the IMG to try to get more clinical exposure, either through electives and attachments or more informally through clinical conferences, morning reports, journal clubs, and didactic sessions with the residents of the program.

Given the trend of USMGs earning intercalated degrees, such as an MBA or PhD, during medical school or even residency, an IMG with an advanced degree is all the more competitive. The disadvantage with this strategy is that it is a considerable time commitment and can be a financial burden.

## DOING NIH-FUNDED RESEARCH

Although this seems difficult, there are numerous such jobs available at major teaching hospitals. Many principal investigators (PIs) find it difficult to find good research staff once they have managed to get funding from the NIH. An IMG often suits these positions very well because the PI can hire a capable, dedicated MD who can communicate well in medical English. The benefit to you is that any publications resulting from this kind of endeavor greatly increase your chances of matching.

## PRESENTING RESEARCH WORK FOR AWARDS

Often, there are opportunities for presenting research work for an award, however small. Many IMG recipients of research awards have matched at very high-caliber programs. Other IMG applicants started in research and ended up excelling and actually benefiting from their own grants. While their numbers are small, these IMGs almost always can match at a residency of their choice.

An additional advantage, if you succeed in your research endeavors, is the possibility of applying for a special category of visas leading to permanent residency. These are based on exceptional ability and achievement, and strong research work is regarded highly.

Even though most IMGs apply to and match at community hospitals, trying for a position at a university teaching hospital is worthwhile, especially if you have done some research or electives or have written some papers. It is important to remember that differences exist between teaching and community hospitals, although both focus on providing excellent patient care.

Overall, an IMG who is very motivated will typically have more success than one who is content to just apply and wait for interviews. The IMG applicant who is willing to sacrifice one to two years doing research may find that it was time well spent, since it led to greater recognition and a match at a good university hospital.

## IMMIGRATION

For detailed current immigration information, please visit the U.S. State Department Web site (travel.state.gov/visa/).

To attend interviews, IMGs must enter the United States. This can be accomplished with the use of a visitor B-1/B-2 visa. These give you ample time (two to six months) to complete interviews. Once it comes time to start a residency, however, things get a bit more complicated.

As an IMG, you need a visa to work or train in the United States unless you are a U.S. citizen or a permanent resident. Two types of visas enable you to accept a residency appointment in the United States: J-1 and H-1B (see Table 5-6). Most sponsoring residency programs (SRPs) prefer a J-1 visa. Above all, this is because SRPs are authorized by the Department of Homeland Security (DHS) to issue a Form DS-2019 directly to an IMG. By contrast, SRPs must complete considerable paperwork, including an application to the Immigration and Labor Department, to apply to the DHS for an H-1B visa on behalf of an IMG.

## THE J-1 VISA

This is a nonimmigrant visa. Key features of this visa include:

- The J-1 visa is one of the most restrictive and inflexible visas on which to come to the United States.

- Also known as the Exchange Visitor Program, the J-1 visa was introduced to give IMGs in diverse specialties the chance to use the training experience obtained in the United States in their respective home countries and improve conditions there.

- To enable an SRP to issue a DS-2019, you must obtain a certificate from the ECFMG indicating that you are eligible to participate in a residency program in the United States. First, however, you must have the Ministry of Health in your country to issue a statement indicating that your country needs physicians with the skills you propose to acquire from a U.S. residency program. This statement, which must bear the seal of your country's government and must be signed by a duly designated government official, is intended to satisfy the U.S. Secretary of Health and Human Services (HHS) that there is such a need.

The Health Ministry in your country should send this statement to the ECFMG. To find out if the government of your country will issue such a statement, you will likely need to contact the Ministry of Health, which, in many countries, maintains a list of medical specialties in which there is a need for further training abroad. A word of caution: if you are applying for a residency in internal medicine and internists are not in short supply in your country, it may help to indicate an intention to pursue a subspecialty after completing your residency training.

The text of your statement of need should read as follows:

> *Name of applicant for visa: _____. There currently exists in _____ (your country) a need for qualified medical practitioners in the specialty of _____. (Name of applicant for visa) has filed a written assurance with the government of this country that he/she will return to _____ (your country) upon completion of training in the United States and intends to enter the practice of medicine in the specialty for which training is being sought. Stamp (or seal and signature) of issuing official of named country. Dated _____*

> J-1 visas can be very restrictive and inflexible.

To facilitate the issuing of such a statement by the Ministry of Health in your country, you should submit a certified copy of the agreement or a contract from your residency in the United States. The agreement or contract must be signed by you and the residency program official responsible for the training. Armed with Form DS-2019, you should then go to the U.S. consulate closest to the residential address indicated in your passport.

J-1 visa applicants must demonstrate to the consulate officer that they have binding ties to a residence in their home country which they have no intention of abandoning, and that they are coming to the United States for a temporary period. As for other nonimmigrant visas, you must prove that you intend to return to your home country. This intent is established in part by demonstrating that you have financial assets and personal ties in your home country. You must also show that all your expenses will be paid. In addition, you may need a certificate of good conduct, which is usually obtained through the medical board in your country.

Usually, after security clearance and authenticating your documents, the U.S. consulate will authorize the visa. Currently, this process can take anywhere between one and six months, depending on your home country. When you enter the United States, be sure to carry all your documents, including your Form DS-2019 and the visa letters you initially submitted to the U.S. embassy at home. Sometimes the INS officers at the port of entry will ask to see these despite your having a visa. You are usually admitted to the United States for the length of the J-1 program, designated as "D/S," or duration of status. The duration of your program is indicated on the DS-2019.

> Allow adequate time for security and immigration clearances when applying for visas.

In the wake of the terrorist attacks of September 11, 2001, a number of new regulations have been introduced to improve the monitoring of exchange visitors during their time in the United States. As of January 30, 2003, all SRPs and students are required to register with the Student and Exchange Visitor Program (SEVP) via the Student and Exchange Visitor Information System (SEVIS). SEVIS allows the DHS to maintain up-to-date information (eg, enrollment status, current address) on exchange visitors. As of January 30, 2002, SEVIS Form DS-2019 will be used for visa applications, admission, and change of status. Non-SEVIS forms, such as Form IAP-66, issued before January 30, 2003, are no longer accepted. Procedural details of this legislation can be obtained from your SRP, the international office at your institution, or the DHS Web site.

## DURATION OF PARTICIPATION

The duration of a resident's participation in a program of graduate medical education or training is limited to the time normally required to complete such a program. The authority charged with determining the duration of time required by an individual IMG is the State Department. The maximum amount of time for participation in a training program is ordinarily limited to seven years unless the IMG has demonstrated to the satisfaction of the ECFMG and the U.S. State Department that his or her home country has an exceptional need for the specialty in which he or she will receive further training. An extension of stay may be granted in the event that an IMG needs to repeat a year of clinical medical training or needs time for training or education to take an exam required for board certification. After the seven years have elapsed, the IMG is required by law to either travel back to his/her home country or pursue a waiver of this requirement. The waiver process can take up to or more than a year, so if you intend to apply for one, start early. More details are provided in the "J-1 Waiver" section below. Please refer to the visa section of the State Department's Web site (travel.state.gov/visa/).

## REQUIREMENTS AFTER ENTRY INTO THE UNITED STATES

Each year, all IMGs participating in a residency program on a J-1 visa must furnish the attorney general of the United States with an affidavit (Form I-644) attesting that they are in good standing in the program of graduate medical education or training in which they are participating and that they will return to their home country upon completion of the education or training for which they came to the United States.

## RESTRICTIONS UNDER THE J-1 VISA

No later than two years after the date of entry into the United States, an IMG participating in a residency program on a J-1 visa is allowed one opportunity to change his or her designated program of graduate medical education or training if his or her director approves that change. The J-1 visa also includes a condition called the "two-year foreign residence requirement." The law requires that a J-1 visa holder, upon completion of the training program, leave the United States and reside in his or her home country for a period of at least two years. Currently, there is pressure from the American Medical Association to extend this period to five years. An IMG on a J-1 visa is ordinarily not allowed to change from J-1 to most other types of visas or (in most cases) to change from J-1 to permanent residence while in the United States until he or she has fulfilled the "foreign residence requirement." The purpose of the foreign residence requirement is to ensure that an IMG uses the training he or she obtained in the United States for the benefit of his or her home country.

## J-2 VISAS/FAMILY MEMBERS

The spouse and children (minors only) of participants in exchange programs may apply for J-2 dependent visas to accompany and join the IMG on the J-1 visa. They must demonstrate that they will have sufficient financial resources to cover all expenses while in the United States. Dependents may apply to the U.S. Citizenship and Immigration Services (USCIS, formerly the Immigration and Naturalization Service) for authorization to accept employment in the United States.

Some individuals may apply for a waiver of the two-year foreign residency requirement. There are five grounds for which the U.S. government may waive the two-year foreign residence requirement:

- If you as an IMG can prove that returning to your country would result in "exceptional hardship" to you or to members of your immediate family who are U.S. citizens or permanent residents;

- If you as an IMG can demonstrate a "well-founded fear of persecution" due to race, religion, or political opinions if forced to return to your country;

- If you obtain a "no objection" statement from your government;

- If you are sponsored by an "interested governmental agency"; or

- If you are sponsored by a designated state Department of Health in the United States.

By far the most commonly used reason and possibly the least rejected application is the "interested governmental agency" sponsoring the IMG.

## APPLYING FOR A J-1 VISA WAIVER

IMGs who have sought a waiver on the basis of the last two alternatives have found it beneficial to approach the following potentially "interested government agencies":

1. **The Department of Health and Human Services.** As of 2003, HHS has expanded its role in reviewing J-1 waiver applications. HHS's considerations for a waiver have classically been as follows:
   - The program or activity in which the IMG is engaged is "of high priority and of national or international significance in an area of interest" to HHS;
   - The IMG must be an "integral" part of the program or activity "so that the loss of his/her services would necessitate discontinuance of the program or a major phase of it"; and
   - The IMG "must possess outstanding qualifications, training, and experience well beyond the usually expected accomplishments at the graduate, postgraduate, and residency levels and must clearly demonstrate the capability to make original and significant contributions to the program."

   Under these criteria, HHS waivers are granted to physicians working in high-level biomedical research.

New rules will also allow HHS to review J-1 waiver applications from community health centers, rural hospitals, and other health care providers. In the past, the U.S. Department of Agriculture (USDA) served as the interested federal government agency that reviewed waiver applications to allow foreign doctors to serve in rural underserved communities outside Appalachia, while the Appalachian Regional Commission (ARC) played that role for Appalachian communities. The USDA is no longer handling applications for J-1 waivers. As such, HHS will now review waiver applications for primary care practitioners and psychiatrists who have completed residency training within one year of application to practice in designated Health Professional Shortage Areas (HPSAs), Medically Underserved Areas and Populations (MUA/Ps), and Mental Health Professional Shortage Areas (MHPSAs). HHS waiver applications should be mailed to:

> Executive Secretary
> Exchange Visitor Waiver Review Board
> Room 639-H, Hubert H. Humphrey Building
> Department of Health and Human Services
> 200 Independence Avenue, S.W.
> Washington, D.C. 20201
> Phone (202) 690-6174; fax (202) 690-7127

2. **Veterans Affairs.** With more than 170 health care facilities located in various parts of the United States, the VA is a major employer of physicians in this country. In addition, many VA hospitals are affiliated with university medical centers. The VA sponsors IMGs working in research, patient care (regardless of specialty), and teaching.

   The waiver applicant may engage in teaching and research in conjunction with clinical duties. The VA's latest guidelines (issued on June 22, 1994) provide that it will act as an interested government agency only when the loss of the IMG's services would necessitate the discontinuance of a program or a major phase of it and when recruitment efforts have failed to locate a U.S. physician to fill the position.

   The procedure for obtaining a VA sponsorship for a J-1 waiver is as follows:

   - The IMG should deal directly with the Human Resources Department at the local VA facility; and
   - The facility must request that the VA's chief medical director sponsor the IMG for a waiver.

   The waiver request should include the following documentation:

   - A letter from the director of the local facility describing the program, the IMG's immigration status, the health care needs of the facility, and the facility's recruitment efforts;
   - Recruitment efforts, including copies of all job advertisements run within the preceding year; and
   - Copies of the IMG's licenses, test results, board certifications, SEVIS DS-2019 forms, etc. The VA contact person in Washington, D.C., should be contacted by the local medical facility rather than by IMGs or their attorneys.

3. **The Appalachian Regional Commission.** The ARC sponsors physicians in certain places in the eastern and southern United States, namely, in Alabama, Georgia, Kentucky, Maryland, Mississippi, New York, North Carolina, Ohio, Pennsylvania, South Carolina, Tennessee, Virginia, and West Virginia. Since

1992, the ARC has sponsored approximately 200 primary care IMGs annually in counties within its jurisdiction that have been designated as HPSAs by HHS. The ARC requires that waiver requests initially be submitted to the ARC contact person in the state of intended employment. Contact information for each state can be found on the ARC Web site (www.arc.gov). If the state concurs, a letter from the state's governor recommending the waiver must be addressed to Anne B. Pope, the new federal co-chairperson of the ARC. The waiver request should include the following documents:

- A letter from the facility to Executive Secretary, Exchange Visitor Waiver Review Board stating the proposed dates of employment, the IMG's medical specialty, the address of the practice location, an assertion that the IMG will practice primary care for at least 40 hours per week in the HPSA, and details as to why the facility needs the services of the IMG;
- A J-1 Visa Data Sheet;
- The ARC federal co-chairperson's J-1 Visa Waiver Policy and the J-1 Visa Waiver Policy Affidavit and Agreement with the notarized signature of the IMG;
- A contract of at least three years' duration;
- Evidence of the IMG's qualifications, including a résumé, medical diplomas and licenses, and IAP-66 or SEVIS DS-2019 forms; and
- Evidence of unsuccessful attempts to recruit qualified U.S. physicians within the preceding six months. Copies of advertisements, copies of résumés received, and reasons for rejection must also be included.

The ARC will not sponsor IMGs who have been out of status for six months or longer. Requests for ARC waivers are then processed in Washington, D.C. (ARC, 1666 Connecticut Avenue, N.W., Washington, D.C. 20009).

The ARC is usually able to forward a letter confirming that a waiver has been recommended to the United States Information Agency (USIA) to the requesting facility or attorney within 30 days of the request.

4. **The Department of Agriculture.** At the time of publication, the USDA is no longer sponsoring J-1 waivers. The scope of the HHS J-1 waiver program has been expanded to fill the gap.

5. **State Departments of Public Health.** There is no application form for a state-sponsored J-1 waiver. However, USIA regulations specify that an application must include the following documents:
   - A letter from the state Department of Public Health identifying the physician and specifying that it would be in the public interest to grant him or her a J-1 waiver;
   - An employment contract that is valid for a minimum of three years and that states the name and address of the facility that will employ the physician and the geographic areas in which he or she will practice medicine;
   - Evidence that these geographic areas are located within HPSAs;
   - A statement by the physician agreeing to the contractual requirements;
   - Copies of all SEVIS DS-2019 forms; and
   - A completed USIA Data Sheet.

Applications are numbered in the order in which they are received, since only 30 physicians per year may be granted waivers in a particular state under the Conrad State 30 program. Individual states may choose to participate or not to participate in this program.

## THE H-1B VISA

Since 1991, the law has allowed medical residency programs to sponsor foreign-born medical residents for H-1B visas. There are no restrictions to changing the H-1B visa to any other kind of visa, including permanent resident status (green card), through employer sponsorship or through close relatives who are U.S. citizens or permanent residents. The overall ceiling for the number of H-1B visas issued to professionals in all categories is 65,000, although certain exceptions listed below exist. It is advisable for residents to apply for H-1B visas as soon as possible in the official year (beginning October 1) when the new quota officially opens up. According to the Web site www.immihelp.com, the following beneficiaries of approved H-1B petitions are exempt from the H-1B annual cap:

- Beneficiaries who are in J-1 nonimmigrant status in order to receive graduate medical education or training, and who have obtained a waiver of the two-year home residency requirement.

- Beneficiaries who are employed at, or who have received an offer of employment from, an institution of higher education or a related or affiliated nonprofit entity.

- Beneficiaries who are employed by, or who have received an offer of employment from, a nonprofit research organization.

## TABLE 5-6

**Differences and Similarities Between the J-1 and H-1B Visa**

| Category | H-1B Visa | J-1 Visa |
|---|---|---|
| Overseeing agency | Departments of Labor and Homeland Security | Departments of State and Homeland Security |
| Required exams | USMLE Steps 1, 2CK, 2CS, and 3 | USMLE Steps 1, 2CK, and 2CS |
| Funding | U.S. employer salary only | Multiple sources allowed |
| Time limit | 6 years | 7 years |
| Return to country | Not required | Must return to home country for 2 years post training unless waiver granted |
| Spousal work allowed | No work permits issued to spouse | Yes, work authorization can be granted to spouse |

- Beneficiaries who are employed by, or who have received an offer of employment from, a governmental research organization.

- Beneficiaries who are currently maintaining, or who have held within the last six years, H-1B status, and are ineligible for another full six-year stay as an H-1B.

- Beneficiaries who have been counted once toward the numerical limit and are the beneficiary of multiple petitions.

H-1B visas are intended for "professionals" in a "specialty occupation." This means that an IMG intending to pursue a residency program in the United States with an H-1B visa needs to clear all three USMLE Steps before becoming eligible for the H-1B. The ECFMG administers Steps 1 and 2, whereas Step 3 is conducted by the individual states. Most states will not allow medical residents to take USMLE Step 3 until they have completed the first year of their residency programs. However, there are 11 states that permit persons to take USMLE Step 3 prior to entering a residency program: Connecticut, Arkansas, California, Florida, Louisiana, Maryland, Nevada, New York, Texas, Virginia, and West Virginia. IMGs interested in being sponsored for H-1B status must travel to one of these states to take and pass USMLE Step 3 before they may be sponsored for an H-1B visa.

You will need to contact the Federation of State Medical Boards (FSMB) or the medical board of the state where you intend to take the Step 3 for additional details.

> More IMGs are obtaining the H-1B visa since it is less restrictive.

## H-1B APPLICATION

An application for an H-1B visa is filed not by the IMG but rather by his or her employment sponsor—in your case, by the residency program in the United States. If an SRP is willing to do so, you will be told about it at the time of your interview for the residency program. If an SRP is unwilling to file for an H-1B visa because of attorney costs, you could suggest that you would be willing to bear the burden of such costs. The entire process of getting an H-1B visa can take anywhere from 10 to 20 weeks.

The physician may not commence employment in the United States until the petition is approved and the physician has either H-1B status or has obtained an H-1B visa and entered the United States. With H-4 visas, a spouse and unmarried children under 21 years old can accompany an H-1B physician and may attend school in the United States, but they cannot work. The initial duration of an H-1B petition is three years, with one additional three-year extension of stay possible. Generally, after six years have elapsed, the physician must either have permanent residence status or depart the United States.

The events of September 11 have led to dramatic changes for all immigrants seeking to enter the United States. The information outlined above as well as in the rest of this book should give you a deeper understanding of the process of matching in the United States as an IMG. That said, just as medicine always changes, so too do procedures for immigration. Do not allow lack of information to prevent your residency dreams from coming true!

## FOR MORE INFO . . .

For information on the ECFMG and on Steps 1 and 2 of the USMLE, including application forms, contact:
Educational Commission for Foreign Medical Graduates
3624 Market Street
Philadelphia, PA 19104-2685
(215) 386-5900
www.ecfmg.org

For general information regarding the USMLE, contact:
USMLE Secretariat
3750 Market Street
Philadelphia, PA 19104-3190
(215) 590-9600
www.usmle.org

For general information on medical licensure and Step 3 of the USMLE, contact:
Federation of State Medical Boards
P.O. Box 619850
Dallas, TX 75261-9850
(817) 868-4000
Fax: (817) 868-4099
www.fsmb.org

For detailed information on the USMLE Step 3 and specific licensure issues, contact the state Board of Medical Examiners in the state in which you wish to practice.

For further information on the NRMP or to request an NRMP application, contact:
National Resident Matching Program
2450 N Street, N.W.
Washington, D.C. 20037-1127
(202) 828-0566
www.nrmp.org
**Please include your USMLE/ECFMG identification number on all correspondence.**

For information on visas and immigration services, contact:
Bureau of Citizenship and Immigration Services
425 I Street, N.W.
Washington, D.C. 20536
(800) 375-5283
www.immigration.gov
American Immigration Lawyers Association
www.aila.org
(800) 982-2839

For IMG resources offered by the American Medical Association, contact:
American Medical Association
Department of IMG Services
515 N. State Street
Chicago, IL 60610
(312) 464-5728
www.ama-assn.org/go/imgs

For additional information about the Exchange Visitor Sponsorship Program for foreign national physicians sponsored by the ECFMG, contact:
ECFMG Exchange Visitor Sponsorship Program
P.O. Box 41673
Philadelphia, PA 19101-1673
(215) 662-1445
Fax: (215) 386-9766

For further information on the Electronic Residency Application Service (ERAS), contact:
ECFMG/ERAS Program
P.O. Box 13467
Philadelphia, PA 19101-3467
(215) 386-5900
Fax: (215) 222-5641
www.aamc.org/audienceeras.htm

For information on Health Professional Shortage Areas (HPSA), contact:
Bureau of Primary Health Care
Division of Shortage Designation
4350 East-West Highway
Bethesda, MD 20814
(301) 594-0816
Online Database of HPSAs:
bphc.hrsa.gov/

For information on ARC, contact:
Appalachian Regional Commission
1666 Connecticut Avenue, NW
Washington, D.C. 20235
(202) 884-7700
www.arc.gov

For information on the VA, contact:
U.S. Department of Veterans Affairs
810 Vermont Avenue, NW
Washington, D.C. 20420
(800) 827-1000
www.va.gov

## REFERENCES

Garibaldi RA, Subhiyah R, Moore ME, Waxman H. The in-training examination in internal medicine: an analysis of resident perfomance over time. *Ann Intern Med* 137(6):505–510, 2002.

Moore RA, Rhodenbaugh EJ: The unkindest cut of all: are IMGS subjected to discrimination by general surgery residency programs? *Curr Surg* 59(2):228–236, 2002.

National Resident Matching Program 2005 Match Data, www.nrmp.org/res_match/tables/table2_05.pdf.

Norcini JJ, Boulet JR, Whelan GP, McKinley DW. Specialty Board certification among U.S. citizen and non-U.S. citizen graduates of international medical schools. *Acad Med* 80(10 Suppl):S42–45, 2005.

Polsky D, Kletke PR, Wozniak GD, Escarce JJ. Initial practice locations of IMGs. *Health Serv Res* 37(4):907–928, 2002.

Whelan GP, Gary NE, Kostis J, Boulet JR, Hallock JA. The changing pool of international medical graduates seeking certification training in U.S. graduate medical education programs. *JAMA* 288(9):1079–1084, 2002.

# Getting Residency Information and Applications

## THE KEY TO SUCCESS: ORGANIZATION!

> A wealth of information is at your fingertips. Begin your search early and remember to organize!

Throughout the application season, you will be gathering and reviewing a lot of information. This information will include the specifics of particular residency programs, housing, cost of living, benefits, and information about the interview itself. As you can imagine, the details can become overwhelming! Many students realize far too late that they have not organized the information appropriately. A lack of preparation could mean missed interviews, overlooked details, and forgotten follow-up letters, with the obvious negative effects on Match Day.

How can you prevent this from happening to you? It's simple: organize early and often! At the end of your third year, purchase a stack of manila folders or expanding folders so that you can create a file system. As you begin to research programs, place all materials concerning each program in a separate respective folder. As you receive interview invitations, include these in the folders, along with interview confirmations, travel plans, and notes created after the interview. If you lose interest in a program, simply toss the entire folder!

Most applicants prefer to keep an electronic record as well. One method is to start a spreadsheet (eg, with Microsoft Excel) that includes columns for the programs, interview dates, dates you sent a thank-you card, brief comments about a program, and any additional information you want to keep track of about each program. Some applicants also rank each program as they progress through the interview trail by adding columns of a program's most important attributes according to the applicant's own values (eg, call schedule, research strength, location, how well you got along with the residents, how academic or clinical the program was, variety of cases, and an overall gestalt feeling). Remember that you should always have a paper backup of your electronic file. This paper backup will also allow you to type up detailed reports on each residency program and insert them into each program's specific folder.

> Be sure to keep copies of interview confirmations! Secretaries can be busy, and you would hate to get lost in the shuffle.

An "interview calendar" should also be set up at this time. You should use the table on the inside front cover to roughly fill in this calendar. Then, as you set up specific interview dates, you can use the calendar to consolidate dates. This can also be done electronically with many common computer applications.

This basic preemptive organization process will serve you well. Once you have a place for everything, you can start putting everything in its place. You can now begin the search for the residency of your dreams.

## LEARNING ABOUT RESIDENCY PROGRAMS

Before you start the application process, you will need to acquire enough information about available residency programs to make a list of programs that fit your needs. Fortunately, there is no scarcity of data available on training programs (see Table 6-1). In fact, you will have to be selective and efficient in your information gathering. Career advisors, for example, can provide a broad perspective on a number of programs, including clinical training and research. On the other hand, junior faculty, fellows, and house staff can draw from their own residency experience

## TABLE 6-1

**Information Resources for Residency Programs**

| Source | Contribution |
|---|---|
| Career advisor (department chairperson, program director, or clinical faculty) | To identify appropriate programs to apply to and inform you of the current status of each. |
| Dean of students | To help you choose between specialties, pick an advisor, and assess overall competitiveness. |
| Faculty and house staff | To provide perspective on training and residency life. |
| Fourth-year medical students | To summarize what's hot/what's not: tips and warnings for prospects in your specialty. |
| AMA Fellowship and Residency Electronic Interactive Database (AMA-FREIDA) Web site (www.ama-assn.org/ama/pub/education-careers/graduate-medical-education/freida-online.shtml) | To provide current contact information for your target programs as well as detailed statistics. |
| *Graduate Medical Education Directory* (the "Green Book") | To provide contacts for residency programs. Next best thing to FREIDA. |
| *NRMP Program Results: Listing of Filled and Unfilled Programs* (available on the NRMP Web site at www.nrmp.org) | To list the programs that did not fill all their spots in the previous Match. |
| *Transitional Year Program Directory* (the "Purple Book") | To give detailed listings of transitional-year programs. |
| Directories published by some specialties | To supplement or update information in FREIDA. |
| San Francisco Matching Program Web site (www.sfmatch.org) | To obtain detailed information on the match process for child neurology, neurotology, and ophthalmology programs. |
| American Urological Association (AUA) Web site (www.auanet.org) | To obtain detailed information on the match process for urology residency programs. |

to give you the nitty-gritty about training at specific programs. However, there is no one source that will tell you everything you need to know as it relates to your goals. Therefore, use enough sources to get the necessary information.

> Resources abound at your medical school. Use them!

## CAREER ADVISOR/MENTOR

Your career advisor/mentor should be aware of your personal and professional goals, and therefore be able to help identify programs that will best fit your needs.

In addition, your advisor often can provide information regarding the "personality" of various programs. For instance, he or she may be able to identify the current department chair, academic and clinical foci, and overall reputation of the research that is conducted at a particular institution. He or she may also be aware of recent graduates from your medical school who are currently training at a given institution. If so, obtain your advisor's contact information and take advantage of the knowledge and insight he or she may have into a specific program. If this is not the case, be proactive and request copies of Match results from the last three graduating classes from your medical school and make phone calls on your own.

## DEAN OF STUDENTS

It is surprising how many students pass up the opportunity to make an appointment with the dean of students, perhaps out of fear that the dean is "too busy" to speak with them or is absorbed with weightier matters. Don't hesitate to schedule an appointment, as this faculty member can be an excellent source of information, advice, and advocacy. Even a brief meeting with your dean can give you inside information about the workings of the Match at your school, advance word on how and when the dean's letter will be written, an early assessment of your academic progress as it might influence your specialty and program choice, and suggestions about who the "hot" advisors are. It is never too early to get some hints about strategies, both academic and personal. Don't forget, many deans have gone through this process themselves, often in the not-too-distant past.

> The dean of students is an often overlooked resource.

## FACULTY AND HOUSE STAFF

Faculty in your desired specialty whom you meet on your junior and senior clerkships can complement information your career advisor provides. You should therefore talk to as many of these people as possible and make an effort to understand their perspectives (eg, geographic, academic versus clinical). The department chair and the program director of your chosen specialty can be an especially useful resource. Senior residents can share their sense of the job market as well as their own job-hunting experiences. Junior faculty and fellows can shed light on the residency programs that trained them. Especially valuable in this regard are junior faculty who trained elsewhere, as these individuals have a recent yet mature perspective on how a particular training program differs from others—or at least how that program differs from the one at your institution. Junior faculty are often enthusiastic about getting involved with students.

> Fellows from other institutions can provide valuable comparisons between programs.

To a certain extent, the same holds true of house staff, who can readily provide information on programs they knew as medical students. Bear in mind, however, that the perspective of house staff is limited to their own program and does not necessarily apply to any others. House staff may also lack the "big picture," just as you do. Interns in their third month of residency, as sleep-deprived and cranky as they tend to be, are unlikely to shed many pearls of wisdom about your future. However, just like senior medical students, they can be a source of information about the "interview trail," having recently gone through it.

## SENIOR MEDICAL STUDENTS

Inasmuch as they have survived their interviews and Match Day, graduating seniors are your best bet for practical application and interviewing tips. Debriefing some of these survivors will give you an additional "feel" for the application process and alert you to potential trouble spots. Most medical schools organize question-and-answer sessions with graduating seniors. Remember, though, that while seniors have considerable "trench" experience, their perspectives are understandably limited when it comes to what programs might be best for you.

## OUTSIDE FACULTY

If your medical school is affiliated with a VA, county, or private hospital, keep the faculty at these institutions in mind as potential sources of advice. Although medical students have historically underutilized such faculty members, many have considerable insight into aspects of medical training that their more academic colleagues in the Ivory Tower lack. For example, they may know of special loan repayment programs offered to VA residents, may be aware of the "job track" at HMOs such as Kaiser Permanente, and may be adept at comparing one county facility with another in terms of training.

## FELLOWSHIP AND RESIDENCY ELECTRONIC INTERACTIVE DATABASE (FREIDA)

FREIDA (www.ama-assn.org/ama/pub/education-careers/graduate-medical-education/freida-online.shtml) is an annually updated, PC-based database of residency programs that is produced by the American Medical Association (AMA). If you use only one resource to gather initial information on residency programs, this should be it. FREIDA contains information on approximately 8600 graduate medical programs and combined programs that are accredited by the Accreditation Council for Graduate Medical Education (ACGME). It is very easy to use and has supplanted the *Graduate Medical Education Directory* (aka the "Green Book") as the most popular source on residency programs. The data within it are derived from the AMA Annual Survey of Graduate Medical Education Programs. These surveys are filled out in the fall and the data are entered in both October and February. Programs can change some of the basic information throughout the year.

> FREIDA is a self-reported database. It does not compare or rank programs.

Accessed through the Internet, FREIDA can search for programs by specialty, region or state, and optional criteria, such as program size, preliminary positions available, and many more, dividing an overwhelming amount of information on each program into eight manageable categories (see Table 6-2). Included in each program's basic information are the name, address, phone number, and e-mail address of the program director and contact person, and the program's Web site address, all of which can help students obtain answers to questions not answered by FREIDA. Each program has a ten-digit identifying number that will be listed in the "Search Results" page as well as under the program's basic information. Writing down these numbers will enable you to bypass the search engine and go directly to that specific program's information in the future.

### TABLE 6-2

**Information in FREIDA**

General program information

Educational environment

Work environment

Compensation and benefits

Clinical environment

Patient population

Medical benefits/institution features

Specialties in institution

FREIDA has two other categories. The category of "Specialty Statistics" provides general information on specialties and subspecialties, such as work hours, work environment, and average compensation. "Physician Workforce Information" provides statistics given by residents and practicing physicians on finding employment, workplace environment, job satisfaction, and the like. There are, however, a few things you should remember about FREIDA. First, the information is sometimes incomplete or outdated. Double check information from FREIDA with information provided on individual program Web sites or the residency program coordinator. Second, all information is provided by the programs themselves, and none of it is verified. Sometimes program directors choose not to answer certain questions that they feel are irrelevant or embarrassing. Other programs do not fill out questionnaires at all and are listed only by name. Finally, keep in mind that as a self-reporting database, FREIDA does not evaluate or compare programs objectively.

## GRADUATE MEDICAL EDUCATION DIRECTORY: THE "GREEN BOOK"

*The Graduate Medical Education Directory* is an annually updated catalog of all training programs recognized by the ACGME. Despite its heft, the directory has very little information for each program other than the contact address and telephone number (see Table 6-3).

> The Green Book is big, but it's no FREIDA.

The Green Book can be obtained at your office of student affairs or medical library. You can order your own copy online at www.ama-assn.org or call toll free (800) 621-8335.

If you are an IMG with no convenient access to FREIDA, you should probably purchase your own copy of the Green Book. Although the program information contained in it is not as extensive as that in FREIDA, the Green Book does feature *some* facts that FREIDA does not cover. These include visa and certification guidelines for international medical graduates seeking graduate medical education in the United States; detailed ACGME requirements for program accreditation by specialty; and state licensure requirements.

## TABLE 6-3

### Information in "Green Book" Program Listing

Program director's name, address, telephone number

Sponsoring institution

Other institutions with a major role in training

Number of training years

Total number of positions in program

Program ID number

## TRANSITIONAL YEAR PROGRAM DIRECTORY: THE "PURPLE BOOK"

The Purple Book lists most transitional-year programs and includes contact information as well as data on required and elective rotations, call schedule, and the like. Given that much of the same information is available in FREIDA, you should use the Purple Book as a secondary resource. It should be available at your office of student affairs and is also available over the Internet (www.ahme.org). A copy can be ordered by calling or writing:

Association for Hospital Medical Education (AHME)
419 Beulah Road
Pittsburgh, PA 15235
(412) 244-9302

## NRMP PROGRAM RESULTS: LISTING OF FILLED AND UNFILLED PROGRAMS

As described in Chapter 1, the NRMP Program Results lists all programs that did not fill their spots in the NRMP Match. If you are a weak candidate in a strong field, you might want to take a closer look at these programs. If this publication is not available at your student affairs office, you can order it for $45 by calling or writing:

Attention: Membership and Publication Orders

National Resident Matching Program

2450 N Street, N.W.

Washington, D.C. 20037-1127

(202) 828-0416

## SPECIALTY-SPECIFIC DIRECTORIES

Several specialty organization Web sites maintain directories of training programs with contact information. In addition, a handful of directories (including those from family practice, internal medicine, psychiatry, physical medicine and rehabilitation, and preventive medicine) rival or surpass FREIDA in terms of comprehensiveness and appropriateness of information. Many of these directories maintain board pass rates for each program. In general, however, the specialty directories are not updated as frequently as FREIDA or the Green Book. See Chapter 4 for a list of specialty organization Web site addresses and contact information.

## EARLY MATCH WEB SITES

For information on child neurology, neurotology, and ophthalmology programs, go to the San Francisco Matching Program Web site at www.sfmatch.org. Information on urology programs can be found in the "Residency" section at the American Urological Association Web site (www.auanet.org).

## HOW MANY PROGRAMS SHOULD I APPLY TO?

Most students want to submit enough applications to yield a healthy number of interviews, which will in turn help ensure a successful match. At the same time, the number of programs you apply to depends on a variety of additional factors, including (1) your competitive standing; (2) the competitiveness of the specialty; (3) the competitiveness of the programs to which you are applying; and (4) whether you're participating in the couples match. Because so many factors figure into this equation, it's best to consult your career advisor or dean to help determine the "right" number for you. If you are even mildly interested in a particular program, however, write or call for an information packet (and an application if it is a non-ERAS [Electronic Residency Application Service] residency program). If you remain unsure, err on the side of submitting too many applications (see Figure 6-1). Don't worry about going overboard at this point, as it is better to decline

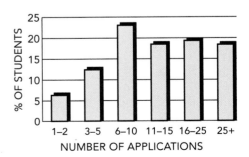

**FIGURE 6-1.** Number of residency applications made by U.S. fourth-year medical students.

> It is far better to apply to too many programs than to too few.

interview invitations later than to realize that you do not have enough interviews to ensure a good match.

You should also consider the "Rule of Thirds" in your efforts to achieve a balanced set of applications and minimize your chances of not matching. A third of your applications should go to your "dream programs" regardless of their competitiveness. Another third should include desirable programs where you have a solid chance of matching. The last third should consist of acceptable programs that can serve as backups. While this category does not necessitate as many entries as the first two tiers, it is good to have a few programs in the "backup" category. The Rule of Thirds works best in the less competitive specialties. Because of the recent implementation of ERAS and the ease of sending out applications, residency programs are receiving a higher volume of applications in comparison to previous years. See Chapter 4 to find a general prescription for a healthy number of applications in each field.

## HOW DO I OBTAIN APPLICATIONS?

The widespread use of ERAS by most specialties has greatly simplified the process of obtaining applications. In fact, for most programs ERAS is the only application you'll need. The application materials are generally available on July 1. Through ERAS, you will complete one common application that can be modified in terms of which letters of recommendation or personal statement you wish to be included for each residency program you apply to.

For those few programs that continue not to use ERAS, use FREIDA or the Green Book to contact programs for applications. Unfortunately, this is the step that triggers an avalanche of paperwork. The great thing is that there are so few of these programs that this shouldn't turn into the huge pile of paperwork it used to be less than a decade ago. To keep yourself sane during this process, **follow two rules from the start**. First, finalize your list of target programs before beginning the application process. Second, try to complete each step of each application at the same time. For example, request all required transcripts in one sitting.

To request applications, purchase prestamped postcards at the post office. If you're using a word processor, it will be worth the effort to create three sets of labels. On the first set, write a brief note requesting information and an application. Type your address on the second set, and enter the name of the program director and the program addresses on the third set. Then, simply attach the three labels to the face of the postcard in the appropriate spots (see Figure 6-2).

You should send for applications and program information **no later than early July**. Allow two to three weeks to receive applications from programs; then follow up with phone calls as needed. If you fall behind on your requests, consider calling all the programs directly for information and applications. It's worth the cost of the phone calls, and you might be able to get answers to some simple questions while you're requesting applications.

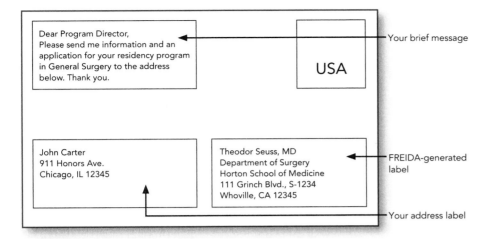

**FIGURE 6-2.** Sample application request postcard.

## WHAT SHOULD I BE LOOKING FOR IN A PROGRAM?

Before you set up your list of programs to apply to, you need to have some idea of your priorities. Although you don't need crystal-ball clarity at this point, you should think through the following issues early in the process, preferably before you start interviewing.

### LOCATION

Location is a critical yet highly personal issue. Some candidates are restricted by the employment requirements of their significant other. Other students want to be near family or wish to use residency as an opportunity to establish contacts in the community where they ultimately hope to practice. If you are adventurous and have no serious "attachments," consider programs that will place you on new terrain. Many students who are doing preliminary or transitional PGY-1 years take advantage of the opportunity to experience another city with a limited time commitment. After all, this might be your last chance to do so before marital and family responsibilities catch up with you.

Experience tells us that once students get settled in a city and become accustomed to a particular program, they are often reluctant to leave. They must then scramble during their busy intern year to find a way to stay put. It is important to consider this possibility when applying to programs, even if you initially intend to stay there for just your transitional or preliminary year.

Some locations are incredibly popular, and programs in these areas may be more competitive (see Table 6-4). If there is a particular location that is desirable to you, be sure to apply to a wealth of programs in that region to increase your chances of matching there. Keep in mind that by limiting yourself geo-

| TABLE 6-4 |
| --- |
| **Some Application Hot Spots** |
| Boston |
| Chicago |
| Hawaii |
| San Diego |
| San Francisco |
| Seattle |

graphically, you may need to compromise on other program attributes that you are seeking.

Finally, regional variations in style and attitudes can affect residency training. During your interviews, you may detect some regional variations in medical training. The most important thing is to choose the style that best suits you!

## SETTING

Most applicants' career plans can be categorized as academically oriented, clinically oriented, or both. You want to find a program that fits your preferences. The majority of programs can be classified into the following settings: university, community, urban/county, or health maintenance organization (HMO). Many of these programs run services at more than one hospital, thus offering their residents exposure to multiple settings. It is worth your while to ask about the amount of time you would spend at each hospital.

**University.** A university medical school affiliation is advantageous for two reasons: (1) medical schools offer teaching opportunities; and (2) the presence of medical students ensures a setting geared toward teaching the residents as well. Teaching conferences are generally of higher quality in university programs than in other settings, although this is not always the case. There are, however, a few drawbacks. For starters, university programs can be more intense, which tends to contribute to a lower level of sociability among the residents. Residents in university programs tend to have greater access to knowledgeable consultants, but some residents complain that because of this wealth of specialists and consultants, they have less autonomy and decision-making responsibility. On one hand, patient populations in a university setting are sometimes not representative of what the resident will encounter in community practice after training. On the other hand, university programs tend to be based in tertiary care centers that give their residents exposure to more unusual or interesting cases.

**Community.** There is great variability among community programs; however, it is often felt that residents receive a kinder, gentler training in these institutions, although this distinction can be specialty specific. In addition, the benefits and salary may also be more generous, and residents are often more relaxed, with less academic pressure and more time for reading. However, some programs may be less academically prestigious, lack formalized educational conferences, and have a large proportion of private patients/attendings. Keep in mind that you may not have the same degree of patient responsibility or diversity of disease experience with less common procedures.

**Urban/county.** If you really want hands-on experience, city and county hospitals will virtually give you blisters. You can forget academic theorization here; you'll be taught to manage a large patient population consisting primarily of urban poor. Most likely, you will also be heavily involved in the decision-making process and will gain experience with a variety of invasive procedures. Unfortunately, county and city hospital personnel are frequently overworked and underpaid. Moreover, these programs often lack the academic prestige and name recognition of their university equivalents, with notable exceptions such as Massachusetts General Hospital and San Francisco General. In addition, ancillary support tends to be weaker, and formal teaching is often uneven and disorganized.

**HMOs.** Health maintenance organizations, or HMOs, often have their own hospitals, especially on the West Coast. A number of these hospitals have their own residency programs in some of the larger specialties such as internal medicine. Several other residency programs at academic hospitals have their residents rotate through these HMO hospitals or clinics so that residents have an idea of how these systems work when it comes time for them to apply for positions after residency. HMOs have become a reality in the United States, and they are a viable residency option for many students who like saner hours, appreciate continuity of care, and have an interest in controlling costs in medicine.

## STABILITY

With graduate medical education facing drastic cuts in federal funding, it is important that you determine how financially secure a residency program is. How much of the program's funding comes from federal sources? How well off is the parent hospital or university? County hospitals in several California cities are on the brink of financial collapse; mergers have changed the rotation options of residents in New York and Boston. Hospitals in Denver have closed entirely, leaving residents there jobless. In addition, many teaching hospitals (especially on the East and West Coasts) are now experiencing unprecedented competition from managed care. Does the parent hospital enjoy a robust patient base, or is it floundering in a rising tide of managed care? Although you can do little to change the fiscal policy of a state or the financial pressures motivating a merger, you can take steps to remain aware of these entities and factor them into your ultimate decision.

> Sweeping changes in health care finances make stability a key issue in county and private programs.

In addition to financial stability, residencies must be accredited in order to train residents. It is therefore worth your while to see if a program has or recently had any problems with accreditation. Probation is a red flag indicating that something is wrong in the residency, but it may or may not indicate that the problem is being addressed. If your program fails to get accredited after a probation period, you may not be board eligible in the field in which you trained.

## REPUTATION

A program's reputation invariably comes into play if an applicant is considering fellowship training or a career in academic medicine. That reputation, whether deserved or not, can greatly influence your ability to secure competitive fellowships or faculty appointments in the future. If a program is too large, however, prestige doesn't matter; you may still have to sweat to get the strong personal recommendations you need to secure a competitive fellowship. The reality in community practice is that most patients will not know or really care what medical school you graduated from, much less where you trained.

## SUBSPECIALTY STRENGTHS

If you're considering subspecialty training after residency, you might want to evaluate programs with strengths in that subspecialty. In addition, it never hurts to have a well-known "name" in a subspecialty write you a strong letter of recommendation. Fellowship directors often trust the strong recommendations of their colleagues, and this can make the difference in competitive fields.

Additionally, it is crucial for all prospective residents—especially those who are thinking about a fellowship—to find out where graduates of a given program are today. This is an appropriate question to ask and is often answered in tabular form during the interview. If not, go ahead and ask; you may not care now, but you'll wish you knew when you apply for some of the more competitive specialties.

## EDUCATIONAL ENVIRONMENT

> People learn in different ways; make sure you understand your own preferences.

Because residency programs are a form of postgraduate education, you will need to appraise the educational philosophy and facilities at the institutions that interest you. Try to obtain as much information as possible regarding education program Web sites and during interview days. Pay attention to the following aspects of residency programs:

**Curricula/conferences.** Residents depend on well-organized conferences and teaching rounds to expand their knowledge base and reinforce what they already know. Most programs have developed an organized curriculum that exposes residents to all major topics in the specialty during their training. This curriculum might include rotations, conferences, and syllabi with assigned reading. Within some specialties, there is a lot of variation in emphasis and formality, so you have to decide which combination best fits your needs. For example, some family practice programs emphasize obstetrics while others practically exclude it. Some medicine programs feature heavy experience and training in HIV; others have next to none.

**Faculty teaching.** The teaching residents receive, as well as the rapport they establish with faculty, can be correlated with many factors, including faculty-to-resident ratio, program setting, the proportion of private attendings, and overall program size. A large program cannot provide as much personal mentoring, but thankfully, you are less at the mercy of a few quirky personalities. When you visit a program, get a sense of how invested the faculty are in the training of its house staff. Also try to get a feel for how important teaching is to the residency program as a whole. Finally, determine if there is an established system for feedback/evaluation of residents and find out how responsive faculty are to this feedback.

**Research and teaching opportunities.** Research and teaching opportunities are almost essential for those who are planning an academic career or subspecialty training, and such opportunities are desirable even if you do not plan to stay within academic walls. So when you assess the research opportunities at a program, ask yourself the following questions: Are well-established researchers available to guide residents? Is time allotted for research, either as a requirement or as an elective? How successful has the program been in securing grants, hospital funding, or internal funding for research? How satisfied are the residents who are currently completing projects? Or, for that matter, how many dissatisfied residents cite a lack of institutional financial support?

# WORK ENVIRONMENT

Don't forget to survey the working environment when you size up a residency program. After all, you'll be putting in a lot of hours in that set of buildings with their cast of characters. So don't overlook the considerations outlined below.

**Work versus education.** Many programs are guilty of exploiting residents' "cheap labor" without providing a rich educational experience. Residency is "learning by doing," to be sure, but be on the lookout for the manner in which service is balanced against education.

**Patient population/load.** The optimal patient load will provide you with enough clinical experience while still leaving you adequate time and energy to read and attend teaching conferences. Patient load is often a function of the program's setting (see above). On your interview visits, ask for an average patient census and the number of admissions residents get when on call, and discreetly ask residents how they feel about the workload. Also, learn what medical problems are common in the population served by the program. For example, an orthopedics program may get more than its share of trauma cases by virtue of its location near several major highways. You should also try to get a feel for other characteristics of the patient population, such as ethnicity/language (is there a large Spanish-speaking population?), socioeconomic status (urban poor?), and attitude (a typical Saturday night ER crowd?). Keep in mind that the best training environment does not have to match that of your future practice. But you must understand how you learn best.

**Patient responsibilities.** The whole point of residency training is to provide you with the experience and skills you need to practice medicine unsupervised. So when you visit a program, find out if the attending allows residents to "run the show" or, conversely, if residents need to obtain approval for major decisions. Is backup assistance readily available if the resident or intern needs help?

**Call schedule.** Call schedules vary widely by specialty, setting, year of training, and training site (for programs with multiple sites). Recognize the range of calls that can deprive you of a good night's sleep. The house officer will often encounter a mix of calls during the year. How much sleep you typically get during a call night and how late you work postcall is almost as important as how often you're on call. For many specialties, call frequency often varies according to training year.

> Don't forget to ask about how much protected sleep time you get and when you go home postcall.

Closely tied to call schedule is the number of work hours you will be expected to work per week. With the new resident work-hour legislation in place, residents are not to work more than 80 hours averaged over a four-week period, should have one day off in seven (averaged over four weeks), should have ten hours off between daily duty periods and after in-house call, and should not work more than 30 hours when on call. When on the interview trail, it is important to ask residents how close they come to meeting the 80-hour workweek requirements. In the end, you must determine your threshold and the workload you are willing to tolerate.

> Know the new ACGME-mandated resident work-hour guidelines.

**Ancillary support.** No one is an island, and your team certainly doesn't go it alone in caring for your patients. Good nursing support, consulting services, phlebotomy, laboratory, hospital information services, transport services, and ER care are keys to a smooth clinical work experience. As an intern, you will often be used as a person of last resort to fill any gaps in ancillary support (unless you scut the poor medical student).

*Esprit de corps.* *Esprit de corps* is a familiar, albeit foreign, term for morale. To gauge it, trust your intuition as well as your powers of observation. Are the residents "happy campers"? Is the atmosphere friendly or competitive? What kind of camaraderie exists among the residents? Among faculty, house staff, and administration? Look for the answers on your visit by asking the house staff and ancillary staff. Quietly divide and conquer. It is usually easier to get an honest answer in private from a departing resident than to ask the chief resident or the program director in front of 20 other interviewees. Afterward, assess the quality of your own experience during the visit.

## SALARY

Residents are paid so little that salary is seldom the central issue. Interestingly enough, most of your paycheck comes from the federal government rather than from the program itself, so you may be fattening the bottom line of a hospital that is not even paying you. The average income of an intern in 2008–2009 was $46,245, but don't bother calculating your pay per hour; it will only depress you. Salary information is readily available on FREIDA. Your income usually rises incrementally during your residency training, but not by much. It is critical to factor in cost of living when comparing salaries; $30,000 will take you much further in Louisville, Kentucky, than $32,000 in Los Angeles (see Table 6-5).

For many, these low figures alone are reason enough to moonlight. Once you are licensed to practice medicine (typically after the first year), you can usually earn anywhere from $20 to $120 per hour working in a variety of settings, including ERs, nursing homes, and outpatient clinics (ie, "doc in the box" settings); doing insurance company physical exams; and even working in prisons. Some programs actually provide in-house moonlighting opportunities, which can be a crucial source of supplementary income. In-house jobs will often take into account your regular

## TABLE 6-5

### Average 2008–2009 Resident Stipends

| Year | All | Northeast | South | Midwest | West |
|------|-----|-----------|-------|---------|------|
| PGY-1 | $46,245 | $48,637 | $44,484 | $45,127 | $46,073 |
| PGY-2 | $48,092 | $50,930 | $45,982 | $46,628 | $48,227 |
| PGY-3 | $50,128 | $53,520 | $47,572 | $48,176 | $50,758 |
| PGY-4 | $52,154 | $55,618 | $49,284 | $50,231 | $53,410 |
| PGY-5 | $54,164 | $57,882 | $50,954 | $51,806 | $55,434 |
| PGY-6 | $56,463 | $60,352 | $53,008 | $53,744 | $57,096 |

Source: AAMC *Survey of Resident/Fellow Stipends and Benefits,* Autumn 2008.

call schedule, making it easier for you to moonlight during residency. On the other hand, many programs either officially ban moonlighting or actively discourage it, so tactfully ask about it on your visit, and someone (usually a graduating resident) will give you the scoop.

> Moonlighting offers the best of both worlds if you can handle the extra work.

## BENEFITS

Although everyone remembers to ask about salary, don't forget about other benefits. While benefits should not be the reason you choose to rank a program highly, you should think carefully about a program whose benefits are below the norm. Many programs offer medical insurance, dental services, paid drug prescriptions, employee health services, and psychiatric counseling (see Table 6-6). So shop around carefully, especially if you have a family. You should also be aware that certain benefits at some programs are available only if a resident pays a portion of the cost. You don't want to end up spending part of your meager salary on benefits that other programs would have provided for free. So when you evaluate insurance, ask yourself (1) who is covered (ie, family); (2) what is covered; and (3) what costs you will have to pay out of pocket.

> Key benefits are $ in the bank.

In addition to asking about health benefits, you should ensure that a program offers adequate life, disability, and liability insurance. After four years in medical school and untold thousands of dollars in expenses, you (and your family) don't want to be left high and dry if you get sick or have an accident.

If you're planning to start a family during residency training, scrutinize the rules on maternity/paternity leave (see Table 6-7). Find out if the policy is written or if it varies with each case (and personality). Currently, of course, maternity leave policies tend to be more generous than paternity leave policies. Other benefits to consider include parking, housing, meals, vacation, education

## TABLE 6-7
### Issues Addressed by a Complete Parental Leave Policy

Differences in maternal versus paternal leave policies

Duration of leaves allowed before and after delivery

Which category of leave credited

Whether leave is paid or unpaid

Whether provision is made for continuation of insurance benefits and the payment of premiums

Whether sick leave and vacation time may be accrued from year to year or used in advance

Whether make-up time will be paid

Policies for adoption

Whether schedule accommodations are allowed

## TABLE 6-6
### Survey of Health Benefits Offered by Residency Programs

| Benefit | % Fully Paid (resident/family) | % Offered/Cost Shared (resident/family) | % Offered/Not Paid (resident/family) | % Not Offered (resident/family) |
|---|---|---|---|---|
| Group medical insurance | 36.4/26.6 | 61.2/66.8 | 0/3.7 | 0/0.5 |
| Group dental insurance | 29.9/19.6 | 53.3/57.9 | 9.8/15.4 | 4.2/3.7 |
| Vision | 29.4/22.0 | 47.7/50.0 | 13.1/18.7 | 6.5/6.1 |
| Drug prescriptions | 38.3/28.5 | 58.9/64.5 | 0/4.2 | 0.5/0.5 |
| Psychiatric benefits | 37.4/27.1 | 59.3/65.4 | 0.5/4.7 | 0/0 |
| Counseling | 41.6/30.4 | 54.2/59.8 | 1.4/5.1 | 0.5/1.9 |

*Source:* AAMC *Survey of Resident/Fellow Stipends and Benefits*, Autumn 2008.

## TABLE 6-8

**Survey of Nonhealth Benefits Offered by Residency Programs**

| Benefit | % Fully Paid | % Offered/ Cost Shared | % Not Offered | % Not Paid |
|---------|--------------|------------------------|---------------|------------|
| Life insurance | 79.9 | 12.1 | 2.8 | 4.2 |
| Disability insurance | 73.4 | 12.6 | 2.8 | 9.8 |
| Housing | 0.5 | 8.9 | 80.4 | 7.9 |
| Parking | 56.5 | 16.8 | 5.1 | 19.2 |
| Meals at work | 22.9 | 27.6 | 23.4 | 23.8 |
| On-call meals | 78.0 | 14.5 | 2.3 | 3.7 |

Source: AAMC *Survey of Resident/Fellow Stipends and Benefits,* Autumn 2008.

leave for conferences, library services (eg, photocopying), and child care (see Table 6-8).

## HOW DO I ORGANIZE THIS INFORMATION?

Great—you know what to look for. But now you need to be able to organize and evaluate all the data. You are already receiving information from multiple sources: from FREIDA, your advisor, and house officers at your medical institution. You will be flooded with even more information on your visits to the programs. All of this information should be going into your centralized manila-folder command center. Additionally, we've included a Program Evaluation Worksheet (PEW) that should allow you to organize information conveniently and evaluate a program objectively (see Figures 6-3A and B and Appendix B). Make a copy for each program on your application hit list, and take these copies with you on the interview trail to record notes and impressions.

> File PEWs into your manila-folder system after your visit.

After this information has been gathered and organized, remember that programs can change rapidly—in many instances, for the worse. All the preparation in the world cannot prevent you from matching at a program whose director suddenly wins the lottery and moves to Tahiti or whose call rooms are flooded by a natural disaster. But a little luck, a thick skin, and a healthy amount of patience will get you through any situation you encounter.

Program Name _____

Date of Visit _____

| Factor | Comments |
|---|---|
| **Location** | |
| Setting | |
| Reputation | |
| Stability of program | |
| Subspecialty strengths | |
| **Education** | |
| Conferences/rounds | |
| Faculty teaching | |
| Postresidency plans of graduates | |
| Research/teaching opportunities | |
| **Work Environment** | |
| Patient population/load | |
| Patient responsibilities | |
| Call frequency/ hours per week | |
| Ancillary support (e.g., nursing) | |
| On-call support (e.g., night float, admission caps) | |
| Health benefits | |
| Non-health benefits | |
| Vacation/sick leave/ parenting leave | |

**FIGURE 6-3A.** Program Evaluation Worksheet (PEW).

**Other Factors/Notes**

Gut feeling

| Advantages | Disadvantages |
|---|---|
| | |

**Preliminary Rank**

☐ Top third        ☐ Middle third        ☐ Bottom third        ☐ Do not rank

**Interviewers and Addresses**

| Name/Address | Topics discussed during interview |
|---|---|
| ☐ Thank-you card or follow-up letter sent | |
| ☐ Thank-you card or follow-up letter sent | |
| ☐ Thank-you card or follow-up letter sent | |
| ☐ Thank-you card or follow-up letter sent | |
| ☐ Thank-you card or follow-up letter sent | |
| ☐ Thank-you card or follow-up letter sent | |

**FIGURE 6-3B.** Program Evaluation Worksheet (continued).

## REFERENCES

AMA Fellowship and Residency Electronic Interactive Database Web site (www.ama-assn.org/ama/pub/education-careers/graduate-medical-education/freida-online.shtml).

American Urological Association Web site (www.auanet.org).

Association of American Medical Colleges. *Survey of Resident/Fellow Stipends and Benefits.* Washington, D.C., Autumn 2008. (www.aamc.org/data/stipend/2008_stipend report.pdf).

Bickel J. Maternity leave policies for residents: an overview of issues and problems. *Acad Med* 64(9):498–501, 1989.

San Francisco Matching Program Web site (www.sfmatch.org).

Steinbrook R. The debate over residents' work hours. *N Engl J Med* 347(16):1296–1302, 2002.

# The Application

7

## WHAT IS IN AN APPLICATION?

There are two categories to which most Match applicants will be applying: Electronic Residency Application Service (ERAS) specialties and early Match specialties (child neurology, neurotology, ophthalmology, and urology). With regard to the former category, your ERAS token should arrive from your school by early summer, usually in June. If you are participating in the early match, you will need to start this process sooner. For all specialties, a complete program application file will consist of several documents or sets of documents that you must assemble, track, and ultimately send off. You will be pulling together the components of this file all summer long and into early fall (see Table 7-1), and you will then be compiling all relevant information either into the file system that you established during the summer or in your dean's office.

## TABLE 7-1

### Common Elements of an Application File

| Document | Function | Quick Advice | More Information |
|---|---|---|---|
| Program application | Foundation of application file | Request by early June. Better to get too many than too few. Most programs participate in ERAS, so requesting applications might be unnecessary. | See pages 161–165 |
| Dean's letter | Compendium of written evaluations compiled by dean of student affairs | Take an active role in helping dean by editing/supplementing content if possible. Clarify any inaccuracies. | See pages 165–167 |
| Letters of recommendation | Written testimonials from faculty familiar with your work | Solicit letters no later than August. Confirm that writer feels comfortable writing a "strong" letter. | See pages 168–170 |
| Transcript | Academic record | Proofread an unofficial copy before having them sent out. | See page 170 |
| CV | Summary of your credentials, activities, and accomplishments | Pull together by late June/early July. Nice to have for preparing personal statement and to accompany requests for letters of recommendation. | See Chapter 8 |
| Personal statement | Opportunity to establish your own voice and distinguish yourself from other applicants | Finish personal statement before applications arrive. Multiple reviewers and revisions are key. Have this completed by the end of June. | See Chapter 9 |

## HOW DO I ORGANIZE THE PAPERWORK?

For ERAS specialties as well as for many early Match specialties, you will fill out one common application. For non-ERAS specialties, however, each program will have its own set of application requirements, which will be outlined either in the program's cover letter or within the application itself. Some programs will ask you to complete the National Resident Matching Program (NRMP) Universal Application, while others will include their own forms. Some programs will want to receive your undergraduate transcript in addition to your medical school transcript. To help you keep track of who wants what, you should photocopy enough copies of the worksheet for application requirements to list all the programs to which you are applying (see Figure 7-1 and Appendix A). Some students will prefer to make an electronic version of Figure 7-1.

> Use a worksheet (like ours) to organize the application process.

**Directions:** Fill in blanks below with requested numbers/names/dates. Under **Application Requirements**, list each requirement by name. Once you have assembled the item for that application, check it off.

| Program Name | Program Director | Program Administrator and Contact Info | App. Deadline | Application Requirements | Notes |
|---|---|---|---|---|---|
| | | | | ☐ ☐ ☐ ☐ ☐ | |
| | | | | ☐ ☐ ☐ ☐ ☐ | |
| | | | | ☐ ☐ ☐ ☐ ☐ | |
| | | | | ☐ ☐ ☐ ☐ ☐ | |
| | | | | ☐ ☐ ☐ ☐ ☐ | |

**FIGURE 7-1.** Worksheet for application requirements.

Fortunately, there are two steps you can take to prevent paperwork from spiraling out of control: (1) do not add any new programs to your list after you have started working on your applications; and (2) try to complete one item (eg, obtaining transcripts) for all applications at the same time.

## WHO EVALUATES MY APPLICATION?

> The program secretary can be a powerful ally . . . or enemy!

As you assemble your application materials, be sure to remember your audience. The residency selection committee is usually composed of the residency director, several faculty members, and a few house officers. All are **extremely busy people** who would rather be doing something other than screening your application on a Saturday afternoon. So try to make their job as pleasant as possible by submitting a neat, professional-looking application with clear, succinct answers.

> Above all: be nice to departmental administrators!

Although faculty members are indeed important, you should bear in mind that departmental administrators and administrative assistants can make or break an application. Many students make the mistake of forgetting their manners when scheduling interviews and asking administrative personnel for further information. Not only is this rude, but it could prove to be detrimental to your application, as the comments made by administrative personnel may well influence the committee's impressions of you. Additionally, the departmental administrator often compiles the list of applicants to be interviewed using screening criteria such as board scores and medical school attended. Therefore, it is not difficult for such people to move your application into the "Do Not Interview" pile or, conversely, from that stack into the "To Be Interviewed" pile. If the departmental administrator likes you well enough, he or she may actually push for your application or direct it to a receptive committee member. If you miss any deadlines, friendly administrative assistants may bend rules to keep your application in the running. Administrative personnel also coordinate complexities such as couples applications and visa issues for international medical graduates (IMGs). We could go on, but you get the message!

## HOW DO THEY EVALUATE MY APPLICATION?

> USMLE scores and class ranks may be used as screening tools!

Once your application lands on the desk of the program director, he or she will direct its contents to a number of readers at different phases in the evaluation process. The typical process can be divided into several stages: screening, the interview, and ranking sessions. Each stage is described below and in subsequent chapters.

### SCREENING

In the initial phase of the evaluation process, your application is usually reviewed by a select few committee members, most of whom screen applications after hours during the week or on weekend afternoons. At this point, some oversubscribed residencies in competitive specialties employ the help of an administrative assistant to divide the applicant pool into a few tiers on the basis of United States Medical Licensing Examination (USMLE) scores or, if available, class rank. Optimally, screeners will read your application, your letters of recommendation, selected portions of your dean's letter, and your transcript. In reality, however, they will likely just scan the highlights of your application package. This is where it can pay off to have an organized CV and a well-written personal statement.

When the committee looks at a dean's letter, members typically focus on junior and senior clerkship evaluations in their field and scan the summary paragraph for crucial code words. Note that the personal statement tends to carry little or no weight at this point in the process, since screeners generally have another 50 files or so to plow through. Screeners then complete an evaluation form, which will toss your application into one of three piles: a recommendation to interview, maybe interview, or not interview. Some programs grant interviews on a rolling basis, so again, it's best to get your application in as early as possible.

> Don't let a poorly prepared interviewer throw you off on interview day.

## THE INTERVIEW

Many conscientious interviewers will review your file before your actual interview takes place. Others, however, prefer to review your file while you're sitting in their office, which is likely to be distracting when you're already under stress. This behavior is difficult to justify, but get over it. Interviewers will still rank you high or low depending on what they think of this meeting.

Busy interviewers zoom in on areas that consistently yield the most informational "bang for the buck," such as your CV, transcript, letters of recommendation from well-known writers, and the dean's letter. The importance of your personal statement will depend on the individual interviewer and on your specialty. The interview day is covered in detail in Chapter 11.

## RANKING SESSIONS

After you have completed all your interviews, there remains at least one highly charged, exhausting session in which the full committee attempts to rank the candidates they've seen. In many cases, not all interviewed applicants are ranked. It should also be noted that the real committee battles are not fought over names placed high on the rank-order list (ROL), as the top applicants are easy to rank. Rather, committee members will squabble over the names in the middle ground.

> Academic factors are only part of the selection committee's criteria.

In general, two rules are often observed during this final meeting. The first is that each and every member has a "right of refusal" for any candidate. This means that while a favorite faculty member cannot guarantee you a high rank, an enemy in the ranking committee can kill your ranking candidacy. This practice is more common in the smaller, more competitive specialties. Committee members all respect each other sufficiently to take one another's opinions seriously. The second rule is that committee members who are not familiar with your application will usually defer to those who are. This may seem obvious, but it goes a long way toward explaining some of the seeming randomness of the process. If your last name starts with an "A" and the person who interviewed you is 10 minutes late to the meeting, you may have no advocate present at that meeting when your application is discussed. Conversely, if the faculty member who interviewed you loves your application, you may have a better chance. It's not fair, but that's how the game works.

As the meeting wears on, application files may be subjected to less balanced assessments. At this point, the committee is likely to overanalyze your personal statement. Anything unusual in your personal statement or in the rest of your application is much more likely to be judged bizarre than to be weighted in your favor. So the bottom line is this: Be smart and assertive, and don't take unnecessary chances.

## SELECTION FACTORS

Throughout the evaluation process, the selection committee tests its pool of applicants against certain criteria that are important to its program. You may think that all programs want is an applicant who has been elected to AΩA, boasts spectacular board scores, and has "honors" plastered all over his or her transcript. In point of fact, however, academic standing is only part of the story. After all, what good is stellar academic performance if an applicant does not interact smoothly with current faculty, house staff, and administration? Program directors want residents who work hard and perform well on a team. According to program directors, the

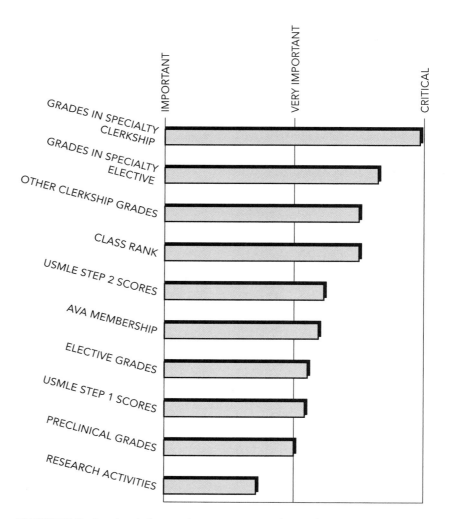

**FIGURE 7-2.** Academic factors important to residency directors.

factors most critical to residency committees tend to be personal (see Table 7-2). This is likely due to the long hours and extended period of time the resident-residency relationship involves. Program directors would prefer to teach someone who doesn't know a lot but is ready to learn rather than cope with a smart but unmotivated resident.

Of course, overall academic performance is important. Among the major academic selection factors, grades in the specialty rotation and electives seem to be the most crucial. Although Figure 7-2 may help you put your performance in perspective, you must keep in mind that selection criteria vary substantially from one field to another. For example, psychiatry residency directors rate AΩA membership as only "somewhat important," whereas general surgery residency directors consider this honor to be a "very important" academic selection factor. See Chapter 4, "Your Specialty and the Match," to learn more about the key criteria in your specialty.

| TABLE 7-2 |
| --- |
| **Factors Most Important to Program Directors** |
| 1. Attitude |
| 2. Stability |
| 3. Interpersonal skills |
| 4. Academic performance |
| 5. Maturity |

## PROGRAM APPLICATIONS

## ERAS APPLICATIONS

Developed by the Association of American Medical Colleges (AAMC), the Electronic Residency Application Service was first employed in 1995–1996 and has four components that make use of the Internet: the MyERAS applicant Web station, the Dean's Office Workstation, the Program Directors Workstation, and the ERAS Post Office. Using MyERAS, applicants complete their applications, select residency programs, and attach any required supporting documents. ERAS is now entirely online; however, not all aspects of the ERAS application are completed by the student. With ERAS, it is theoretically much easier to keep track of all the documents and forms in your application, as you will always know exactly what went to whom. The intuitive and user-friendly student software automatically guides you through a series of windows to create your application. It's so easy that many students do not even consult the instruction manual (see Table 7-3).

| TABLE 7-3 |
| --- |
| **Major Steps in ERAS** |
| Fill out common application form |
| Create a personal statement |
| Request letters of recommendation |
| Release USMLE transcript |
| Select residency programs to receive applications |

Applicants can use ERAS on any computer (PC or Mac) with World Wide Web access using Netscape 4.77, Internet Explorer 5.0, or AOL 5.0 or greater. In addition, you must have a modem that is 56 kbps or faster, 32 MB of RAM, and an e-mail address. Most medical schools have student computer workstations containing ERAS.

The first step is to create an ERAS account using the "token" supplied to you by your dean's office, usually between early June and late July. Once your account has been created, you can start to work on your application. The ERAS application consists of four basic areas: "My Account," "My Application," "My Documents," and "Programs." In "My Account" you will find a profile section, checklist, a section for messages from residency programs, and a password section. The profile is where you enter demographic information, USMLE ID (so scores can be released), ACLS/PALS certification, AΩA membership, and/or Sigma Sigma Phi status. The other sections are all self-explanatory. In "My Application," you essentially enter your CV. Be sure to scrutinize every detail of this document because it is the one document that interviewers will peruse prior to interviews. In addition, once submitted, it cannot be edited. So, you want to be sure it is free of errors! In "My Documents" you create your personal statement and shells for letters of recommendation, and release USMLE/COMLEX transcripts. Further, this section allows you to customize your applications. Moreover, you can individualize your personal statement for each program. Also, you can designate as many letter writers as you would like and assign different letters to different programs. Thus, if one of your letter writers did his residency at a program that you are applying to, you can be sure to send that letter to that program. But keep in mind that you can assign a maximum of only four letters, not including the dean's letter, to any program. Finally, in the "Programs" section you are able to search allopathic/osteopathic programs, select the programs that you would like to apply to, apply to programs (after the September 1 deadline), and visualize and obtain a copy of your invoice. Of note, both your program selection list and the total number of programs to which you are applying are confidential information that remains between you and the dean's office.

Your completed application will then be transmitted to the ERAS Post Office, where your chosen residency programs can download it at any time via the Program Directors Workstation (except for the dean's letter, which is held in the ERAS Post Office until November 1). It is important to note that additional items may be attached to your application as the application process proceeds. For example, if a letter writer has not yet finished writing your letter of recommendation, it can be picked up by the program directors at a later date. The same holds true of programs with late AΩA elections. So **do not let a missing letter of recommendation delay your application!** Simply get the application in and the letters will be added as they come in to the ERAS Post Office.

ERAS is used by most residency programs in anesthesiology, dermatology, diagnostic radiology, emergency medicine, family practice, general surgery, internal medicine, obstetrics and gynecology, orthopedic surgery, ENT, neurosurgery, neurology, pathology, pediatrics, physical medicine and rehabilitation, psychiatry, and transitional-year programs. It is also used by all Army and Navy GME-1 positions as well as by combined family practice/psychiatry, internal medicine/emergency medicine, internal medicine/family practice, internal medicine/pediatrics, internal medicine/psychiatry, and internal medicine/physical medicine and rehabilitation programs. Some programs in the above specialties may not be using ERAS, so you may need to contact these programs separately for applications.

As mentioned earlier, U.S. medical students, including osteopathic students, will receive their ERAS token through their student affairs office. IMGs who are interested in using ERAS should contact the Educational Commission for Foreign Medical Graduates (ECFMG), which acts as the dean's office for foreign graduates. The ECFMG will attach deans' letters, transcripts, and letters of recommendation and will transmit USMLE scores on behalf of IMGs. The ECFMG can be reached at the following address:

ECFMG/ERAS Program
P.O. Box 11746
Philadelphia, PA 19101-0746
www.ecfmg.org

> The ERAS system allows you to create multiple applications for different programs.

Canadian medical school graduates interested in applying to U.S. residency programs should contact the Canadian Resident Matching Service (CaRMS) at the address below:

Canadian Resident Matching Service

2283 St. Laurent Boulevard, Suite 110

Ottawa, Ontario, Canada K1G 3H7

(613) 237-0075

www.carms.ca

If you decide to apply to additional programs, you can modify portions of your application for these programs before you send your application to each. Although ERAS imposes an absolute deadline of December 1, be sure to check with the individual programs to ascertain their application deadlines. Applicants can also check the status of their documents via the Applicant Document Tracking System (ADTS). This service tells you which documents a given residency program has "picked up" from the ERAS Post Office.

## ERAS/MISCELLANEOUS FEES

**ERAS fees.** Current ERAS fees are as follows: For each specialty, the application plus up to 10 programs selected will cost $60. An additional $8 will be assessed for programs 11–20, $15 for programs 21–30, and $25 for programs 31 and up (see Table 7-4). IMGs will be charged an additional $75 by the ECFMG, since it will serve as their dean's office.

**Miscellaneous fees.** Applicants are currently charged a $60 fee for an unlimited number of USMLE/NBME (National Board of Medical Examiners) transcripts, which include your Step 1 and Step 2 scores. Once your request reaches the ERAS Post Office, the NBME will begin processing it within one week. Your Step 2 scores will not be automatically sent to residency programs unless you include a transcript request with your application, send an electronic request separately from the application, or mark the box on the application that automatically sends your updated transcript. Osteopathic applicants may request an unlimited number of COMLEX transcripts to be sent via ERAS for $60 as well.

## REGISTERING FOR THE MATCH

Do not forget to register for the Match if you want programs to find your name when they enter their ROL. The AAMC runs both the application process (ERAS) and the matching process (NRMP), and it would seem obvious that people applying for residency might be interested in matching to one. In point of fact, however, the two processes are separate. To register for the Match, you must enter your AAMC ID and pay $40 to the NRMP at www.nrmp.org/res_match/index.html. This fee allows you to rank up to 15 programs. If you wish to rank more than 15 programs, additional fees will apply when you certify your rank list.

## SAN FRANCISCO MATCH

The San Francisco Match application is handled and processed by the Central Application Service (CAS). Bear in mind, however, that while CAS is manda-

> Don't let the fees discourage you from submitting enough applications.

## TABLE 7-4

### ERAS Fees

| Number of Programs per Specialty | AAMC Fees |
|---|---|
| Up to 10 | $60 |
| 11–20 | $8 each |
| 21–30 | $15 each |
| 31 or more | $25 each |

> Filling out ERAS forms does not register you for the Match.

tory for ophthalmology programs and for some programs in neurotology and child neurology, it is optional for others. CAS materials are generally sent to registered applicants by early July. The CAS process is similar to that of ERAS in that you fill out one common application. After you obtain one copy of each supporting document, you must mail the entire application packet to CAS. Overnight delivery is recommended so that you can track your document's receipt. The application will then be copied and sent to your selected programs. Application fees are currently $60 total for the first 10 programs. An additional $10 each will be charged for programs 11–20, $15 for programs 21–30, $20 for programs 31–40, and $35 for program 41 and up. For more information, go to www.sfmatch.org. In addition, you will be charged a nonrefundable $100 fee for registration and matching.

The Urology Match is very similar to the SF Match and NMRP. Applicants who wish to pursue careers in urology must register with the American Urological Association ($75 fee). Once they have received their ID number, they can register with ERAS or utilize ERAS to contact programs that do not participate in their services, so that they may request applications. Applicants must keep in mind that the deadlines are earlier than common ERAS deadlines; therefore, they must be on top of things early! However, this means that rewards come early as well. The Match is typically finished by late January. For more information, visit www.auanet.org.

## PAPER (NON-ERAS) APPLICATIONS

Although there are very few programs that do not use ERAS as their application, some programs continue to require paper applications. The NRMP Universal Application was created to simplify the application process for non-ERAS programs. The idea was that you would complete this application once and would then send photocopies of it to programs that accept it. Unfortunately, however, a few programs insist on using their own forms. The writing process for non-ERAS programs can thus be very frustrating, since these "custom" applications, while often differing only slightly from the Universal Application in content, use unique layouts—forcing applicants to go back to their typewriters or word processors for yet another round of cut and paste.

If any of your prospective programs request the Universal Application, **fill it out first,** as much of the material that it calls for will resurface in other application forms. Some students find it helpful to hire a secretarial service to handle the paperwork and produce top-quality, customized application materials. If you are on busy clinical rotations or don't have the skills or compulsiveness to track all the details yourself, these services can preserve your sanity.

When you receive a program application, **make at least two photocopies of the blank application.** Neatly write the necessary information by hand on one of the photocopies before typing on the original. That way, if you mortally mess up the original and have no time to request another, the second photocopy will serve as a backup. As you complete the application, keep the following tips in mind:

- For information to be filled in on the form itself, use a good electric typewriter with good error correction. Alternatively, if you are experienced and ambi-

> Give them what they want where they want it.

tious, you may elect to use a word processor. This second method involves the risky process of feeding applications into laser printers or photocopiers (the overlay method)—a true test of your alignment skills. Word processing is best reserved for the personal statement, for which looks count and a nice, proportionally spaced computer font is more compact and readable than most typewriter fonts. If you can't do it right, get help from a computer-savvy friend or a secretarial service.

- Avoid filling a blank on an application with "See CV" or "See Personal Statement." These abbreviations may make sense to you but can annoy residency directors to no end, since the personal statement or CV is often a loose piece of paper located elsewhere in your application file. In addition, these shorthand terms bespeak a certain lack of motivation. You can, of course, abbreviate specific titles or similar terms in the information requested if necessary (eg, "U" for "University," "Schl" for "School"). If the space provided is too small, fill it in with the most important information; only then should you add "Also see CV" or "Also see Personal Statement."

- When you are finished, **make and file a photocopy of the complete application.** Applications do get lost in the mail, so you might need to fax a copy or send a replacement by express mail to the program if the post office fouls up. Also, having your copy handy right before your interview serves as a helpful memory refresher. Reviewing what you wrote in your application will help you anticipate questions while also eliminating possible inconsistencies between what you put down on paper and what you may say in person.

If a program that ranks high on your list gives you the choice of the NRMP Universal Application or its own form, use the latter. Resist the urge to take the easy way out, especially if a program expresses a preference for its own application form.

## THE DEAN'S LETTER

As we mentioned earlier, the letter from your dean is a key item at the screening and interview stages of the application process. Deans' letters convey a range of information about you to committee members (see Figure 7-3). Although the dean's letter is supposed to be an objective evaluation of your medical school performance, most deans' letters come across as enthusiastic letters of recommendation, thus bolstering many average or weak applications while possibly diluting strong ones. For this reason, the dean's letter is often used less as an objective criterion than as a way to get to know you as an applicant. This is the only document that brings together the diverse experiences that have made up your medical school career.

Although deans' letters can vary substantially, they typically contain the following components:

- **Personal background information.** This includes pertinent and noteworthy information from your undergraduate career and medical school application (eg, graduating magna cum laude, leadership positions).

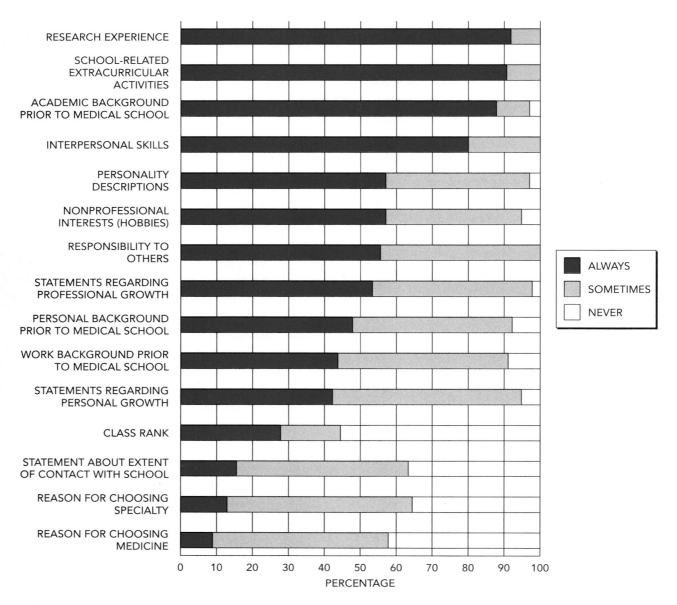

**FIGURE 7-3.** Information that commonly appears in deans' letters.

- **Preclinical evaluations.** This section will tell the committee about your preclinical honors or, conversely, about any irregularities in progress or required remediation.

- **Clinical evaluations.** This is typically the longest portion of the dean's letter. The majority of deans' letters will include quotes from your clinical evaluations. Some letters cite such evaluations verbatim, while others use abridged versions or just choice positive excerpts. Some deans' letters include histograms that depict the grade distributions in courses and rotations, with the student's position marked on each.

- **Special activities.** Here the dean has an opportunity to highlight your extracurricular activities and any outstanding achievements. These passages often read like portraiture or—at worst—caricature.

## TABLE 7-5

**Examples of Buzzwords Used in Deans' Letters**

| Best ↕ Worst | | | |
|---|---|---|---|
| Best | Recommend in highest terms | Outstanding | Strongest of year |
| | Recommend very highly | Excellent | Very strong |
| | Recommend highly | Very good | Strong |
| Worst | Recommend | Good | Good |

- **Summary paragraph.** This section is usually the one that the residency selection committee reads first. It is typically a concise synopsis of the dean's letter and often provides a comparative analysis of your performance, whether through a class rank, a class percentile, or buzzwords that function to cluster or single out students (see Table 7-5).

In some cases, the dean's letter can be written without your input. At the other extreme, your school might ask you to proofread the letter for typos and factual errors or even allow you limited editorial privileges with regard to its content. Other schools will consider it a federal offense if you so much as sneak a peek at your dean's letter. If your dean's office calls you in for a talk with the dean, be sure to bring along your CV or personal statement. In any event, ask savvy seniors and your student affairs office about the structure of the typical dean's letter from your institution and try to find out what role you can expect to play in its final development.

> Be aware of the level of input you have into the dean's letter!

If you are given an opportunity to review your dean's letter, check it carefully for accuracy, grammar, and spelling as well as for the presence of all your clerkship evaluations (there is no need to point out any weak ones that might be missing). If you have not already done so, do not hesitate to visit your dean of students to discuss any evaluations that you believe to be unfair, inaccurate, or even inappropriate. If your school gives you the opportunity to edit the content of your dean's letter, **grab it!** Medical schools want their graduates to do well, and few can market you as well as you can. Make sure the dean's letter emphasizes your strong points while tactfully expressing concern about negative material that may have made its way into the collection. Everyone has suffered a premature or harsh judgment made by someone who doesn't really know them. If you have one or two isolated "pans" in your record, a sympathetic dean may be willing to soften or delete them. You would much rather have your dean's letter be bland than negative.

Many deans swear that they are not "ranking" students with the last paragraph of the dean's letter. If you have some editorial privileges as to the final version of your dean's letter, this is the place to use them. Tell the dean that if no ranking is being done, you would rather be referred to as "outstanding" than "good" if it's all the same to him or her. At least it's worth a try.

Most deans' letters are mailed out on November 1, a date agreed upon by the Council of Deans. A few deans send out their information earlier. The dean's letter will automatically be attached to your application at this time, not beforehand. You don't have to do much about it other than wait and check the ADTS in early November to verify that it has been picked up by your programs.

## LETTERS OF RECOMMENDATION

Along with your dean's letter, your letters of recommendation are vital to the success of your application. You should thus take the time to select your letter writers wisely and provide them with all the materials they may need to refresh their memories when they write their recommendations.

### WHEN SHOULD I START REQUESTING LETTERS OF RECOMMENDATION?

You can ask for letters of recommendation after you have completed any significant clinical or research experience. Most students start collecting letters during the third year of medical school. If you did well on a third-year clerkship, ask the attending to write a letter while you are still fresh in his or her mind, keeping in mind that the letter can subsequently be modified to reflect your specialty choice and career goals. In general, whenever you ask for a letter, give the writer at least four weeks to write and mail it off. Treat a letter writer the way you yourself would want to be treated: Supply him or her with your CV, your personal statement, envelopes, and postage. Note that if you are participating in ERAS from a U.S. or Canadian medical school, your dean's office will likely receive and scan these letters into ERAS for you. If you make it easy, the letters are more likely to get done accurately and on time.

> Always meet with your letter writers in person before they write the letter.

### HOW DO I GET A STRONG LETTER OF RECOMMENDATION?

When you solicit letters of recommendation, there are a few steps you can take to maximize your chances of getting the strongest possible response. First, go to the clerkship office and read the evaluations that your potential reference wrote about you during your rotation. The strength and eloquence of the writer's evaluation will certainly be reflected in any subsequent letter he or she may write on your behalf.

Second, when asking for a letter of recommendation, phrase your request carefully. This precaution may reduce your vulnerability to weak letters. Tact and discretion are even more important late in the game, when clerkship evaluations may not be available to you. You can, for example, ask the person, "Do you think you know me well enough to write me a strong letter of recommendation?" If the potential reference does not feel comfortable writing a strong letter about you, he or she can take the graceful exit you provided by saying, "Actually, I don't believe I know you well enough. Perhaps you should ask someone else." Then you are free to request a letter from another attending or faculty member who may give you a better reference.

Third, meet in person with the writer **before** he or she sits down to compose the letter so that you can discuss your choice of specialty and your career goals. Provide your letter writer with a copy of your personal statement, your CV, and the names of the programs you will be considering if it is possible to do so. Medicine is a small world, and many people know one another; your letter writer may be old friends

## TABLE 7-6

**Signs of a Strong or Weak Letter**

| Strong | Weak |
|--------|------|
| Typewritten on official letterhead and personally signed | Handwritten on plain paper and photocopied |
| Handwritten postscript a big plus | Signed by an assistant or signature photocopied |
| Lengthy | Short |
| Detailed description of fund of knowledge, clinical skills, and past performance | Vague; focuses on marginally relevant personality traits or work habits (eg, "He was punctual and well dressed.") |
| Frequent personal references | Lack of familiarity |
| Unconditional praise | Lukewarm praise; qualifications of any kind (but, except, etc.) |

with a few of the program directors you will encounter on your interview trail. If a letter writer cannot meet you despite your reasonable best efforts, you might not get the strongest letter and may consider someone else who can make the time.

Some attendings will draft a letter of recommendation and offer you the chance to read it and either decline or accept it. If the letter is not as strong as you had hoped, you may decline it as long as you have better letters coming (see Table 7-6). If the attending does not offer to show you the letter, you may tactfully try the direct approach and ask if he or she would mind if you saw it. However, while you have the right to see your letters under the Family Education Rights and Privacy Act (FERPA), most letter writers will include a line stating whether you have or have not waived the right to review your letter. It is considered a red flag by many residency program directors if you did not waive the right to see your letter, as they feel the writers may not have felt free to be completely honest. Therefore, it is standard practice in U.S. medical schools for students to waive their right to view their letters. Again, the best way to get strong letters is to work hard and to ask the faculty member if they would be able to write you a strong letter.

Alternatively, you may opt to be less direct and ask to receive a copy for your files. Many writers view this as a reasonable request, since letters of recommendation often get lost, and you may end up having to fax a copy of the missing letter to the program at the last minute to complete your file. If you are applying in a competitive specialty or if you are a marginal candidate, you may also want to keep copies of your letters for the Scramble in the event that you do not match. Despite all this, some attendings maintain that their letters should remain strictly confidential. If you do see the letter early and it is unfavorable (see Table 7-6), you may decide to withhold program addresses. However, make sure you have someone else to ask for a letter. Even if your letters have been sent, you should be aware of their content just in case an issue pops up during the residency interview.

## WHOM SHOULD I ASK FOR LETTERS OF RECOMMENDATION?

There are a number of characteristics you should look for in each of your letter writers. If possible, he or she should be someone who:

- Will write you a strong letter

- Knows you well in a clinical setting

- Is well established in the field (in order of desirability: chairman, professor, clinical instructor)

- Works in your specialty choice or in a related field

- Trained at or is well known at your top-choice program

If given the choice between a letter from a well-connected figure who does not know you well and one from a lesser-known attending who is familiar with you and your work, give priority to the person who knows you better. Unfortunately, many students request letters from less-than-optimal sources (see Table 7-7). Letters from research mentors are acceptable if you already have two clinical letters and have a strong interest in doing research in the future. However, make sure the letter is from someone with whom you have done considerable work (ie, more than one summer). By the same token, not having a letter from a research mentor or PhD advisor you have spent substantial time with may be viewed as a serious omission and thus a red flag. Letter selection also depends on the type of program to which you are applying. Although it borders on excessive, some applicants actually pick and choose from among five or more letter writers, depending on the characteristics of each program on their list.

### TABLE 7-7

**Suboptimal Sources for Letters of Recommendation**

Residents

Preclinical professors

Family, friends

Community figures

Previous employers

## TRANSCRIPTS

Before you have your medical school and, in some cases, undergraduate transcripts mailed out, request a student copy to review for errors and completeness. You can often obtain an unofficial transcript from your school's Web site. Try to get your official transcript requests to the registrar's office a few weeks before you send out your applications (September for most NRMP applicants). If you receive excellent grades after the transcripts have been mailed, send out updated transcripts.

> Proofread your transcript; it may contain errors.

## PHOTO

Most applications as well as ERAS reserve a space for a passport-size photograph. Others will ask you to bring a photo when you interview. Although it is illegal to require a photograph with the application, it is better to comply. This photo will follow you throughout your interview process. Each interviewer will have a copy of your file, including the photo. This is so that they can identify you, but also so that when they go to make decisions about candidates, they will have a picture to help remind them of the interview. Consider going to a studio for professional photography, and have color prints developed unless specified otherwise. Residency program directors and the faculty reviewing your application will expect you to look professional in your photo. Dress in a suit or a professional shirt, including a tie for men. A photo in which you are dressed casually or that is very poor in quality will reflect negatively on your overall application.

## APPLICATION STATUS

ERAS applicants can track the status of their applications through the ADTS. The ADTS will show you a list of your selected programs along with the dates the documents were uploaded by the dean's office and downloaded by the residency program. Early Match applicants will receive a letter from CAS detailing the documents it has received and the programs to which the application has been sent.

Non-ERAS residency programs have a variety of methods for acknowledging receipt of your application material, ranging from no response at all to a letter acknowledging receipt of the application form that checks off any missing materials. Overall, it's up to you to track your application materials. This can easily be done by including a stamped, self-addressed postcard that notes receipt of your application and includes a checklist for missing material (see Figure 7-4). To ensure that the acknowledgment postcard does its job, make arrangements for all other materials well before you send in your applications. The exception is the dean's letter, which is usually mailed out on November 1.

> Do not expect programs to notify you of missing materials. Double and triple check yourself.

Unfortunately, enclosing a postcard works only if the overworked program secretary is in the mood to mail it back. Return-receipt service from the post office and express mail with tracking numbers are better but more expensive ways to track your applications. If you prefer, wait a few weeks after your application has been sent in, and then call the program to check on your file (especially if you did not receive an "application completed" postcard). Not only will the contact person

This is to acknowledge receipt of your application.
____ Your application is **complete.**
____ Your application is **not** complete. We are missing the following item(s):

    ____ Dean's letter
    ____ Transcript
    ____ Letter from Dr. Alpha
    ____ Letter from Dr. Beta
    ____ Letter from Dr. Gamma
    ____ Other _____

    *(You fill in the blank)*
_____    _____
Program                                           Date

**FIGURE 7-4.** Sample application status postcard.

at the program verify if your file is complete, but he or she may have advance word on your interview status. Most programs don't mind a phone call as long as your manner is courteous and professional. Remember: The impression you make on the office staff may tip the balance toward or against your application.

## REFERENCES

AAMC-ERAS Web site (www.aamc.org/students/eras/start.htm).

Greenburg AG, Doyle J, McClure DK. Letters of recommendation for surgical residencies: what they say and what they mean. *J Surg Res* 56(2):192–198, 1994.

Hunt DD, MacLaren CF, Scott CS, Chu J, Leiden LL. Characteristics of dean's letters in 1981 and 1992. *Acad Med* 68(12):905–911, 1993.

Leiden LI, Miller GD. National survey of writers of dean's letters for residency applications. *J Med Educ* 61(12):943–953, 1986.

San Francisco Matching Program Web site (www.sfmatch.org).

*Vanderbilt School of Medicine Guide to Residency Applications*. Nashville, TN: Vanderbilt University, 1994.

Wagoner NE, Suriano JR. Program directors' responses to a survey on variables used to select residents in a time of change. *Acad Med* 74(1):51–58, 1999.

Wagoner NE, Suriano JR, Stoner JA. Factors used by program directors to select residents. *J Med Educ* 61(1):10–21, 1986.

Zagumny MJ, Rudolph J. Comparing medical students' and residency directors' ratings of criteria used to select residents. *Acad Med* 67(9):613, 1992.

# 8

# The Curriculum Vitae

Medicine is a profession that heavily values experience. Much of what you will achieve in medicine will be a direct result of your past accomplishments. Whether applying to residency or applying to become the chair of your department, the medium for showcasing your achievements will be your curriculum vitae, or CV.

In the world of applications and interviews, the CV is the equivalent of the one-minute bullet-point patient presentation. A well-written CV places a succinct summary of your academic, career, and extracurricular accomplishments at the fingertips of the interviewer. However, your CV is more than just a quick road map to your residency application. Preparing your CV gives you the opportunity to shape the message you wish to send about yourself as an applicant to your recommenders and your interviewers.

In applying for residency, your formal CV will be embedded in the Electronic Residency Application Service (ERAS) application, and it works with the rest of your application to win you an interview. ERAS requires that applicants enter CV information directly into the program, without the option to change fonts, styles, or margins. However, you should also prepare a formal and professionally formatted CV. First, many letter writers will require a CV that they can use as a reference while working on your recommendation. Second, when you are attending interviews, it never hurts to have a copy in case an interviewer wants to glance at it. Finally, maintaining an up-to-date CV will help you in all future application processes.

For these reasons, we recommend creating a CV early in the application process. Finishing a preliminary draft by May or June will help jump-start your application process and allow you to make updates easily. Furthermore, for those students applying to specialties with Match processes outside of the National Resident Matching Program (NRMP), such as ophthalmology and urology, your professional CV will be a part of your formal application.

> Your CV is a snapshot of your application.

> Start early! A thorough preliminary CV can help both you and your letter writers!

## WHAT'S IN A CV?

A CV typically will include the following elements:

- **Name and address.** Stick with the same name that you use in your applications, dean's letter, transcripts, and correspondence with programs and the matching service. Make sure you include an address, a phone number, and an e-mail address through which program directors can reach you during the entire interview season. Give a secondary address and phone number (eg, a cell phone number) if no one is at your primary address when you are away during the interviewing season.

- **Objective.** In a traditional CV, this should consist of a terse, one-sentence statement of your goals. An objective should be included in your residency CV **only** if your career goals are not readily apparent to the residency director (eg, applying in a medicine and pediatrics joint residency program).

- **Education.** List all major or medically related educational experiences from college through to the present. Dual graduate degrees (eg, MD/PhD, MD/MPH, MD/JD) are particularly impressive and should be highlighted. Include the name and place of the institution, your area of study, dates of enrollment, type of degree received, and honors bestowed at graduation (eg, graduating *cum laude*), and any applicable grade point average (GPA) or class rank. However, if your GPA or rank are not very remarkable, it may be better to leave them out of your CV, as including them could draw attention to a deficit that the interviewer may otherwise not have noted. If you are a senior medical student in the United States, list your expected graduation date.

- **Honors.** Include any awards and scholarships that you have received during your med school years as well as the most important awards and scholarships you received during your undergraduate years.

- **Scores.** If your board scores are particularly good, include them on your CV. This will help the interviewers notice them. However, if they are not a strong point of your application, leave them out of your CV, as the interviewer can always find the information in other parts of your application.

- **Publications.** Catalog any abstracts and papers you have published or submitted for publication. Format each publication as a detailed bibliographic reference. Also list research presented or talks given at conferences or poster sessions.

- **Work experience.** List all major or medically related work experiences, whether paid or volunteer (eg, paramedic work, nursing). Include dates of work experience. Leave out the summer job at the country club.

- **Extracurricular activities.** Include the most important long-term activities in which you were involved during medical school (or more recently if you have already graduated). This category should include activities such as community service projects, committee work, and participation in student organizations.

- **Professional memberships.** Be sure to mention professional organizations to which you belong (eg, American Academy of Pediatrics).

- **Personal information.** In a short line at the end, list hobbies and interests that define you. Also mention any special qualifications or skills that might enhance your effectiveness as a house officer (eg, foreign language training, knowledge of American sign language, computer skills).

The phrase "references available upon request," seen in most nonmedical CVs, is redundant in the application process, as letters of recommendation are a required element of the application. Sometimes, however, it helps to list your references by name in the CV, especially if those references are particularly illustrious and widely respected.

Note that certain information is not appropriate for a medical professional CV (see Table 8-1). However, you may have to consider including information about citizenship or visa status if you are an international medical graduate (IMG).

## TABLE 8-1
### Information Not Appropriate in a CV

Birthplace and date

Citizenship status (except IMGs)

Marital status

Names of spouse and family members

High school education/accomplishments

## TABLE 8-2

### CV Writing Tips

Organize categories to highlight strengths.

If you're an older applicant, try to avoid unexplained gaps in your timeline by highlighting intervening jobs, experiences, etc.

Use terse, precise, and vivid language.

Create parallel structure in lists (eg, each item in a list starts with a verb).

Follow consistent punctuation rules.

Follow consistent capitalization rules.

Consult a style manual or a professional editor.

When it comes to the appearance of the CV, you should try to blend in. When it comes to the content, you should try to stand out!

Prioritize! Organize your CV to highlight your strengths.

# HOW DO I PUT TOGETHER MY CV?

Study the sample CVs at the end of this chapter to get a feel for the appearance you want in your finished CV (see Figures 8-1 through 8-4). Using the examples below or a template on a word processor, fill in the information in the categories listed above. If you have nothing to say under a category, do not include it. Note that most CVs start with "Name/Address" and "Education" and end with "Personal." In the middle, however, feel free to rearrange the order of the remaining categories to emphasize your strengths and downplay your less impressive areas.

After you have input this basic information, edit your document into a professional and attractive format and style using the sample CVs as a guide. See Table 8-2 for specific writing tips. You should also make sure your CV is pleasing to the eye (see Table 8-3). Remember to keep your language terse. Use vivid nouns and active verbs to demonstrate strength, enthusiasm, and initiative (see Tables 8-4 and 8-5). Also pay careful attention to style and punctuation. Medicine is a detail-oriented specialty, and sloppiness can be interpreted as evidence of carelessness or lack of motivation. If you have any further doubts, refer to the sample CVs, show your draft to a friend with good writing skills, and consult a manual of style such as Strunk and White's *The Elements of Style*.

Once you have a good draft of your CV, ask your career advisor and at least one other person to read it and provide feedback on appearance, legibility, ease of reading, grammar, punctuation, and style (see Table 8-3). After making any necessary revisions, print the CV onto high-quality, heavy cotton bond paper that is white or neutral in color.

## TABLE 8-3

### CV Layout and Design Tips

Allow for generous margins (1–1.5 inches).

Limit CV to two pages.

Avoid splitting a section when going from page 1 to page 2.

Try a serif font (eg, Times Roman) as the base text font for better legibility. Save sans serif (eg, Arial) for section headers.

Do not go below 12 points for the general font size and 14 points for headings.

Stick with one or, at most, two fonts. Too many can be distracting and gaudy.

Be consistent with section headers in style and formatting.

Boldface your name in any publications cited.

Use boldface, small caps, italics, and bullet symbols sparingly. Avoid underlining.

Print your CV on a laser printer at 300 dpi or more.

Print your CV on a heavyweight, cotton bond paper. Use a neutral color (eg, ivory).

Make sure the printed CV photocopies well.

## TABLE 8-4
### Action Verbs for CVs

| | | | |
|---|---|---|---|
| accelerated | directed | lectured | reorganized |
| accomplished | effected | led | restructured |
| achieved | elucidated | maintained | reviewed |
| adapted | established | managed | revised |
| administered | evaluated | mastered | scheduled |
| analyzed | examined | motivated | set up |
| approved | expanded | operated | solved |
| attained | expedited | organized | streamlined |
| clarified | facilitated | originated | structured |
| completed | found | participated | studied |
| conceived | generated | performed | supervised |
| conducted | improved | pinpointed | supported |
| controlled | increased | planned | synthesized |
| coordinated | influenced | proposed | taught |
| created | implemented | proved | trained |
| delegated | initiated | provided | translated |
| demonstrated | instructed | recommended | used |
| designed | interpreted | reduced | won |
| developed | launched | reinforced | wrote |

## TABLE 8-5
### Concrete Nouns and Positive Modifiers for CVs

| | | | |
|---|---|---|---|
| ability | competent | proficient | technical |
| actively | consistent | qualified | unique |
| capacity | effectively | resourceful | versatile |
| competence | pertinent | substantially | vigorous |

## ERRORS TO AVOID

Finally, here is a list of "no-no's" for CVs. Any one of these can be a killer. To repeat advice given earlier, have your advisor and another competent person read your CV, paying particular attention to the following:

- **Inaccuracies or exaggerations.** This is the most important error to avoid! Present your talents and accomplishments in the best possible light, but do not misrepresent them. If you took two semesters of a language in college, do not state that you are fluent. You run the risk of the interviewer speaking to you in that language and looking foolish if you cannot respond. Residency directors have many ways to verify your claims. Even a minor "misrepresentation" can have a major impact on your credibility. You must always be 100% truthful.

- **Unprofessional appearance.** Do **not** write your CV by hand or use a typewriter. Do not print it on a dot matrix printer. If you find a mistake on your CV, no matter how minor it may be, print out a new, corrected version. Do **not** make corrections, handwritten or typed, on the CV itself. Use only high-quality, heavyweight bond paper. Appropriate colors are white, ivory, beige, and light gray. Other colors, such as pastel pink, only attract negative attention.

- **Too lengthy.** Do not exceed two pages in length unless you have really stellar experience and an impressive list of publications to justify more space. Remember that this is a capsule summary of your career to date, not an extended autobiography.

- **Misspellings, poor grammar.** These unspectacular mistakes will only contribute to an image of carelessness or incompetence, particularly since word processors make it easy to check spelling and grammar.

- **Weak writing.** Verbosity kills, so keep your sentences short and succinct. Specifics count; the more precisely you can describe your experience, the better the reader can picture—and appreciate—what you say. Stay away from bland nouns and passive verbs.

> Avoid brightly colored or patterned paper.

## SAMPLE CVS

Figures 8-1 through 8-4 are sample CVs to give you ideas about formatting and arranging your text on the page. Depending on your strengths (research, extracurricular activities, or awards) and your application goals (academic or community program, highly competitive or less competitive specialty) you should highlight different areas.

This applicant has a well-rounded CV. He is applying to several academic training programs, so he chooses to list his research experience first, followed by his posters and publications.

**WILLIAM BRADFORD THOMAS**

325 Drummond Lane
Louisville, KY 40322
(512) 555-7457
**wthomas@medschool.edu**

## *EDUCATION*

| | |
|---|---|
| 2007–Present | **University of Louisville School of Medicine.** MD anticipated May 2011. |
| 2003–2007 | **Centre College of Kentucky.** BS, Biology and Psychology, *magna cum laude.* |

## *RESEARCH*

| | |
|---|---|
| Summer 2004 | **Summer Research Fellow.** Stefan Maguire, PhD, Hormone Research Institute. Elucidated the role of glutamic acid decarboxylase in the autoimmune pathogenesis of insulin dependent diabetes mellitus. |
| Summer 2005 | **Research Assistant.** Richard Woodbridge, MD, University of Kentucky Medical Research Building. Analyzed flow characteristics of IV infusion pumps to evaluate their accuracy in removing outflow of spent dialysate and ultrafiltrate. |

Do not forget to list your principal investigator

## *PUBLICATIONS*

**W. Thomas** and S. Maguire. "Is GAD65 localized to synaptic-like vesicles in β-pancreatic cells?" 2005 School of Medicine Research Poster Session.

R. Woodbridge, **W. Thomas**, D. Arnold, J. Funk. "Accuracy of IV Pumps in CAVHD." *American Society for Artificial Internal Organs: 2006 Abstracts,* 2006, p. 78.

Text is indented to keep clean, vertical look

## *HONORS & AWARDS*

| | |
|---|---|
| 2006 | **Michael Ryan Biology Prize.** Centre College. |
| 2006 | **Jeffrey Scott McBride Leadership Award.** Centre College. |
| 2007 | **Phi Beta Kappa** |
| 2003–2007 | **Centre College Trustee Scholarship.** Half tuition merit scholarship. |

**FIGURE 8-1.** Sample CV no. 1.

**WILLIAM BRADFORD THOMAS**

Use "action" verbs to give an active tone

| | |
|---|---|
| 2007–Present | **Faculty Student Network Committee.** Organized events and meetings for faculty advisors and medical students. |
| | **School of Medicine Representative, Registration Fee Committee.** Allocated student fees to student organizations and services. |
| 2008–2009 | **Peer Counselor, Campus Health.** Provided counseling and support for first-year medical students. |
| 2008–Present | **Homeless Health Clinic.** Evaluated and treated homeless patients as medical volunteer in homeless shelter. |
| 2008–2009 | **Vice president, AMA—Medical Student Section Chapter.** Organized health fairs and guest speakers for medical school chapter. |

*PROFESSIONAL MEMBERSHIPS*

| | |
|---|---|
| 2007–Present | **American Medical Association, Medical Student Section** |
| 2008–Present | **American Academy of Pediatrics, Medical Student Section** |

*PERSONAL*

Proficient in American sign language.

Hobbies include volleyball and jogging.

**FIGURE 8-1.** Sample CV no. 1 (continued).

This CV emphasizes the applicant's considerable research accomplishments. If she were applying to clinical programs, she might choose to highlight her strong extracurricular activities. Since her CV cannot fit on one page, she has spread out the sections so that they completely fill two pages, rather than just fill one and one-half pages.

---

## Sarah Lin

| | |
|---|---|
| ***Permanent Address*** | ***School Address*** |
| *P.O. Box 271 MDSC* | *234 Wisteria Lane* |
| *Clarksville, IN 47160* | *Nashville, TN 37215* |
| *(812) 555-3952* | *(615) 555-5456* |
| | *slin@medschool.edu* |

### EDUCATION

**Vanderbilt University School of Medicine**            *2007 to Present*
Nashville, TN
    MD EXPECTED IN MAY 2011

**St. Louis University**            *2003 to 2007*
St. Louis, MO
    BA, BIOLOGY AND PSYCHOLOGY, *magna cum laude*

### RESEARCH

**Research Assistant**            *Summer 2005*
University of California, San Diego
    SAMUEL STOCKTON, MD, PHD. Developed a rat model to study the inflammatory process in asthma.

**Research Assistant**            *Summer 2008*
Vanderbilt University School of Medicine
    SHELLEY PISA, MD. Characterized the interactions between anesthetic drugs and the erythrocyte B and 3 anion exchange channel.

**Research Assistant**            *May 2009 to December 2009*
St. Louis University
    ANTHONY HILL, PHD. Explored the medicinal value of the plant *Rhamnacea* used by South American Indians in wound healing.

**Research Assistant**            *January 2009 to October 2009*
St. Louis University
    TIMOTHY ROBERTS, PHD. Developed protocols for the use of mutant strains of *Chlamydomonas* in transformation experiments.

Alternative way to keep dates separated from text

**FIGURE 8-2.** Sample CV no. 2.

Include a header if your CV has two pages →

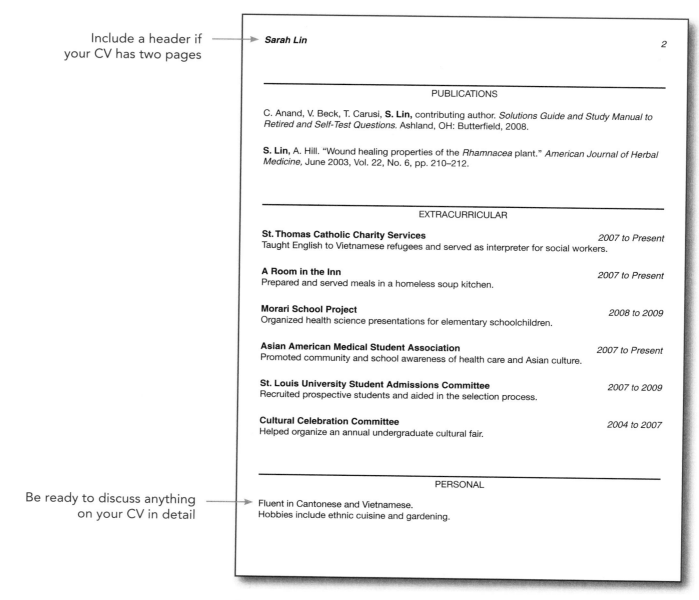

Be ready to discuss anything on your CV in detail →

**FIGURE 8-2.** Sample CV no. 2 (continued).

---

The content of the CV page shown:

**Sarah Lin** 2

---

### PUBLICATIONS

C. Anand, V. Beck, T. Carusi, **S. Lin,** contributing author. *Solutions Guide and Study Manual to Retired and Self-Test Questions.* Ashland, OH: Butterfield, 2008.

**S. Lin,** A. Hill. "Wound healing properties of the *Rhamnacea* plant." *American Journal of Herbal Medicine,* June 2003, Vol. 22, No. 6, pp. 210–212.

---

### EXTRACURRICULAR

**St. Thomas Catholic Charity Services** *2007 to Present*
Taught English to Vietnamese refugees and served as interpreter for social workers.

**A Room in the Inn** *2007 to Present*
Prepared and served meals in a homeless soup kitchen.

**Morari School Project** *2008 to 2009*
Organized health science presentations for elementary schoolchildren.

**Asian American Medical Student Association** *2007 to Present*
Promoted community and school awareness of health care and Asian culture.

**St. Louis University Student Admissions Committee** *2007 to 2009*
Recruited prospective students and aided in the selection process.

**Cultural Celebration Committee** *2004 to 2007*
Helped organize an annual undergraduate cultural fair.

---

### PERSONAL

Fluent in Cantonese and Vietnamese.
Hobbies include ethnic cuisine and gardening.

This applicant has an impressive number of awards and honors. Because she is entering family practice, she emphasizes her community service experience and lists her research on the second page. Her CV could be stronger if she listed a brief description of all of her awards, rather than just some of them.

---

### Jacquelyn H. Lemmon

**School Address**
576 London Road, Apt. #5
Tucson, AZ 85719
(602) 555-7456
jlemmon@medschool.edu

**Permanent Address**
2145 Red Valley Drive
Danville, TN 37205
(615) 555-5760

**Education**

| | |
|---|---|
| 2007–present | UNIVERSITY OF ARIZONA SCHOOL OF MEDICINE<br>M.D. expected in May, 2011 |
| 2003–2007 | WASHINGTON UNIVERSITY<br>B.S. in Engineering & Policy |

All caps is an alternative to boldfaced text.

**Honors & Awards**

| | |
|---|---|
| 2009 | SUMMER RESEARCH GRANT<br>Awarded by American Society for Lasers in Medicine and Surgery. |
| 2008 | DIABETES SUMMER RESEARCH GRANT<br>Awarded by Diabetes Research and Training Center. |
| 2007–2008 | MICROBES AND DEFENSE SOCIETY |
| 2006–2007 | MORTAR BOARD HONOR SOCIETY |
| 2006 | BRISTOL-MYERS SQUIBB SCHOLAR |
| 2005–2006 | JUSTIN POTTER SCHOLARSHIP<br>Merit award based on leadership potential. |
| 2003–2005 | JOHN B. ERVIN SCHOLARSHIP |

**Extracurricular**

| | |
|---|---|
| 2008–Present | STUDENT NATIONAL MEDICAL ASSOCIATION<br>Promoted health care and minority issues. Served as co-chairperson and treasurer of Arizona chapter. |
| 2007–Present | TUCSON CARES<br>Made lecture presentations on HIV/AIDS to the general public on behalf of agency, which serves HIV/AIDS population. |

---

**FIGURE 8-3.** Sample CV no. 3.

*Jacquelyn H. Lemmon*

*Extracurricular, continued*

A good way to present multiple small activities.

2007–Present     SERVICE ACTIVITIES
Participated in several community service activities including Inn for the Homeless, Habitat for Humanity, wheelchair ramp construction, and role model activities for black youth.

*Research*

March–August 2009     RESEARCH ELECTIVE, CENTERS FOR DISEASE CONTROL AND PREVENTION
Preceptor Richard Woodbridge, MD. Designed methods for collecting and organizing for international importations data.
Collected and analyzed 2008 data with comparison to data collected from 2000 to 2007.

2008     RESEARCH ASSISTANT
Preceptor George Sherman, MD. Characterized lymphocytic migration in RSV-infected mice. Results presented at National Medical Fellowships Research Seminar in February, 2009.

Summer 2007     SUMMER RESEARCH FELLOW
Preceptor Lou Ritter, MD. Tested various pulse structures of the electron laser to evaluate its efficacy in bone ablation.

Summer 2006     RESEARCH ASSISTANT
Preceptor Lou Ritter, MD. Developed optimal laser firing patterns to achieve minimal thermal buildup in a collagen-based target. Results presented to the Arizona Diabetes Research Training Center.

2004     SUBSTANCE ABUSE AND PREVENTION PROGRAM
Counseled high-risk youth.

*Personal*

Hobbies include jogging, playing piano, and swimming.

2

**FIGURE 8-3.** Sample CV no. 3 (continued).

Both a one-page CV and a two-page CV are acceptable. This applicant was able to fit everything on one page. In this format, the order of categories is not as important.

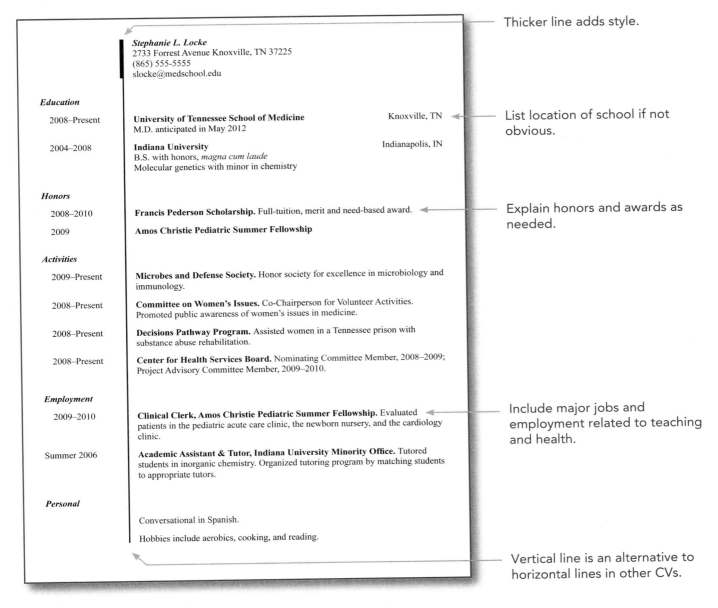

Thicker line adds style.

**Stephanie L. Locke**
2733 Forrest Avenue Knoxville, TN 37225
(865) 555-5555
slocke@medschool.edu

*Education*

2008–Present  **University of Tennessee School of Medicine**     Knoxville, TN
M.D. anticipated in May 2012

List location of school if not obvious.

2004–2008  **Indiana University**     Indianapolis, IN
B.S. with honors, *magna cum laude*
Molecular genetics with minor in chemistry

*Honors*

2008–2010  **Francis Pederson Scholarship.** Full-tuition, merit and need-based award.

Explain honors and awards as needed.

2009  **Amos Christie Pediatric Summer Fellowship**

*Activities*

2009–Present  **Microbes and Defense Society.** Honor society for excellence in microbiology and immunology.

2008–Present  **Committee on Women's Issues.** Co-Chairperson for Volunteer Activities. Promoted public awareness of women's issues in medicine.

2008–Present  **Decisions Pathway Program.** Assisted women in a Tennessee prison with substance abuse rehabilitation.

2008–Present  **Center for Health Services Board.** Nominating Committee Member, 2008–2009; Project Advisory Committee Member, 2009–2010.

*Employment*

2009–2010  **Clinical Clerk, Amos Christie Pediatric Summer Fellowship.** Evaluated patients in the pediatric acute care clinic, the newborn nursery, and the cardiology clinic.

Include major jobs and employment related to teaching and health.

Summer 2006  **Academic Assistant & Tutor, Indiana University Minority Office.** Tutored students in inorganic chemistry. Organized tutoring program by matching students to appropriate tutors.

*Personal*

Conversational in Spanish.

Hobbies include aerobics, cooking, and reading.

Vertical line is an alternative to horizontal lines in other CVs.

**FIGURE 8-4.** Sample CV no. 4.

# REFERENCES

"Resume Guidelines." West Springfield, MA: Southworth Paper Company, 1995.

Ireland S. *The Complete Idiot's Guide to the Perfect Resume*, 4th ed. New York: Alpha Books, 2006.

# 9

# The Personal Statement

For many residency applicants, writing a personal statement is the most daunting aspect of their application. The formula for a great personal statement can be enigmatic, and program directors provide little guidance for applicants. How will your personal statement be used? How can it enhance or harm your application? Will it even be read? The answers to these questions may vary from program to program, but one fact remains true: It is the only component of your application in which your individual voice and personality can be showcased. Therefore, it needs to be both well thought out and well written.

> Your personal statement injects personality to your application.

## HOW A PERSONAL STATEMENT CAN HELP YOU

The personal statement is your opportunity to declare a total commitment to the specialty for which you are applying. Whether a program director hangs on every word you write or chooses to glance at it, your words must convey love for the academic and personal aspects of the specialty. The essay should leave the reader with the impression that you are dedicated to the specialty, that you will be an upbeat member of the team, and that your enthusiasm will continue. Correctly conveying your enthusiasm and this sentiment in an honest and direct fashion will elevate your application. Failure to accomplish these goals can make an otherwise glowing application appear unprofessional and disingenuous, which is a kiss of death in trying to gain a coveted interview.

> A poorly executed statement shows a lack of professionalism.

## WHAT BELONGS IN A PERSONAL STATEMENT?

A good personal statement will strive to capture current enthusiasm, past accomplishments, and future goals. A great personal statement will unify these three components with a theme and cohesive story arc. For example, many medical students will experience moments of clarity, inspiration, and growth while on the wards or clinics. Others have had personal experiences with illness that have inspired them. If you have had such an experience, by all means describe it. These are true sources of inspiration that fueled your enthusiasm for a specific field or professional calling.

Discussing the origins of your enthusiasm can also provide the foundation for introducing your accomplishments into a personal statement. After all, the personal statement is a time to elaborate on your strengths. For example, if you were able to channel your enthusiasm for radiology into clinical research, or your interest in pediatric diabetes into volunteering at a juvenile diabetes camp, be sure to discuss it! Your personal statement is not your CV; rather, it is an opportunity for you to introduce a select few activities, accomplishments, or accolades into your unique narrative.

Your enthusiasm and accomplishments should not be the end of your story. They should lead into an important part of your personal statement: what you hope to accomplish. You must address your career goals. Do you hope to stay in family practice? Work in an underserved community? Would you like a career in academics? Do you envision yourself on the forefront of health policy decision making?

While interviewers understand that plans frequently change during residency, they like to know that you have thought about the future and have some career aspirations that excite you. Before you conclude your personal statement, try to indicate what you will bring to the residency program in the short term and to the field as a whole in the long term. It shows that you have thought through not only your specialty choice, but also what you can do to enhance that specialty.

> A personal statement should read as a cohesive personal narrative—the story of your decision to enter a field of medicine. It should not be a list of reasons why your chosen specialty is the best.

## WHAT DOESN'T BELONG IN A PERSONAL STATEMENT?

To discover what does not belong in a personal statement, imagine the dark extreme of each of three categories listed above: hyperbolized emotion, falsified events, and exaggerated understanding of what you strive to accomplish. When writing about emotional experiences or events, try to maintain a realistic tone to your description. Emotional exaggerations are obvious to the reader, who most likely has had similar experiences as a physician. To that end, falsified experiences for the sake of having a "pivotal medical moment" are equally transparent. If you write that caring for your brother with diabetes has given you deep insight into the disease, be prepared to describe those insights in your personal statement. If a summer research experience showed you the beauty of science, express that beauty— but be sure you remember what you actually did in the laboratory!

Lying about or exaggerating your achievements in your personal statement is unethical as well as foolish. Your personal statement will be used as a template for questioning during your interviews. Do not write about anything that you do not wish to discuss—especially if it will expose an embellishment. If you write that you speak fluent Spanish, be prepared to conduct the interview in Spanish if the interviewer happens to also be fluent. If you claim to be an avid opera fan, be sure you can discuss the topic intelligently with an interviewer who may be an opera aficionado.

Another egregious error is utilizing the personal statement to discuss application weaknesses. Drawing attention to a failed USMLE attempt or to a low clerkship score with an explanation of illness or personal distraction is rarely helpful. Describing oneself as great on the wards, but a poor test taker, is also worrisome. The personal statement should be a time to celebrate a great medical school and appreciation for an excellent education. Any experiences that reflect poorly on your school or your education should not be included. (For example, "My shelf exam scores are low because we received no guidance on what to study.") If the interviewer wants you to elaborate on any weaknesses in your application, he or she will ask you about them. Do not volunteer the information needlessly.

You should also avoid any negativity in your personal statement. For example, if you went to graduate school and switched to medical school because you hated your time in graduate school, do not say so overtly. Focus on what you learned through the experience of going to graduate school and how it motivated you to pursue medicine. Discuss how you feel medicine is a better fit for you, but do not dwell excessively on the negative aspects of your experiences.

Finally, your personal statement must be well executed technically. Some program directors will read your statement quickly and are not likely to evaluate punctuation. However, a poorly written statement replete with spelling mistakes and other errors reflects poorly on the applicant. We are members of a profession

## TABLE 9-1

### Personal Statement Tips

**DO**

Get an early start. A well-written statement requires a significant investment of your time and energy.

Have a high-quality draft ready when you contact potential letter writers. Most will want a copy of your personal statement.

Catch the readers' attention—use a strong opening.

Consider including your motivation for choosing the specialty, your ideal residency program, and/or future aspirations in the specialty.

Highlight your strengths and accomplishments; expand on significant extracurricular and community accomplishments.

Make every word count. Use terse, precise, and vivid language to tell your story.

Make it "flow." Smooth transitions keep your reader engaged.

Make it personal. Consider discussing your interests outside of medicine if they pertain to qualities that will make you a good resident.

Tie it all together with a strong finish.

Limit the length of your essay to about one page. Too short a statement conveys a lack of effort and interest.

Have your advisor, other faculty, and program director review your statement.

Be familiar with your essay. Any material contained within it is a fair topic for discussion in interviews.

**DON'T**

Blow it off. You have no way of knowing which programs will weight your statement heavily and which will merely glance at it. Prepare your statement as if every program will read it carefully. An inferiorly written statement can only hurt your application.

Simply recap all of the information in your CV. Pick a few items of significance and expand on them to develop an idea or point central to your strengths as an applicant in your desired specialty.

Use worn-out clichés, metaphors, and analogies.

Start every sentence with "I."

Be shy. Go ahead and express lofty career goals or high expectations (within reason). Programs will admire your future aspirations.

Make excuses. The personal statement is not the place to call attention to weaknesses in your application. Save the explanation of failed boards or a poor clerkship grade for the interview.

Make grammar and spelling mistakes. These errors demonstrate carelessness, a quality unbecoming in a future resident.

Embellish, inflate, or lie under any circumstances. It is definitely not worth the price you will pay if you are discovered.

Be too verbose. Keep it short, sweet, and to the point. Your audience will thank you.

Come across as arrogant. This is the place to showcase your strengths, but in a humble way.

that does not tolerate mistakes well. So read and reread your statement, and have others look at it. Whether English is your first language or your third, have several other people review your personal statement critically. Swap it with other medical students, send it to your mentors or advisors, and ask your parents for a favor. It can only help you to have many people give their perspectives and check for spelling or grammatical errors.

> Your weaknesses will be apparent from your application—don't use the personal statement to highlight them.

## SAMPLE EXCERPTS

Below are excerpts from actual personal statements as examples of "do's and don'ts" for certain issues. Names and locations have been changed to protect the writers' identities, but otherwise most essays appear as they were submitted in their applications. The applicants behind these statements matched at excellent institutions across the country. Many of the comments that accompany our examples are derived from the observations of several residency directors, admissions committee members, and professional editors. These critiques should help you acquire a "feel" for good form as well as good content. Keep in mind, however, that no two residency directors (even in the same specialty) read a personal statement with the same opinions and preferences.

## OPENINGS

### EXAMPLE 1

This applicant in emergency medicine draws on rich family and cultural traditions and values. A residency director reading this introduction is not only making the acquaintance of an applicant; he or she is also learning about the applicant's value system. However, the applicant's metaphor is slightly drawn out, without the creation of a direct link.

> My great-grandfather once told me that everyone's life is like a book, full of chapters that are continually written and revised. Each life, each book, is unique, made so through the experiences and the actions of the person living. My personal anthology is no exception, having been enriched by the many people whom I have met. Through these experiences, I have strengthened my desire to enter a training program that will lead to a career in emergency medicine. **Thus begins a new chapter in my book.**

← Careful word choice enlivens an overused analogy.

← Excellent transition to background info.

### EXAMPLE 2

This family practice applicant presents a well-done teaser for the rest of the statement. He weaves his sense of social responsibility and worldview through a number of vivid experiences. Carefully, without arrogance, the introduction draws the reader in using personal anecdotes.

An enticing invitation to any director who has seen too many formulaic statements. ——→ I have always been interested in people's stories. This and a deep-seated desire to help make the world a better place have drawn me to the work I do. From working on a crew harvesting filberts to sitting down for a bowl of soup with a homeless friend, I have met many

Major cliché. ——→ people, each one with a story, each story having something to teach me. Some of the wisest people I have met are very poor with little access to housing, education, or health care. I get a lot out of listening to their stories; what do I give back? I first began to question the ethics of being a responsible listener when I went to Nicaragua as a Spanish interpreter. I was with a group of agronomists on a struggling agricultural cooperative nestled deep in the mountains of Matagalpa. The life was hard, but the work was fascinating and the setting beautiful. I finally got up the courage to ask the cooperative leader if I could stay longer. He smiled, "You gringos eat a lot. Now, maybe if you were a

A noble reason to become a doctor. But why medicine versus other altruistic vocations? ——→ doctor. ..." I chose to become a physician as a way to work intimately with people and hear their stories. But, just as importantly, it is a way to tangibly improve their lives.

## EXAMPLE 3

In this personal statement, an applicant in anesthesiology recycles a familiar travel theme with vivid imagery. The opening paragraph introduces a traveler enriched by his adventures. However, travel metaphors can be clichéd. This one, in particular, shows meandering without purpose.

One hopes his choice of specialty was more deliberate. Rewrite to show some method to this madness. ——→ While driving in the Mojave Desert, I turned off Highway 14 onto a dirt path. The road was crisscrossed by many other trails. Small hills blocked my view of what lay ahead on each road. Unable to see what each road led to, I randomly chose to drive along one road, then another, and then another. Every new direction possessed its own

Vivid! You feel as if you're there. ——→ beauty and worth. One road revealed towering, sand-carved cliffs with striated bands of crimson, orange, and tan spotted with turquoise. Another road led to a lone Joshua tree standing majestically in the des-

Weak tie-in to medicine. ——→ ert grass. Each new path inspired a new thought. I have had a similar experience in medicine.

## EXAMPLE 4

This applicant in orthopedic surgery wants to return to the Midwest after having trained at an East Coast medical school. He combines the family legacy of an immigrant background with the traditional values of Middle America. By playing up the Midwest, however, he runs the risk of turning off East and West Coast directors in a highly competitive specialty in which applicants must often apply coast to coast in order to match.

Growing up in the small farming community of Vernon in east-central Indiana, I have experienced a spectrum of attitudes unique to a rural population. Folks here are down to earth, with simple, relaxed life-styles. It was here where I have lived almost all my life, moving from Birmingham, Alabama, my birthplace, at nine months of age. It was here where my father set up his urology practice 30 years ago, having come from abroad with little more than a dream for a successful future. It was here, amidst the cornfields and cattle, which I could see from my bedroom window, that I grew up with my older sister and younger brother under a strict, coherent value system of hard work, motivation, dedication, and perseverance.

← Back off a little on the rural imagery here. We get the point.

← Nice way of associating yourself with a set of values. Stating the same directly can come off as presumptuous.

## EXAMPLE 5

In her personal statement for pediatrics, this applicant describes an endearing picture of herself as a child. The information itself is not particularly monumental, but the tone of the paragraph communicates her excitement about the field and leaves the reader wanting to know more about her character.

My first inkling of a career in pediatrics came to me as I perched on my toes on the baseboard, gripping the windowsill for stability, and peered into the Duke Hospital nursery. As a kindergartner, occasionally accompanying my mother to her job as a hospital administrative assistant, I would wander the halls of the hospital and faithfully find my way to the nursery to examine the newborns and their caregivers through the glass. I passed the time imagining my future self, clad in a white coat, examining the neonates up close.

← A catchy beginning, leaving the reader wanting to know more about her.

## EXAMPLE 6

The opening line "I will never forget the…" is somewhat overused and clichéd. This opening sentence sparks some interest because of the large amount of money he describes. However, the author then goes on to start every sentence with the word "I." This gets repetitive and sounds self-centered. Try to compose sentences with a variety of structures and lengths and avoid excessive use of the first person pronoun.

I will never forget the day we made four million dollars at Lehman Brothers. I was 21 years old with a Cal-Tech engineering degree under my belt working on the Nasdaq trading desk. I was poised to launch into a lucrative career in banking, but fortunately I had the foresight to choose a different career path. I know being a physician will allow me to look back at age 50 and know that I made a difference.

← Sounds interesting, but …

← I … I … I … I … It is a personal statement about you, but don't start every phrase with "I."

## EXAMPLE 7

While this author doubtless has interesting stories to tell, the opening line is long and feels awkward. Aim for a succinct, catchy opening sentence. You have the rest of the page to delve into details and flesh out your ideas.

A mouthful! ———→ A 5-year-old boy with multiple skin and respiratory infections from de-layed immunizations, and a 9-year-old girl with chronic stasis ulcers, to-gether etched an indelible impression upon me through their innocent yet dire calls for help. I met Eshetu as the community services chair for my fraternity at Claremont College. At the time, I had put forward the idea of sponsoring an impoverished child's health and education in Ethiopia. Although straightforward, I believed that an act of service, solely financial in nature, would be empty and ineffective.

## REASONS FOR ENTERING SPECIALTY

### EXAMPLE  1

The following comes close to being a model illustration of good organization and presentation of motivations for pursuing a specialty. The applicant is obviously comfortable discussing the specialty and appears sincere in his enthusiasm without being patronizing. The writing is spare but is neither dry nor flat.

A bit of a cliché. ———→ I grew up with surgery in my blood, but it was not until the middle of my third year of medical school that I discovered that I wanted to prac-tice orthopedic surgery. It was at this time that I was first exposed to orthopedic surgery at Springfield Memorial Hospital. My love of being

Note the number of concrete ———→ in the operating room, combined with the very precise mechanical reasons orthopedics and technical nature of orthopedic surgery, sparked my interest in the appeals to him. field. Perhaps the feature that fascinates me the most about ortho-pedics is that it is both a craft and a science. I enjoy the "hands-on" nature of orthopedic surgery, both in clinic and in the operating room. I am also attracted to the diversity of orthopedic cases and the vast amount of direct patient contact. Treating patients of all age groups and both sexes, with a wide variety of problems encountered at work, in accidents, or during recreation, makes orthopedic surgery a very exciting specialty. Above all, although very demanding, I found my orthopedic surgery experiences to be the most rewarding and exhila-

A good paragraph that ———→ rating in medical school. One can almost always do something specific plays to the classic and helpful for each patient, usually leading to a complete resolution strengths of the specialty. of the patient's problem, so they can resume an active lifestyle.

### EXAMPLE 2

This is a tightly written paragraph in which the applicant clearly delineates her reasons for entering the specialty. The writing is fast-paced and precise, like the specialty she aspires to enter.

ER docs should be excited ———→ Although I have found all my clinical rotations interesting, I experi-about their work but also cool enced the most excitement from my time in the emergency depart-under fire. ment. Emergency medicine offers me the opportunity to be at the forefront of medicine and to participate actively in making decisions right from the onset of patient care. The fast pace and the constant demand for rapid and clear thinking have always been attractive, as is the chance to be the first to see a patient, to gather all the relevant information, and then to ferret out the diagnosis. It is in the ED that I find a balanced mixture of the deliberative side of medicine with the more hands-on approach of surgery. But most of all, I enjoy relating to patients of different backgrounds and eagerly look forward to the opportunity to care for the great variety of patients seen in emergency and acute settings.

⟵ Text flows well.

## EXAMPLE 3

The following personal statement offers an interesting combination of professional and personal reasons for selecting the specialty. However, the writer risks conveying the impression that he chose ophthalmology more as the result of a process of elimination than for its intrinsic attractiveness.

Although I have long been interested in ophthalmology, my choice of the specialty was not an easy one. Only after sampling what many other specialties had to offer did I realize that none suited me as well. The chance to combine extensive patient contact in a clinical setting with the need for surgical precision, attention to minute detail, and aptitude in the most advanced technology medicine has to offer is an obvious attraction of the specialty. Of all of my clinical experiences as a medical student at UCSF, however, none rivaled the pure emotion I felt during my senior clerkship in ophthalmology, as I watched the vision of a patient with a dense cataract I had examined in clinic be transformed from mere detection of hand motion to near normal the next day as a result of the ophthalmologist's expertise.

⟵ Long sentences.

⟵ Feelings seem disproportionate to event.

## EXAMPLE 4

In an application for internal medicine, this author presents her twofold motivation: the patient care aspect of medicine, and the scientific aspect. Starting with a quote from a patient adds a personal dimension to her writing, but does come across as clichéd.

"Do not lose the empathy behind your eyes," my patient's wife said as she thanked me for caring for her husband. My motivation to pursue a career in internal medicine is embodied by her words. Medicine is a field in which my love for pathophysiology and my commitment to serving others can continue to grow. I have a strong desire to use my problem-solving abilities while helping people through their most difficult times. I have found caring for patients with multiple, complex medical problems to be both challenging and incredibly rewarding.

⟵ A well-presented balance between the humanistic and scientific sides of medicine.

## EXAMPLE 5

This author presents several good reasons why she has chosen internal medicine. However, the tone is somewhat melodramatic. Beware of grandiose-sounding statements as in the first sentence and the repeated use of the first person.

> I love internal medicine because it stands alone above all other special-ties due to its versatility and broad range of the field. I will be trained to master all situations, from serious patients urgently admitted to the medical intensive care unit fighting for life to patients visiting the clinic for minor health maladies. I will be trained to diagnose and treat dis-orders ranging from cancer to renal dysfunction to cardiac problems, allowing me to take care of my patients completely.

*Really? It seems pretty similar in versatility and range to many other fields such as pediatrics, family practice, or surgery.*

*Medicine is always a team sport, so avoid sounding like you plan to single-handedly save the world.*

## MEDICINE AS A SECOND CAREER

### EXAMPLE 1

In contrast to some second-career candidates, this applicant emphasizes the com-mon ground between pediatrics and his previous career. In fact, the paragraph does not explain why he decided to make the career change—something that should be done in the rest of the personal statement, in a way that highlights the positive nature of the decision.

> For five years prior to medical school, I taught computer science in grades 2–12 at a private bilingual school. I loved working with children and their families and had the joy of seeing my students learn and grow over a number of years. These same preferences led me to an interest in pediatrics as a specialty. Pediatrics is a heady mixture of the exotic and the mundane, of glowing health and desperate illness. It offers a wide variety of patients, a mix of common and uncommon disorders, a practice based in growth and development, and the possibility to make a real difference in the lives of patients and their families.

*Smooth transition.*

*This sentence does not give any new information, and comes across as word-filler.*

### EXAMPLE 2

Like many second-career applicants, this student also felt that something meaning-ful was missing from his career. However, he makes one misstep; in contrasting his future career in psychiatry with his past work in mathematics, he puts the latter down unnecessarily. You should retain a positive attitude toward past experiences, even if you did not enjoy them. Instead, point out some of the things you learned through the experience and how it led you to a career in medicine. While it is true that making a career change is not easy, characterizing a career change as a monumental achievement may sound overblown.

> My pure math activities were enjoyable for themselves, yet I had a growing sense that community service was what gave my life mean-ing and direction. Did I want to get to the end of my life and answer "What have I done?" with "I proved theorems"? Hoping to use science

*Don't denigrate previous accomplishments.*

to help others rather than merely to create more science, I concluded I might be happiest in the long run in medicine, and courageously decided to change careers. So far, medicine has more than fulfilled my expectations as a context to combine the heart and the head. I am particularly intrigued by the doctor-patient relationship, which impresses me as a seamless blend of problem solving, hypothesis testing, trust building, and appreciation of the patients' individuality.

## EXAMPLE 3

This is a well-written paragraph that demonstrates remarkable insight and maturity of thought. The first half of the paragraph is a concise description of the applicant's activities during the year off. In the latter half, the applicant shares what he has learned without portraying it as an unprecedented revelation.

After my third year of medical school, I pursued my interest in policy issues by studying for a master's degree in public health at Emory. I spent the year exploring the epidemiology of infectious diseases, options for health care reform, and the empowerment of low-income communities. I learned useful skills in biostatistics and qualitative evaluation, and gained a global perspective on our health care system. At times, however, our discussions of abstract ideas and numbers felt too far removed from the realities of people's lives. I became convinced that debates about health care delivery should be rooted in concrete clinical practice, in the stories of patients and providers. My experience in public health taught me that doctors have a special role in society because they are trusted by patients and respected by policy makers. This combination allows physicians to be potent advocates for their patients and their community.

*← Good summary.*

*← Nice tie-in with his interest in family practice. Clear, concise, and thoughtful.*

## EXAMPLE 4

After switching from a career in teaching to one in medicine, this applicant is applying in pediatrics. She presents one way in which her teaching experience has helped equip her for a career in pediatrics. She also highlights some of her volunteer experience, which is a good launching point for discussions during an interview.

Given that the word "doctor" is derived from the Latin word for "teacher," I do not find it all too surprising that teaching has made a large impact on my decision to enter pediatrics. I spent a year during medical school giving lessons to eighth-graders on health education as part of the Brothers and Sisters in Science program. My volunteer work clearly prepared me with the skills I needed to build a solid rapport with my adolescent patients and, more importantly, to better care for them through their trust in me.

*← A good way to demonstrate her long-standing interest in children's health education, and her commitment to the field.*

## EXAMPLE

This applicant had experience as a classical singer before entering medical school. His opening two lines leave the reader interested and wanting to know more about his prior career and his reasons for changing. However, he then launches into a somewhat rambling paragraph that does not have a tight tie-in to psychiatry. It could have been improved by making the analogy shorter and more succinct, and by linking it to medicine more clearly. He also uses "one" repeatedly, which gives the paragraph an awkward feel.

> **"One ... one ... one ..." is almost as bad as "I ... I ... I ..."**

I have not always known that I wanted to be a psychiatrist or even a physician. In fact, I spent eight years studying a very different field—classical singing. I did not realize that many of the things I loved about making music were preparing me for a career in psychiatry. In classical singing, one is taught to create a character and tell a story with each piece of music. One must find a way to identify with experiences that may be very different from one's own. To give a character and a performance depth, one must be able to convey the text in a way that is emotionally meaningful, but it is not only the text that matters, it is the story behind the story—the subtext that can truly bring a character to life. There are few experiences that are more precious to me than being entrusted with the story of another person's life.

## STRONG EXTRACURRICULAR/COMMUNITY ACCOMPLISHMENTS

### EXAMPLE 1

This applicant has an impressive list of extracurricular activities and achievements, but it is the richness of detail that convinces you that she has diverse interests and is involved in her community.

> **This sentence preempts any concern that the writer's extracurricular activities would interfere with her duties as a resident.**

Self-motivated, I work vigorously at my research, teaching, and patient care. However, it is also very important to me to continue furthering my personal interests, including the creative preparation and presentation of gourmet foods, wreath making, and horse training. Especially rewarding is my weekend volunteer work with the Stony Brook Riding Club for the Handicapped, which entails rounding up the herd at 6 A.M., feeding, grooming, tacking, and assisting the physically and/or mentally disabled riders in any way necessary. Annual CPR organization and instruction to the public brings important education to the community and keeps me abreast of the layman's current fund of medical knowledge. Additionally, my family background of being the eldest daughter of an architect and a nuclear medicine technologist

> **Be careful not to digress; they need a house officer, not an illustrator.**

from Indonesia has led me to a longtime interest in the integration of drawing and science, namely medical illustration. My aspiration is to obtain formal training in illustration technique when my medical education is complete; in the meantime, I hope to continue publishing my drawings and using them in presentations during my residency.

> If you discuss an extracurricular activity in your personal statement, be sure you can discuss it intelligently in your interview.

## EXAMPLE 2

It is not enough to list your academic accomplishments in the style of a CV. This student highlights the significance of his academic activities in clear, well-organized expository writing.

Computer consulting work has provided me with close contact with creative researchers in science and medicine. A two-year thesis project with Dr. Elizabeth Rutter challenged my skills in relational databases, clinical record-keeping systems, and exploratory statistical techniques. In the laboratory of Dr. Jeffrey Greenberg, I applied innovative real-time video microscopy and image processing techniques to fundamental growth and cell-division questions in cell biology. Through my lab work I have developed interests in improving the quality and utility of medical technology for clinical decision making. I have supplemented medical school by being an active participant in basic biomedical science. In addition to medicine, I am familiar with the tools and vocabulary of modern molecular biology. I read a wide variety of clinical and scientific journals, and use literature searching extensively.

← Emphasizes professional skills developed during the project.

← Attempts to connect basic science to clinical research.

← Applicant seeking a research-oriented residency skillfully weaves in additional academic activities.

## EXAMPLE 3

This applicant in radiology had experience as a professional dancer and presents some interesting ideas about how she would combine dance and radiology. These would be great starting points for conversations during the interview.

I see tremendous opportunities in radiology to combine my passions for dance and medicine. Currently, radiology is an undeveloped field within performing arts medicine. There are no radiologists in the entire International Association of Dance Medicine and Science, and I believe that my calling is to be a pioneer in the radiological aspects of performing arts medicine. I envision myself helping dancers and other artists in ways that have not yet been discovered. For example, as a Fulbright scholar I garnered unique clinical knowledge about musculoskeletal injuries of dancers and musicians, which correlates directly with musculoskeletal imaging. Subtleties at the metatarsophalangeal and subtalar joints, which may be considered clinically insignificant radiographic findings in the normal population, can have profound effects on a dancer's ability to continue dancing at the level expected of him or her.

← An interesting and unique combination.

← This sounds interesting but vague. She could have written that she hopes to help dancers and other artists in concrete ways through her research.

## PERSONAL EXPERIENCES

### EXAMPLE

This applicant uses a bare-bones description of a patient experience to demonstrate her appreciation of the unparalleled access physicians have to their patients' lives. A program director might not fully appreciate how a simple statement from a patient might affect a medical student.

Functional summary of volunteer experience. →

In my second year of medical school, I spent one afternoon each week with a primary care physician in San Francisco. The practice specialized in caring for HIV-positive men. In addition to learning about the health care and social issues of this population, the patients and I grew comfortable with each other as I worked to earn their trust. The privilege of health care providers to share difficult times and confidential information with patients was clearly illustrated to me when after an interview a patient remarked, "You know, you're the only woman I've ever talked to about this."

Choice quote at end adds warmth. →

### EXAMPLE 2

This applicant in family medicine makes a basic cultural and human observation through a touching yet humorous experience in an overcrowded Kenyan hospital. The richness of prose is matched by the complexity and maturity of thought underlying her observations.

Note the lush and perhaps excessive detail. →

I found the explanation for my surprising happiness one night in an unusual way. At 3 A.M. I was called to the wards to admit a young woman and arrived to find her comatose, moaning, and rocking on her half of a rickety cot. I examined her, hung IV quinine for likely cerebral malaria, did a lumbar puncture, and put down an NG tube as the entire ward of sick women gravely watched the proceedings, their faces eerily illuminated by my penlight, the only source of light. Last to do was the Foley catheter, but try as I might I could not locate the woman's urethra. One of the nurses began to giggle—just a little giggle. I began to giggle.

Very powerful. →

The women on the ward began to smile through their fevers, then chuckle. Soon the entire ward was laughing, great guffaws resounding through that miserable ward. I understood immediately. There was nothing vindictive or belittling in our laughter. On some unspoken group level, really a cultural level, we were pulling together to survive, transcending the almost unbearably hopeless human suffering. No one of us as an individual could hope to escape, but together, as a group, through this laughter—symbolic of some human universal, some common denominator—we stood a chance of retaining our dignity, our perspective, our optimism. Thinking about this moment afterwards, and, indeed, about my whole experience at

Mogashi Hospital, I have come to realize the crucial role that cultural constructs—shared belief systems, mutual ways of reacting to circumstances, family, friends, rituals, society—play in an individual's life.

← Observations that bespeak intelligence and insight.

## EXAMPLE 3

Anecdotes about patients are commonly used to highlight an applicant's compassion and sensitivity. Such accounts should, however, be used with discretion. The following example is a particularly overused theme. Try and decide what is a "standard" medical encounter and what is truly unique, and focus on the latter. This is not to say that "standard" encounters are not meaningful or inspiring. However, the reader has probably seen a dozen other personal statements describing similar patient interactions.

During the first week of my outpatient medicine clerkship I met Miss G., a 65-year-old woman who came to the clinic for a routine health assessment. During the course of her evaluation, I obtained a screening mammogram, which unfortunately revealed a spiculated mass suggestive of malignancy. For the first time in her life, Miss G. faced the possibility of a diagnosis of cancer and realized she must come to terms with her own mortality. For the first time in my life, I found myself looking into the eyes of a patient, trying to be honest and kind while conveying bad news. It was a moment I remember well. I saw Miss G. in clinic on several occasions over the ensuing weeks. Although she usually came to see me for health maintenance needs, we invariably turned to her concerns about breast cancer. She approached her fears with remarkable courage and stoicism, finally surrendering to tears of relief when her biopsy was found to be benign. I experienced both a sense of loss and a wonderful feeling of fulfillment when the months in the clinics came to an end. In retrospect, Miss G. taught me more about illness, therapy, and what makes a patient "feel better" than I had learned in all of my classes.

← Writer must have made a connection with the patient, but the message is not clear.

← Avoid criticizing "all my classes," as the reader probably teaches one.

## EXAMPLE 4

The opening sentence is catchy and striking. The author clearly describes her experience, which is one that would evoke universal empathy. In other parts of her personal statement, she could try to incorporate a sense of hope and optimism to keep the tone of her statement from becoming too bleak or depressing.

Reality caught me unprepared: within the first few weeks of my arrival in India, 11 infants and one mother died on the small desert island of P—. Most of these deaths occurred in people's homes. I called a meeting with the only care providers in the area, the traditional midwives, to investigate why these deaths occurred. We discovered a complete lack of prenatal care, no malaria prophylaxis during the rainy season, and care by untrained midwives for deliveries. The most tragic and

← A dramatic introduction describing an intense, meaningful experience.

telling case was 20-year-old Rhada, a wiry woman who tilled her farm in the heat and carried gallons of water atop her head up until she went into labor. At the moment of delivery, all attention turned to her newborn son and Rhada silently bled. When the midwife realized that Rhada's placenta had not delivered, she attempted manual extraction and failed. She panicked as Rhada became faint, and sent her to the nearest hospital, two hours away. Rhada died en route. Bearing witness to these senseless deaths affected me deeply. What separated me from these young Indian women?

*This does not come across as cliché, given the nature of her experience and the way it was described.*

## FINISHES

### EXAMPLE 1

This is an example of a strong finish, although it is somewhat compromised by overuse of the first person singular. The applicant efficiently states his professional and personal goals, highlights notable personal qualities, and sets forth his expectations for residency training—all within five sentences. Unfortunately, each one starts with an "I."

*Very concise.*

At UCSF I have experienced tremendous personal growth and have clarified my professional goals. I am committed to developing pragmatic multidisciplinary approaches to improving the quality and delivery of health care in the United States. Personally, I desire to provide compassionate and technically excellent medical care to patients from all walks of life. I will bring to residency energy, enthusiasm, integrity, and ability. I expect a challenging, rich environment in which to learn and practice good medicine.

*Written with conviction and sincerity.*

### EXAMPLE 2

Many applicants finish with a "ready for anything" type of statement without convincing the reader that they understand what they're getting themselves into. This applicant takes an honest look at the challenges ahead and her ability to meet them. In addition, she balances discussions of her career plans with a glimpse into her personal life. We see how the interplay between work and leisure maintains her balance and stamina.

*Dose of humility makes applicant seem more human.*

I know I have set high goals for myself: clinician, educator, and health advocate. The majority of the time I find working with underserved populations extremely rewarding; however, it can also be emotionally demanding. I have profound admiration for family physicians who have devoted their life to this work. I often grapple with the question of what will enable me to sustain this commitment for a lifetime. The combination of working at an individual level to address health needs and at a more macroscopic level to affect health policy is synergistic

*Reality check shows forethought about career plans.*

for me—each inspires my work in the other. On a personal level, I find my time away from medicine rejuvenating as well. Spending time backpacking, gardening, or being with friends and family enables me to return to work refreshed. Being a physician entails personal sacrifice and dedication, and I am eager to begin the challenge.

## EXAMPLE 3

This applicant uses a good quote for his ending paragraph. However, there is no need to state that he had used it in his personal statement for medical school. It sounds as though he is rehashing the same material. It would have sounded much more succinct and fresh if he had left the opening statement out.

> In my personal statement for medical school, I quoted Paul Farmer saying, "I don't know why everyone isn't excited about [medicine]." Medical school has been a great source of joy for me, and I have no doubt that I am doing what I was put on this earth to do. Now that I have decided to pursue orthopedics, I have a renewed passion for medicine. It excites me, it stimulates me, and I cannot imagine doing anything else.

It's good that he is sure of his choice, but this sounds melodramatic!

## EXAMPLE 4

This is a solid ending to a general surgery personal statement. It communicates her excitement in a way that displays humility despite the repeated use of the first person pronoun.

> As I stand ready to transition to the next level of my professional development as a surgeon, I am every bit as enthusiastic as I was standing before the operating table during that first case. I anxiously await the unique privilege of participating in such a rewarding and exciting field of patient care.

A good tie-in from her first experience in the OR to the rest of her career.

## SAMPLE PERSONAL STATEMENTS

In the following pages, we have reproduced some successful personal statements in their entirety, edited only to protect the applicant's identity. The applicants behind these statements matched at top institutions across the country. Once again, much of the commentary is based on the observations of several residency directors, personal statement coaches, and professional editors. Remember that your personal statement must reflect your own unique style and personality.

### PERSONAL STATEMENT #1

The writer of the following statement left a career in neuroscience research to pursue pediatric neurology. Her statement effectively discusses her reasons for delaying medical school, disliking graduate training, and then ultimately entering medical school—thereby directly addressing the questions a director might have

> Use the personal statement to tell your story. This is your chance to stand out from the crowd!

about an older applicant. The essay reads very naturally, and her enthusiasm for the specialty is evident. The essay would have been improved, however, if the applicant had toned down her remarks about her love for the specialty.

Good motivation. ——————→

When I first entered Oberlin College in 1980 I wanted to go into medicine—it took me 11 years to get there. When I first applied to medical school I thought about pediatric neurology—fortunately, it has not taken me another 11 years. During my third-year pediatrics clerkship, I told one of my best friends from college (who is now a primary care attending) that I absolutely loved going to work every day and that I was amazed at how much fun it was to "play with" your patients. Her response was that I could have children of my own and I didn't need to go into a field of medicine just to "play with kids." As I continued to love every minute of my other pediatric rotations, I began to realize that, of course, I didn't need to, but that I certainly could if it was what I enjoyed the most and what I seemed to do the best.

Appropriate exploration of reasons for entering first career. ——————→

When I was in college, I initially put off medicine for entirely the wrong reasons: I hated the competition of the premeds, I could not imagine studying nonstop, and I did not want to stay up all night every three to four days for years of my life. Instead, I knew that I wanted to study the brain. I had two wonderful role models in my psychobiology career: I got my thesis published, and I headed to graduate school looking forward to a career in neuroscience research. But I feel fortunate now that my six years in a graduate program in experimental neuropsychology at UCSD showed me that a career in research by itself was not enough.

Dramatizes her shift in values. ——————→

The turning point was deeply personal. My four-month-old niece was diagnosed with a grade 4 glioblastoma multiforme at the start of my fourth year. I remember sitting in the ICU waiting room at Denver Children's trying to concentrate on a paper related to my dissertation and realizing that what I was studying would never be directly helpful to this beautiful little child or to the rest of my family. It was then that I focused on why I had not been truly satisfied with my graduate experience—something was missing. And I came to realize that what was missing is the very thing that I need and want most from my career—direct application of my work. My personality needs more instant gratification than full-time research was bound to give me. In fact, the only gratification that I did seem to be getting routinely in graduate school was through teaching. I loved the interaction with students, the challenge of being an effective communicator, and the sense of responsibility toward the students, all of which are integral parts of being a successful teacher. I received the Distinguished Teacher Award in 1992 and was subsequently appointed to the teaching assistant consultant position responsible for training all the new TAs in the Psychology Department. Unfortunately, in much of academia, teaching is not as valued a commodity as it should be, and I was constantly made to feel that I was spending "too much time and effort" teaching. As for my research efforts, I am fortunate enough to have experienced the thrill that comes from finding the predicted effects during the final data analysis of my dissertation project, but I know that this thrill would have been magnified ten times if the research had been clinically applicable. I also realized that ultimately I wanted more out of my interaction with patients than having them as research subjects. My experience in medical school has taught me that I was right, there is nothing more rewarding than direct patient care—no matter how challenging it can be. The fact that a career in academic medicine combines the patient care, teaching, and clinical research that I value so much makes me realize how lucky I am to have found this path.

> Integrates awards into paragraph on interests.

Despite the fact that it was a little disconcerting to turn 30 during my first year of medical school in a class whose mean age was 23, and that it may seem a little harder for me to stay up all night than for my 25-year-old classmates, I have never regretted my path. I feel that the life experience gained from my year as a social worker working with pregnant and parenting teens, and my years in graduate school have contributed immeasurably to my learning of medicine. I knew better during first and second year what was really important—not the grades that I received, but rather how well I could learn to apply that knowledge to a clinical setting. I can also look at the frustrated and angry parents of a sick child and understand a little better what they are going through by applying my experience with my sister and niece.

> Lighthearted acknowledgment that medicine is a second career.

> Demonstrates how maturity works in applicant's favor.

For a short time during my third year I allowed myself to be steered toward adult neurology by eminent senior faculty members, but I knew there was something in my heart that would not let me make a final career decision until I had experienced child neurology. I went into it with mixed feelings. Another friend who was finishing her pediatrics residency had told me that she had considered doing a neurology fellowship, but thought that it was "too depressing" ... so she went into oncology instead. I must admit that this scared me. But I knew after only a few days that this was what I was meant to do. I enjoyed every patient interaction I had—the 14-year-old with a static encephalopathy

> Humor works surprisingly well here.

and an intractable seizure disorder, the perfectly normal four-year-old who came for follow-up after a "bonk" on the head, and the eight-year-old with sudden onset of cranial nerve palsies of still unknown etiology. My learning curve was vertical, and I went to sleep every night with Dr. Bruce Silverstein's text on my bed, and then was fortunate enough to have the opportunity to ask him questions in clinic in the morning. Many people have told me how lucky I am to have found a field that I am so enthusiastic about, that to fall so completely in love with something is what everybody hopes for. I knew that day that I went to Toys R Us (postcall) to buy a koosh ball to test visual fields and small plastic toys to test manual dexterity, and the night at 4 A.M. when I sat in a rocker to console a methadone baby in the nursery before going to bed for that all-important two hours' sleep, that they were right.

*You can chill; we know you like the specialty.* →

## PERSONAL STATEMENT #2

The applicant has done a terrific job making her enthusiasm and convictions apparent to us. The introduction is unevenly written, but the decision to launch the essay with a set of reasons for specializing in pediatrics makes the essay focused and direct from the start. In the middle two paragraphs, the applicant's extensive community activities are well described. Overall, the essay is solid and persuasive.

*The writer scraps a superfluous introduction.* →

Of the many contributing factors in my decision to pursue a career in pediatrics, the opportunity for patient education stands out as the most influential. During my clinical clerkships, I discovered many fields to be intriguing and learned from, as well as enjoyed, many aspects of each. It became clear, however, that the rotations providing more patient contact and continuity of care were the most fulfilling. My memories of third-year clerkships are of explaining cardiac catheterization to help allay fears, diagramming reasonable schedules of discharge medications, and discussing puberty with girls beginning their development.

*Good motivation.* →

Thus, choosing a field became not merely a determination of what I found to be intellectually challenging, but a selection of the role I wished to play in delivering health care to my patients. Pediatrics as a specialty allows the most interaction with patients and their families and affords perhaps the broadest role for the physician, including that of child advocate/social activist, health educator, family friend, and role model. Here, colleagues are interested in a patient's adoption history and school performance, and time can be scheduled solely for the purpose of STD teaching.

In my own educational experiences I have been blessed with supportive teachers who were also excellent role models. I was awarded the opportunity to enter a research laboratory as a high school student largely due to the commitment of a chemistry teacher and the generosity of a pharmacologist. This led to an aspiration to run my own laboratory with a program for future students. In college, a biochemistry professor's encouragement allowed me to pursue an individual project resulting in a publication. Perhaps as a means to reciprocate, I became involved in the local community. I performed the majority of my volunteer work through Alpha Phi Omega, a coeducational service fraternity affiliated with the Boy Scouts of America. Typical activities of the organization were Easter egg hunts for the county's foster children, creating a haunted house every Halloween at the Salvation Army, and providing aid in the aftermath of a local earthquake. Other community-oriented projects included tutoring of Chinatown youths on academic warning. As examples of Asians in college, the tutors also assumed roles of "big siblings" to help the students bridge cultural gaps and to encourage exploration of life opportunities outside the inner city. These activities eventually led me to realize that medicine, with its emphasis on service, would be the more satisfying career for me.

In medical school, I continued my community activities as time permitted. The two most rewarding experiences were that of teaching at a middle school and of organizing a series of talks for fellow preprofessional students. A few classmates and I taught middle schoolers through a program (Med Teach) coordinated by the medical school and the local school district. We had tremendous fun creating lesson plans for three classes each week, selecting different topics and styles of presentation for each age group. In addition to short traditional lectures, we often added interactive sessions such as class "Jeopardy" or "pin the organ on the body." One of our lessons on the eye even included group dissection of bovine eyeballs. This interest eventually grew to include the education of fellow classmates. As the community outreach chairperson for the Asian Health Caucus, I wanted medical professionals to learn about the special cultural as well as medical characteristics of the Asian patient (eg, population differences in disease prevalence and drug tolerances). This idea of hosting a single lecture on an Asian health topic was discussed with friends, many of whom voiced wishes for similar talks on other cultural groups. Thus sprouted the daylong Multicultural Health Forum, which explored various cultures and their relevant health issues with speakers from different institutions. Moreover, I was able to secure sponsorship from the Department of Psychiatry and develop the forum as a credited class with

Laying it on a bit thick with the community activities.

"Most rewarding experiences": Good way of organizing paragraph.

The writer describes a project from start to finish, showing that she can follow through.

availability to all preprofessional schools, including those of pharmacy, nursing, dentistry, and medicine.

I am eager to maintain my interest in teaching, both through patient education and through involvement with medical student training—knowing well the difference an interested resident can make in the medical student experience. Because of this factor, there was never any doubt that I would be best suited for a university-based/affiliated pediatrics residency program. I currently anticipate a career in general pediatrics and therefore desire a well-rounded program with strong training in primary care. However, infectious disease and genetics are two areas that I wish to further explore, with the option of possible advanced training.

*Balanced and realistic discussion of career goals and training aspirations.*

## PERSONAL STATEMENT #3

This applicant in plastic and reconstructive surgery does a particularly good job detailing research interests without overloading the reader. Note that he rarely has to discuss his interest in plastic surgery in abstract terms—specificity makes this essay work. Through careful attention to his prose, the applicant shows that he cares about his future career in plastics.

As a volunteer anatomy and pathology laboratory instructor, each year I am faced with a new set of students, unpredictable new group dynamics, and ultimately new challenges for presenting material. At times such as these, I truly appreciate the remarkable plasticity of the human mind. A principle taught to me by my college anatomy instructor, who influenced my career by teaching me how to teach, often comes to mind: "Answering a confused student's question with the same words repeatedly is like trying to cut paper by hitting it with a hammer over and over. Instead, trash the hammer and get a pair of scissors," she said, "or start tearing." Through the years, I have learned that effectual communication entails transmission of the understanding that you possess to others, so that they now also understand and are stimulated to think. This requires flexibility and patience, a good understanding and organization of the material, and a high degree of enthusiasm on the part of the teacher. While some of these attributes are inherent in my character, others have been learned and improved upon with every new enterprise.

*Effective use of an anecdote to illustrate a point.*

It is a similar challenge that attracts me to the field of plastic and reconstructive surgery, where often there are situations when operative procedures are modified to accommodate a patient's situation. Whether there is a paucity of soft tissue in one area, an abundance of skin in another, or a lack of bone due to destruction or congenital ab-

*Interesting analogy— plasticity as a parallel between teaching and reconstructive surgery.*

sence, the human body can be made plastic much like the mind modifying the procedures. I welcome and look forward to a lifetime career of meeting these types of challenges creatively in both the adult and pediatric populations, always keeping in mind aesthetics, prognosis, functionality, and the patient's wishes.

Creativity extends to the area of research, which, together with teaching, draws me toward a career in academics. To offer a patient an objective list of therapeutic alternatives requires an active hand in contributing to basic and clinical sciences while keeping abreast of the most recent advancements. As an undergraduate in kinesiology at the University of Miami Biomechanics Laboratory, I investigated the recruitment pattern of the medial and lateral gastrocnemius heads in the cat across a continuum of postural and movement demands. To further study pathophysiologic mechanisms of diseases in light of a surgical subspecialty, I completed a post-sophomore fellowship with the Florida State Department of Anatomic Pathology, gaining familiarity with frozen biopsy criteria and processing, histologic examination of surgical specimens, special stains, cytologic interpretation, and fresh anatomic dissection during autopsies. Interested in diseases of the musculoskeletal system, I researched a new monoclonal antibody, O13, directed against the p30/32 gene of Ewing's sarcoma and its cross-reactivities with other small round blue cell tumors. Possessing a special interest in pediatric orthopedics, I participated in many of the Toland Hospital for Crippled Children activities over the course of three years, including an anesthesia clerkship, contributing to research conducted in the Gait Laboratory, participating in rounds and conferences, and observing a variety of orthopedic surgeries, the majority involving congenital hand abnormalities. It was here that I met Dr. Kathryn Douglass of Baylor University, who introduced me to the notion of approaching a possible hand fellowship from the direction of plastic surgery. Now, with my current interest in plastic and reconstructive surgery, I am presently exploring with Dr. William Schrock at Baylor University the potential of capitalizing upon the angiogenic properties of fibroblast growth factor in the creation of flaps for larger wound coverage secondary to burns or other major trauma.

Plasticity also is a key virtue during any residency. I am quick to learn new theories and techniques, and able to work well with a wide variety of patient and medical staff personalities. These attributes, coupled with patience and a good sense of humor, have been instrumental in

← Good use of specific details.

← The writer's name dropping is effective because he substantiates the references and explains their significance.

my growth thus far and will continue to be the basic foundation of my philosophy for success in plastic and reconstructive surgery.

## PERSONAL STATEMENT #4

In her personal statement for general surgery, this applicant effectively communicates her excitement about the field, as well as some of the personal characteristics that make her suited for it.

A good introduction, conveying her enthusiasm, though the sentence is somewhat long and unwiedly.

Exhilaration, anticipation, and a heightened awareness of myriad details—these were the emotions I experienced the first time I scrubbed into a case, a revision sternotomy and ASD repair, early in my third year of medical school. Hundreds of cases later, I am every bit as enthusiastic each time I step into the OR. In light of this and several other reasons, I am confident about my pursuit of a future career in surgery.

Although my interest in general surgery solidified during my recent clinical years, it began to develop far earlier. The thrill and personal satisfaction I perceived while shadowing a community surgeon was an early formative experience leading me to medical school in the first place. During my preclinical years, I marveled at the elegance and clinical relevance of human physiology and anatomy. Attending the Society of Thoracic Surgeons conference was an exciting introduction to the world of academic surgery.

By the end of my third-year surgery clerkship, I had a number of rich experiences reinforcing my interest. On the cardiothoracic service, I was enthralled by the intricate and immediate connection between anatomy and physiology, brought to life through surgical manipulation. During pediatric surgery, I was fascinated by the seamless integration of intraoperative technology, from HIDA scans to thoracoscopy, as well as the capacity to definitively cure patients of their pathology. My experience on the UCSF trauma service highlighted the unique role of the surgeon as "the whole doctor," caring for patients in their most critical hours, assuming full medical management and employing surgical interventions when indicated. Excited by the opportunity to effect drastic changes in patients' bodies and lives with such brief and elegant interventions, I knew that I wanted to pursue a career in surgery.

My unique personality and aptitudes make me a strong candidate as a future surgical trainee. I fully commit myself to my academic and personal endeavors with enthusiasm and passion; I enjoy hard work and take great personal satisfaction from seeing the immediate results of my efforts. My meticulous attention to detail and natural ability to work as part of a team have been among my strongest assets during my clinical clerkships, evident through my zeal for taking on challenging and often critical patients, coordinating efficiently with nursing staff and consulting services, and educating my ward teams by including the relevant literature with both unusual and "routine" patient presentations. These personal traits have no doubt benefited from years of teaching martial arts and playing soccer, even through the rigors of my third-year rotations and recent subinternships, highlighting my capacity for multitasking. I tend to be somebody who does not waver on important decisions, but rather, will deliberate seriously, resolve on a course of action, and move forward confidently. As I have embraced new technologies throughout my life, the rapid innovation prevalent in all fields of surgery is tremendously appealing to me.

Important traits for a surgeon.

I will likely further specialize, though I am not yet certain in which field. The ideal training program is one that can foster my growth into a seasoned surgeon with broad experience, comfortable operating autonomously and prepared for the rigors of fellowship and practice. I have always been passionate about teaching and mentoring, and therefore, I envision a future practice at an academic center. As such, I consider the availability of meaningful research and the opportunity to teach fellow residents and medical students important facets of a training program. Advancing patient care through clinical research and technological progress, from device design to translational research, has been one of the proud traditions of American surgery, one in which I plan to actively participate. The old adage that "no man is an island" rings true here, and, recognizing this, I will ideally practice in a university setting that can support this endeavor and offer important interdisciplinary and industry connections.

After discussing her own personal strengths, it is good to see that she recognizes the importance of working on a team.

As I stand ready to transition to the next level of my professional development as a surgeon, I am every bit as enthusiastic as I was standing before the operating table during that first case. I anxiously await the unique privilege of participating in such a rewarding and exciting field of patient care.

## PERSONAL STATEMENT #5

This candidate's statement is well written, presenting a cohesive story of a number of different experiences and influences that have steered her to emergency medicine. She also cites a number of experiences in which she has demonstrated her ability to flourish in leadership roles.

Saturday night news of a large fire flooded the airwaves. Fueled by the summer drought and the strongest winds in years, seven "uncontrollable" fires began blazing around our city. Over 500,000 people were under mandatory evacuation orders, many of whom sought refuge at Park Stone Stadium. Without hesitation and compelled by the situation, I threw on my white coat, slung my first-aid bag over my shoulder, and rushed to the stadium.

Controlled chaos best describes the scene that first day. With a small staff of health care workers and volunteers, we managed to put together "Centercomm Hospital," complete with fully functioning triage, acute care, pharmacy, and specialty teams. We assumed responsibility for 520 patients displaced from skilled nursing facilities, and 97 acute-care patients. Every night until the fires were out, I returned to Centercomm to work the graveyard shift, helping out every way I could.

I was always interested in emergency medicine, but this was my first taste of it outside of the ED—when the hallway became patient triage, the bar turned into a pharmacy, and the lounge served as an acute-care facility. The EM doctors took charge, and their knowledge, composure, and decision making was inspiring and ensured there would be no casualties. As I worked shoulder to shoulder with them, my aspirations to specialize in EM quickly solidified. I want to be the doctor who can see patients inside the hospital or in a parking lot if need be. I want to develop the skills, understanding, and experience to handle any situation.

Less than a year later, I found myself aboard the USNS Med-Help ship, a 1000-bed floating hospital on a humanitarian mission in the South Pacific. Working alongside EM residents and attendings on the shores of Papua New Guinea and Micronesia, we would see upwards of 600 patients a day. There, I was challenged to recall details of microbiology and dermatology (without referencing the Internet) while seeing everyone, from infants to the elderly, in the seemingly endless line. Patients often presented with vague symptoms and were limited by language barriers, further complicating my detective work. I experienced firsthand how a broad knowledge base is essential in EM.

I have been an organizer and leader throughout my life, able to multitask, motivate, and excel in many settings. During medical school I became the class president, helped begin the Border Health Project medical outreach, created the school's lending library, started an out-

---

She comes across as a good potential ER doc, ready to jump into the action whenever she is needed.

Another interesting experience, where she has been in the middle of the action, not an observer from the sidelines.

She describes a number of great accomplishments, as well as the characteristics that allowed her to achieve them.

door retreat for incoming students, helped shape the school's curriculum reforms, edited the Human Condition literary magazine, and was copresident of the EM Interest Group. I am proud to say that when I leave medical school, I will have left it a better place than when I began though new programs and lasting changes. I take on each commitment with enthusiasm and passion, supported by a strong work ethic and perseverance. I am an action-oriented person and see projects though to the finish. When challenges arise, I pride myself in my ability to think through the issues rationally, deliberate effectively, and act confidently.

Emergency medicine is where I find my passion, and it is a true fit for me in both personality and professional goals. I am ready for the challenges of EM and inspired to be a part of future solutions and improvements in the field. Seeing patients at first presentation promises to keep me mentally engaged and clinically sharp. My hands-on nature and effective leadership skills will be well served in the ED. Furthermore, it makes me proud that the ED practices true community medicine, where patients are helped regardless of ability to pay.

> An important facet of an ED physician's character.

The firestorm in my city was contained within 19 days, but the impressions made and lessons learned will be everlasting. A spark was lit inside of me, exposing me to a new side of emergency medicine and drawing me to a specialty I will soon call my own. I look forward to residency training to prepare me such that when the day comes, I will be able to manage the controlled chaos and help those in need.

> A good tie-in to the beginning of her statement, making it feel organized and polished.

## PERSONAL STATEMENT #6

This is a strong, well-written personal statement from a candidate in emergency medicine. He begins and ends describing the story of a meaningful patient interaction. However, he does it in a way that does not sound clichéd and that shows his empathy. His tone throughout the essay is comfortable and genuine. He lays out the qualities he thinks are important in an emergency medicine physician and then demonstrates he has developed those qualities.

As my cardiothoracic surgery fellow and I hurried to the ED, we learned that the Lifestar helicopter was transporting Mrs. M, a patient suffering from a Type A dissection with extension into her carotids. She was 81 years old and intubated, and unknown to the surgeons or the ED doctors was her baseline status and functioning. Whether to operate was now the question. This was the first family meeting I had attended that had such an urgency to it, yet it needed to be in a setting where time could stand still. Mrs. M's grandson pulled me aside and asked,

A good application of the experience to his future role as an ED physician.

"If she had the surgery, would she ever wake up?" I began to realize the power of information and just how important decision making in the emergency room was upon outcomes for patients. Finally, Mr. M decided we should go forward with the surgery, and within minutes we were in the OR and starting to open.

He comes across as genuine and humble, while still listing a number of accomplishments.

To me, emergency medicine is about leadership, teamwork, and humility. Contributing to my teams and leading them to success has always been important. I have served in this capacity many times, whether it was teaching as a Human Biology Course Associate, working on our student LCME committee, or being part of clinical teams on the wards. Our struggles and triumphs as groups have taught me leadership skills and made me a stronger teammate, knowing how to trust in others and when to ask for help. As an emergency physician, I hope to be a colleague in the truest sense of the word so that patients will be best served by our medical care. The emergency department is also a place that reflects the pulse of a community—it is a place where patients of all backgrounds and cultures arrive, and for me, this is something I desire as part of my practice. Having so much of my family in India and spread around the globe has given me the opportunity to travel broadly and interact with different cultures. Working as a clinician at our student-run free clinic has taught me about the impact doctors can have in underserved populations and the medical needs of my own community. Caring for a diverse population of patients is something that drives me and draws me toward a career in emergency medicine.

I first learned through my undergraduate research the value of contributing new knowledge to the fields of which I am a part, and I have had the chance to broaden my research experiences during medical school. My time working in a pediatric cardiology lab showed me how an understanding of signaling in heart development could relate to the presentation of a young infant with cyanosis. Now, as I embark on a clinical research project to assess risk stratification among ED patients with sepsis, I will have the chance to take ownership of a project from the IRB stage through data analysis and completion of a thesis. This opportunity to directly contribute toward evidence-based medicine is something I find intellectually interesting, challenging, and rewarding.

After the surgery, I was not sure whether Mrs. M would make it through the night, but the next morning she was extubated, and the first thing she asked me was, "Doctor, do you watch Grey's Anatomy on TV? I watch every week." Mrs. M is a patient I won't forget easily. She taught me the importance of listening to patients and families, the need for critical decision making sometimes without clear evidence, the sense of teamwork and responsibility that comes with caring for emergency department patients, and the feelings of reward when we, as physicians, are able to provide the care that patients need.

A great return to the original story, with a very natural, human interaction and a happy ending.

## PERSONAL STATEMENT BY DISCIPLINE

The examples below of personal statements from a range of fields can be used to see how some personal statements address issues particular to a specialty choice. Students use these statements to describe why they chose the particular specialty. You can see from the examples that there are many and varied reasons for students to become attracted to a particular career. For more examples of personal statements, got to Firstaidteam.com.

### ANESTHESIOLOGY

I have met each challenge in my life with hard work and dedication. Whether it was training for a marathon, working full time while going to school, or starting a family, I knew that by working hard I would succeed. That's why when I had to take time off during my undergraduate education due to the financial strains of living in New York and starting a family, I knew this would be a momentary delay in achieving my lifelong goal of becoming a doctor. After my wife and I were able to obtain some financial security, I finished my BS in physiology at the University of Arizona and was accepted into St. Lucas University School of Medicine.

St. Lucas University is located on the beautiful island of St. Kitts in the British West Indies. Most of the classes are taught by retired professors from U.S. medical schools. Besides the excellent education I received, the life experiences my wife and I gained living in a foreign country without the amenities of the United States were priceless. We will never forget washing our clothes in the sink or searching for propane gas to cook with on our stove.

I finished my basic sciences with a 3.96 GPA. I went on to score a 246/95 on the USMLE Step 1. My high score placed me at Douglas Medical Center (DMC) in Fresno, California, for all of my clinical rotations. DMC is an excellent county hospital affiliated with University Hospital School of Medicine, which accepts the best students from St. Lucas University into its clerkship program. DMC provided me with a well-rounded clinical experience and prepared me well for the USMLE Step 2, on which I scored a 255/98. Also, during my surgery core rotation my beautiful baby girl was born.

Although I have found all my clinical rotations interesting, I experienced the most excitement from my time in anesthesiology. Anesthesiology offers me the opportunity to integrate my basic science knowledge with clinical care. In no other rotation did I have the hands-on application of basic sciences; every OR case was a mini-experiment in pharmacology and physiology. The fast pace and the constant demand for rapid, clear thinking made my time in anesthesiology nothing but exhilarating. My rotation also showed me the various duties of anesthesiologists beyond the OR and the integral part they play in labor and delivery, the emergency room, the intensive care unit, and the management of pain.

On a personal level, I find my time away from medicine rejuvenating as well. Spending time running, mountain biking, surfing, and being with my wife and daughter enables me to return to work refreshed.

My career goal is to enter a university-based anesthesiology program. I believe my strong science knowledge base, clinical experience, and ability to make quick decisions are well suited for anesthesiology. I am highly detail oriented and enjoy being part of a cohesive medical care team. I look forward to the education, practice, and research opportunities available in anesthesiology.

# DERMATOLOGY

During medical school I became involved in research with Dr. Flynn in the Department of Anatomy and Neurobiology at Medical State University. I utilized the skills I had obtained through my bachelor's degree in visual arts toward our project. The manual dexterity I acquired through artwork allowed me ease in performing microscopic, stereotactic surgeries; my work with chemistry in photographic development proved useful in immunohistochemical staining of our injection sites; and my illustrative abilities were applied in mapping the axonal projections of the nuclei. My background in art has provided me a breadth of knowledge that enriches my approach to medicine. I continue in my tradition of challenging myself in new areas: entering medicine with a background in art, presenting and publishing research, and now endeavoring to become a dermatologist.

Dermatology is the field in which many of my interests and skills converge. The pattern, texture, and color of artwork are discussed in a similar manner as skin pathology is described. I am confident in my ability to appreciate and interpret the visual manifestation of disease. I enjoy creating a precise image of primary and secondary lesions in order to develop a thorough and accurate differential diagnosis.

Comprehension of histopathology is essential to the study of dermatology. Through my prior work in a surgical pathology lab and experience performing biopsies in my dermatology rotations, I have acquired an appreciation of the processes involved in and the necessity of obtaining adequate samples of tissue for diagnosis and treatment. I have refined my procedural skills through my experience in microscopic surgery and in suturing Mohs repairs.

As with most areas of medicine, relating to patients with understanding and empathy is a priority in dermatology. I have developed my interpersonal skills by interacting with a variety of people through my study of art, my residence abroad within a different culture, and my current work in medicine. Open communication with others has come with ease. I value the mutual respect and trust that develops between physician and patient; I witness the healing effect that such a relationship has in treating patients.

As a field that continuously changes through medical and technological advances, dermatology encourages the ability to engage in research. Having completed a study observing trends in basal cell carcinoma in an individual surgery practice, I am currently coauthoring a chapter on different types of skin cancer, to be published in a medical journal designed for general practitioners. I anticipate continuing in research throughout residency and my career in academic dermatology.

One of my greatest motivations in studying medicine is the opportunity to study and learn throughout my career. My introduction to dermatology in medical school generated great interest and a desire to learn much more about its practice and new developments. I appreciate the expanse of material involved and knowledge yet to acquire in the study of dermatology.

Dermatology is a field in which I can continue to challenge myself. Through my rotations in surgery and general dermatology, I have discovered that it is the field of medicine to which I am best suited. I eagerly anticipate engaging in and contributing to the study of the skin and its manifestation of disease. My studies in art and involvement in research have enriched my medical education and will continue to provide a unique and enlightened approach to the practice of dermatology.

## EMERGENCY MEDICINE

During my junior year at UCLA, I became certified as an emergency medical technician (EMT), a decision that had a profound effect on my life. I was subsequently hired by UCLA Emergency Medical Services (EMS) and staffed the campus ambulance, serving as a first responder for all medical aid calls on the UCLA campus and neighboring communities. There was a tremendous sense of responsibility in being the first medical provider on scene to assess and provide treatment for potentially unstable patients in unpredictable environments. In addition to cementing my desire to attend medical school, my experience with UCLA EMS introduced me to the field of emergency medicine.

At the completion of my first year of medical school, I was awarded the Student Research Committee Fellowship. This fellowship supported a research project designed to evaluate the safety and efficacy of external cardiac pacing of patients with symptomatic bradycardia by paramedics in the prehospital setting. This two-and-a-half-year project was supervised by the medical director of the San Francisco Fire Department. The data demonstrated a trend toward increased survival among patients treated with external cardiac pacing compared to those treated with conventional therapy alone. Based upon this data, the State of California Emergency Medical Services Commission approved external cardiac pacing as first-line therapy for this patient population, permitting EMS providers throughout the state to perform this procedure.

Throughout medical school, I was aware of my interest in emergency medicine but made a conscious effort not to prematurely exclude other specialties. I thought I might find one clerkship to stand out among them all, calling me to devote my life to it. Instead, I found them all incredibly challenging and fulfilling, particularly those experiences requiring immediate decisions to be made, procedures to be performed, and, most of all, trips to the emergency department. My greatest sense of achievement, regardless of the clerkship, was when I was caring for patients with an acute illness, exacerbation of a chronic disease, or a traumatic injury.

I am eager to begin my residency training and look forward to expanding my knowledge base, becoming more adept in assessment, diagnosis, and treatment in the acute setting, and gaining the experience necessary to become a well-rounded, confident physician. I hope to train in a facility with a culturally diverse patient population and a broad variety of trauma, medical illness, pediatric emergency experience, EMS exposure, and clinical research opportunities. In addition to supporting my growth as a physician, I want to train at a program that supports my development outside the hospital, encouraging continued participation in my personal interests, such as exercising, camping, and traveling.

My long-term goals include attending in a high-acuity, academically oriented, Level 1 trauma center that conducts high-quality clinical research. I am also interested in pursuing a fellowship in emergency medical services to enhance my ability to promote quality prehospital care. My understanding of the field of emergency medicine has vastly matured from my days as an EMT. I now realize that the realm of the emergency physician extends well beyond the back of an ambulance or the entrance to a hospital. Emergency physicians are regularly faced with the entire spectrum of medical and surgical disease, requiring immense skill, diagnostic acumen, and empathy for both the frightened patient and concerned family members. In this era of managed care and cost containment, emergency physicians must be conservative in their diagnostic evaluations, yet remain aggressive in their pursuit of excluding acutely life-threatening illnesses. More importantly, emergency physicians serve as powerful patient advocates and valuable liaisons between the medical community and general public.

I feel I have proven myself capable of compassionate, competent care during my clinical years and have no doubt that I will greatly benefit from residency training in emergency medicine. I eagerly await the next phase of my education and welcome the challenges and excitement it will bring.

## GENERAL SURGERY

"Far and away the best prize that life offers is the chance to work hard at work worth doing." —Theodore Roosevelt

My parents carefully measured out their wisdom like coffee grounds: shake hands firmly … look everyone in the eyes … never complain … work harder … smile and enjoy … always do the right thing. The experience of living has been the water that percolates through these lessons, ultimately defining my cardinal principles of work and life.

Passion, beneficence, and excellence are fundamental to these principles and drive my pursuit of general surgery. Passion. Every day I strive to deserve the privilege of practicing surgery. From my earliest research experiences with cardiac surgery in dogs, I have aspired to learn enough, work enough, and care enough to earn the trust of my future patients and colleagues. This passion is my sustaining force. It is the excitement that kept me up through four emergency appendectomies starting at midnight. It is the calm that steadied my hand to insert a chest tube and drop a central line at a 4 A.M. trauma. It is the sympathy that gave me patience to hear Mr. H.'s story detailing each evening's mighty struggle to stuff a volleyball-sized hernia back into his abdomen for 22 years before coming in for surgery.

This passion motivates me to be a great surgeon. Beneficence. I am devoted to improving the way things work; I believe that basic scientific research and medical education are essential for enhanced patient care. However, administrative efforts outside the immediate realm of medicine are also important to forging advancements in health care. After identifying a deficit in funding of student research, I developed a proposal for an endowed fellowship for scientific investigation. Resulting from a combination of numerous meetings, letters, and a big piece of my heart, the alumni trustees, medical center administrators, and university financiers agreed to endow over half a million dollars for a fellowship to support medical student research. This fellowship is funded for perpetuity and provides $25,000 to one student annually to pursue independent research. The first fellowship was awarded this past spring to a promising second-year who wants to cure cancer. Whether or not she achieves her goal, it is the spirit and talent of thousands of students and scientists like her that impel progress in medical science. My desire and ability to produce tangible improvements will benefit the field of general surgery.

Excellence. I am always searching for ways to improve myself as a human being and as a surgeon. Because a problem-based curriculum afforded a flexible schedule, I was able to regularly participate in service projects, most often visiting elementary schools to discuss safe sex and drugs with high-risk children. Frequently, later in the evenings, I helped treat sexually transmitted diseases at an indigent clinic. I chose to explore fields related to a career in surgery through a year of independent research. By putting my head down to get through the daily grind, I overcame the obstacles of gel exposure snafus, cell culture contamination, and editing for publication, to be productive in basic and clinical projects. My achievements in this previously unfamiliar territory—I was a philosophy major in college—have given me the experience, confidence, and motivation to support research as I move on to my next stage of training.

This commitment to self-improvement maximizes my abilities and opportunities. By remaining true to my cardinal principles I will enthusiastically strive toward, and hopefully lead, the promotion of patient care as a surgeon. Benefiting from my experiences and equipped with knowledge, effort, and spirit, I am prepared to continue such work worth doing.

## INTERNAL MEDICINE

Choosing a specialty in medicine, like medical school in general, is a unique experience that will make a tremendous impact on the rest of your personal and professional life. Many students are dead set on specific careers before they even make their first shaky incision in gross anatomy. Others think they know which field they ultimately want to pursue, only to discover later on that everything about their chosen specialty disagrees with them. Then there are students like me, who go to medical school armed with the knowledge that ultimately they'll become doctors, but not really knowing which kind.

When I began my medical education, I was honestly surprised to learn that many of my new classmates were already committed to specific paths, some of them with extensive research and experience in their fields of choice. My older brother, who changed his mind at least three times before he applied for residency, had advised me to wait until the clinical years so that I could make an informed choice, and that had been my plan from the beginning. But as more and more of my friends began narrowing down their choices in the first two years of school, my plan to wait to make a decision suddenly felt like procrastination. Nevertheless, with limited clinical exposure and plenty of studying to keep me busy, I resigned myself to following my brother's advice and to wait until my third year.

Making the abrupt shift from bookworm to third-year clinical clerk was both a nerve-wracking and exciting prospect. Although we had discussed the doctor-patient relationship and the art of medicine during the first two years of school, the opportunities to practice those concepts were few and far between. Interviewing patients for an hour once a week didn't seem like a realistic picture of things to come (it wasn't). I was nervous about balancing a schedule that I knew would be hectic, being responsible for patients while trying to read about diagnosis, pathophysiology, and treatment. Mostly, I was excited that I'd finally have the chance to learn how to care for people and to explore possible future careers. My introduction to clinical medicine was cut short, though. That fall, my mother was scheduled for extensive spinal surgery in an effort to relieve years of discomfort, and I was granted a leave of absence by the school and returned to Los Angeles to be with her for the next six months. When I returned in the winter to begin my clerkships, I realized that it was impossible to finish all the necessary requirements in time to graduate in 1999, and I became a member of the class of 2000.

In retrospect, taking the extra time was a serendipitous blessing in disguise. It allowed me to objectively approach the clinical clerkships without rushing to make a career decision. As I rotated through the various specialties, I began to get a better understanding of what I found interesting. Initially, radiology was one field that intrigued me, combining technology and intuition to clarify disease pathology. I signed up for electives and became involved in research, hoping to further stoke my interest and solidify my desire to possibly pursue radiology as a career. Instead, it had the opposite effect. I quickly realized that although I found the images and technology amazing, I sorely missed the direct one-to-one patient contact that we had talked about during the first two years and that we had been introduced to during the third year.

People often say that the lessons learned along the way are what make a journey worthwhile, that the opportunities to gain insight and acquire knowledge can be easily missed if you simply focus on traveling from point A to point B. It is this idea that embodies my experiences in medical school and that has led me to my decision to pursue internal medicine as a career. What I've realized is that the things I find most rewarding are developing relationships with patients and being in an environment that fosters continuity of care. Caring for patients from admission to discharge and following up long term to provide for their health care needs is what I ultimately want to base my career as a physician upon. Everyone who goes to medical school has unique experiences that lead them to discover their own personal niches. To me, internal medicine covers a wide spectrum of disease pathology while allowing personal relationships to develop with patients, offering the ideal blend of academic challenge and personal fulfillment. In this way, I can share in the lessons learned from other people's journeys while I continue on my own.

## INTERNAL MEDICINE–PEDIATRICS

During a clerkship in my third year of medical school in my hometown of St. Louis, I was struck by a comment made by a nurse one morning before rounds. She recognized my name as being the same as two previous physicians who had cared for her and her family. These physicians were my grandfather and great-grandfather. She then went on to tell me that my great-grandfather had delivered her, and that my grandfather had cared for her during her childhood at his office. What moved me most about what she said was how tangible my relationship to my grandfather had become, and the very meaningful impact they had made on this nurse's life. I chose to go into medicine during college on my own accord, yet the fact that I have two previous family members who were a part of this profession gives me a profound sense of integrity and responsibility.

Throughout my schooling, working directly with people has always interested me. My experience while attending Loyola University in New Orleans, where I worked as a health assistant for two years, helped me realize that I would succeed in medicine. A month-long trip during my senior year of college to a village in Nicaragua challenged my ability to communicate and work with people, and solidified even more my desire to study medicine. Multiple involvements during medical school, such as coordinating a student-run clinic on several Saturdays, supported my interest in primary care and at the same time fostered leadership skills and a better sense of team spirit.

My rotation in internal medicine at a Veterans Administration hospital, the first of my third-year clerkships, initiated a desire to pursue the specialty of internal medicine. I was exposed to patients with conditions ranging from asthma to resistant HIV, which I found to be intellectually challenging and professionally fulfilling. Later in the course of my third year, my exposure to pediatrics paralleled my experience in internal medicine, and my learning curve took off even more. Now I find myself using the medical literature more frequently to support my rising interests. I find clinic to be a rewarding interaction and a wonderful chance to counsel parents/guardians. My interest in combined internal medicine and pediatrics as a specialty solidified at the end of my third year of medical school. Primary care is my interest. Seeing and helping patients of a wide age range and of various clinical presentations is what I want to focus on. My enthusiasm for internal medicine and pediatrics is both complementary and synergistic. I intend to take full advantage of the training offered and become an extremely competent, well-trained, and respected physician. In short, I want to be a resource for my patients and a source of appropriate medical care. The variety of patients in this setting draws me toward this field and will keep me continually interested and enthusiastic throughout the course of my career. The fact that I will comprehensively train in treating children and adults alike compels me to pursue internal medicine/pediatrics.

The bridge and relationship between the two areas, in my perception, are well connected. In my student experience, both internal medicine and pediatrics hold a common approach to patients. Their corresponding knowledge funds are both diverse and comprehensive. I look forward to being able to employ that knowledge competently and effectively throughout the course of my career.

## NEUROLOGY

Among many other things I have learned in medical school, I have come to the opinion that the role people assume in the somewhat conservative field of medicine involves wearing a relatively thick professional mask. This is not necessarily negative, as there is no denying that an air of competence and compassion is certainly inspiring to patients. However, perhaps in part because I have never been a particularly accomplished actor myself, I find it all the more interesting when that mask is taken off and the true self emerges through all the layers of professionalism. When one truly enjoys his job, the most fun and energetic part of his personality emerges. When a patient presents with a rare and interesting disease, or when there is a captivating diagnostic problem, physicians who love their jobs bring their full intellect and attention to bear. Then, amazingly, all the layers of formality and pride are peeled away to reveal an enthusiasm to solve the problem and share their knowledge and excitement, which I find extremely infectious. In that moment when a diagnostic test is performed, or when a novel scientific result is on the brink of revealing itself, we are all transformed into a curious child all over again, whether we are students, attendings, or Nobel laureates.

I have chosen neurology as a specialty because it is a field that fascinates me to that point of enthusiasm—an enthusiasm that I wish to share with my patients, future colleagues, and students. I believe that the central nervous system has so much intrinsic interest that it draws a higher proportion of physicians who are genuinely captivated by their field. An important benefit from this is that it provides for the opportunity to work with others with similar enthusiasm, enabling a more enjoyable and educational experience. The clinical work is interesting and satisfying to me because of the close association of findings on the history and physical exam with the lesion location and etiology. I also find some of the more subtle cognitive deficits from brain pathology to be extremely interesting, shedding light on the function of arguably the most important, complex, and uniquely human organ of the body.

I feel that neurology remains a final frontier of biomedicine, with many clinical and scientific truths yet to be unraveled and translated for the benefit of human health and knowledge. In an era when molecular genetic approaches are rapidly revolutionizing the field of medicine, neurology stands poised to gain significant therapeutic benefit, as many cerebral disorders appear beyond our present ability to cure. It is especially fulfilling for me to be able to offer help in these areas where it is sorely needed, and I anticipate a day when we have the power to prevent or cure intractable diseases like ALS or Alzheimer's disease as research efforts from the Decade of the Brain yield fruit. During my third year of medical school, I had the exciting opportunity to work on a basic problem in neurophysiology at the National Institutes of Health with a fellowship from the Howard Hughes Medical Institute. From my experience at the NIH, I have gained an enormous appreciation for the scientific efforts in elucidating the workings of the nervous system and the process involved in finding treatments for specific disorders. I was able to meet very accomplished physicians in the research arena who serve as my role models. The experience has been instrumental in shaping my career aspirations to pursue a biomedical research career, which appeals to the creative side of my personality. In addition to medical and scientific impact, neurology and neuroscience are fields whose questions have far-reaching implications for apparently unrelated fields such as religion and philosophy. By providing insights into mechanisms of behavior and consciousness, it addresses critical questions related to our essential humanity, which I find extremely intellectually stimulating.

I hope that with my sincere passion for the field, a diligent work ethic, and a good-natured team attitude, I will be able to help alleviate suffering from neurologic disease and simultaneously learn about how our minds work. For the future, I hope to be a part of the forefront of our advancing understanding of the neurological sciences and use that knowledge to heal our patients and train others interested in the field. For these reasons, I have chosen to specialize in neurology, with an eventual goal of practicing, teaching, and conducting research at an academic hospital.

## NEUROSURGERY

Very few matriculating medical students can realistically determine their future career choices. We all enter with the altruistic goals of becoming caring physicians and making a significant contribution to medicine. As laypersons, we do not grasp the breadth of medicine and often are unaware of its specialization. I myself come from a medical family background and therefore had a somewhat greater exposure to medicine, but I was in no way qualified upon entering medical school to reach a conclusion regarding a career in a particular specialty. In spite of this, I always entertained the notion of becoming a neurosurgeon.

The central nervous system represented to me the most intriguing and complex human organ system. During my first two medical school years, I was fascinated by the study of the central nervous system, including its intricate three-dimensional anatomy, physiology, and pathology. During my third year of medical school, I gravitated toward the surgical specialties. I had the opportunity to become a member of the University of Mississippi neurosurgical team and participate in many neurosurgical procedures, an experience that I greatly enjoyed. The meticulous surgeries and the application of intricate anatomical knowledge and physiology markedly impressed me. Neurosurgery offers the challenge of not merely maintaining a patient's life, but sustaining their spirit, intelligence, and personality. Unlike almost any other field, neurosurgery deals with the elements that contribute to our consciousness and make us human. These experiences led to the coalescence of my decision to pursue a career in neurosurgery.

My professional goals include the completion of a comprehensive neurosurgical residency training in conjunction with basic science research experience and subsequently pursuing a career in academic neurosurgery. The academic discourse and the intellectual stimulation afforded in an academic environment are appealing as well as the opportunity to participate in the endeavor of furthering the scope of our knowledge. I will strive to follow the clinician/scientist model that I admire and hope to develop a research program complementary to my clinical interests. On my part, I bring the desire to work hard, participate actively in my own education, and make a positive contribution to my residency program and neurosurgery.

I believe that my credentials to pursue a career in neurosurgery include my strong academic background. I began my undergraduate education at Clemson University, where I was elected to the Phi Eta Sigma freshman honor society before transferring to Georgia Tech University because of my desire to be closer to my family secondary to an illness in the family. At Georgia Tech University, I was elected to the Phi Beta Kappa honor society and received the College of Liberal Arts and Sciences (CLAS) Outstanding Scholar Award, an award conferred on the graduating CLAS student with the highest grade point average. At the University of Mississippi School of Medicine, I was awarded the Board of Trustees Academic Scholarship and continued my strong academic performance. Additionally, I was honored with the Basic Science Research Scholarship on the basis of an original research proposal involving the synaptic integration and information processing carried out in a single nerve cell. The research culminated in a poster presentation at the Eastern Student Research Forum. I have used that experience to pursue neurosurgical research relating to spinal cord injury that is currently in progress.

Aside from academics, I have been active in the Mississippi Medical Association and have visited that state capital on several occasions to observe and participate in the lobbying process. Currently, I am serving on the Mississippi Medical Association's Public Relations Council and am participating in the planning of programs designed to increase membership in our professional medical associations and raise physician awareness concerning current medically related political issues in the rapidly changing managed care market. For recreation, I am an active participant in pickup basketball games and make an effort to weight lift on a consistent basis. I have also maintained an interest in the area of technology applications and recently published an article concerning the Internet's medical applications. I am also currently in the process of constructing a home page for the University of Mississippi's Neurosurgery Department.

## OBSTETRICS AND GYNECOLOGY

While my path to becoming a physician has always been a straight one, my interest in the field of obstetrics and gynecology has come full circle. During vacations from college, I worked in the office of an obstetrician-gynecologist in Washington, D.C. Excited by the breadth of patients that he saw, I was also impressed by the surgical nature of the field. Thus, I began medical school believing I would one day be an obstetrician-gynecologist. During my first two years of medical school, I drifted from this belief and considered the areas of medicine and pediatrics. However, the experiences of my third year helped me to better focus my interests. While I was impressed with the thought processes involved in the evaluation of patients during my medicine rotation, I was often frustrated by the inability to physically do something to help. During my pediatrics rotation, I was amazed by the young body's ability to heal, although I often felt this healing had less to do with the medical team than with the body's natural defenses. The resiliency of my patients, coupled with the opportunity to practice preventative medicine and primary care, initially left me thinking I would enter the field of pediatrics. I began obstetrics and gynecology excited to see babies delivered, but otherwise completely naïve that this was my calling. After just a short time on the rotation, I found myself feeling not obligated to read at home, but excited to learn more about the problems I had faced that day. As in pediatrics, it was refreshing to see a generally young, healthy patient population. However, unlike in pediatrics, in obstetrics and gynecology there was often the opportunity to physically do something that would lead to beneficial outcomes. I look forward to the opportunities to combine prevention and treatment strategies to keep my patients healthy.

I see my career occupied not just with medicine, but with health care policy and management. During medical school, I have come to appreciate the quantity and complexity of health care issues today. I realize that as a medical student and resident I must focus on learning the facts and skills needed to be a successful clinician, but I also believe that knowledge of and participation in the vast number of health care decisions being made each day is imperative for a clinician. For this reason, I plan to constantly continue my education, both in the professional setting and by earning a degree in either public policy or business administration. With knowledge and credentials, I will become actively involved in creating and implementing health care policy that focuses on the needs of patients rather than of insurance companies or administrators.

I have always had an interest in education and community outreach, and my goal is to make a difference in the policies of the health care system. Access to health care in rural and urban communities is a serious problem that our nation faces, and I feel obligated to use my knowledge and background to help, whether on a local or national level. My desire to improve communities in need is long-standing. An important influence on this interest began with my high school sociology teacher and friend, Mr. C. Progressive in his requirement of 20 community service hours per semester, he stressed the importance of reaching out to others. Because of his hands-on approach, I learned about my responsibility to help others.

Unfortunately, Mr. C. died of complications arising from AIDS in February 1994. At his memorial service, a speaker asked the mourners to look around the crowded auditorium full of people whose lives Mr. C. had touched, a group that represented just a fraction of the whole. The speaker reminded us that if each of us could touch just one other person in the same way, and that person would touch one more person, and so on, the memory of Mr. C. would never be lost. I choose medicine as my way to impart knowledge, to give hope, and to touch others with love and understanding.

## OPHTHALMOLOGY

A person who feels a specific calling in his life is a fortunate person. While we never know what the future may hold for us, having a definite direction in which to travel is a real blessing and a rare occurrence. My calling to pursue a career in ophthalmology came after three years of dedication to studying the human body, interacting with patients, and "trying on" various medical specialties in my third year of rotations. My interest in the eye, however, began in my second year, during the ophthalmology section of the mechanisms of disease class. I found the intricacy and vastly varied pathology of the visual system to be fascinating. Even more interesting was the small amount of clinical exposure to ophthalmology in our third-year curriculum. Except for four afternoons spent in ophthalmologists' clinic during the general practice clerkship, the eye was not discussed much, but I thirsted for more knowledge in this area.

My firsthand experience with ophthalmology came under the guidance of a second-year ophthalmology resident, whom I greatly respect spiritually, personally, and professionally. I met him at a church youth-group function, and he invited me to visit the triage area of the emergency department. I spent a day in the emergency room with him, where he showed me patient after patient, each case more interesting than the one before. The patients were very concerned about their vision. As he went through the general exam with me, pointing out the varying pathology, he calmed each patient by explaining the details of their illness and treatment. After watching him during a few more visits to the ER, I knew I wanted to be this type of physician. Furthermore, after a day in the OR with an attending physician and a few discussions with my student advisors, I knew I wanted to treat these types of patients.

During medical school, my family and friends, who remain a very important part of my life, complemented my influences in the medical field by providing support and fellowship in a nonacademic arena. My mother, a school psychologist, and my father, a retired USAF pilot, continue to provide counsel from my hometown in Florida. My brother, a lawyer (in a firm that represents doctors and hospitals), also encourages me from his home in Florida. Following their example, I have been able to establish a strong work ethic and moral basis from which to guide my career. I have also been fortunate enough to pass along my experiences and advice to the youth at my church during church functions, including the annual youth choir trip. Throughout medical school, I believe I have learned the value of hard work, punctuality, discipline, knowledge, and a good attitude. These values are contagious, and I look forward to bringing them to whatever work environment I encounter.

Ophthalmology contains all of what I love about the medical profession: medicine, surgery, treatment of both the old and the young, primary care, and specialized procedures. Ophthalmology is also a dynamic field, with frequent new advances in preserving or improving people's vision. I will enjoy the challenge of keeping up with new developments and will take satisfaction in contributing to that growth. Having a calling that will grant me the opportunity to positively impact people's eyesight and health while offering them compassion during a stressful time will be a rewarding experience and a rich personal blessing.

## ORTHOPEDIC SURGERY

Running has been an integral part of my life since high school, when I became involved in cross-country and track. During college and medical school I have continued running and have completed several road races and two triathlons. Running has taught me the value of patience, dedication, and perseverance; provided an outlet for stress; and kept me physically and mentally fit. It was also through running that I began to appreciate the importance of the musculoskeletal system. I would periodically sustain various sports-related injuries, which led to my first exposure to the field of orthopedic surgery.

While I believe the traits I developed as a runner prepared me for the rigors of surgery, my interest in orthopedic surgery stems from my fascination with the effects of structure on function. From fashioning various creations out of Legos as a child to constructing electronic circuits and building off-road remote control cars as an adolescent, I have always enjoyed learning about how things work. As a young teen, I built a cabin with my cousin and uncle. I was enthralled during each step of the process: drafting the plans, setting the foundation, constructing the walls, laying the roof, and weatherproofing the exterior.

The opportunity to visualize and mentally construct objects in three dimensions combined with an interest in how the building blocks of life are put together attracted me to organic chemistry and biochemistry. In these courses I learned how minor changes in molecular structure could have drastic effects on chemical properties. While exploring the structure and function of cells and molecules through research, I became increasingly fascinated with the anatomy and physiology of the human body. During medical school, I conducted research using a rat model to investigate the effects of interleukin-10 on inflammation associated with venous thrombosis. This experience allowed me to gain familiarity with operating on rats under a low-power microscope, examining and preparing surgical specimens, and taking gross and histologic photographs. I particularly enjoyed operating on the rats, which enhanced my interest in surgery.

In addition to acquiring new knowledge via research, I also enjoy sharing knowledge with others through teaching. My mentors demonstrated time and time again how the combination of hard work and talent could allow a person to reach his or her fullest potential. My father, one of my greatest mentors as well as a physician, has shown me that happiness and tremendous personal satisfaction can be acquired by making a difference in patients' lives. It is these principles as well as factual concepts that I strive to share with students. As a senior in college I helped other prospective medical students prepare for the MCAT by teaching classes for Kaplan Educational Centers. In the year before I began medical school, I was a teaching assistant for an honors organic chemistry laboratory and discussion group.

In medical school I have experienced tremendous personal growth and have focused my career objectives. Key elements that I have used to achieve continued success include maintaining a good sense of humor, learning how to work effectively with a variety of different patient and medical staff personalities, spending time with friends and family, and having interests outside of medicine. I will bring to my residency energy, enthusiasm, a strong work ethic, and a constant desire to learn new things and share ideas with others. I am seeking a challenging, engaging environment in which to learn and deliver high-quality care to patients. I hope to help myself and others fully develop our talents so that our patients can achieve optimal health, mobility, and function. I am looking forward to a challenging career in orthopedic surgery involving patient care, teaching, and future discovery.

## OTOLARYNGOLOGY

I have always been driven by meeting new challenges, and it is that aspect of otolaryngology that is most attractive to me. The spectrum of ENT, ranging from microsurgical procedures of the ear to large head and neck cancer surgery, is one enjoyed by few medical specialties. ENT also encompasses allergy, infectious disease, and endocrinology, to name a few areas, and it is this broad scope of possibilities that has drawn me to the field. I am excited about working in a surgical specialty that gives me the opportunity to provide both primary and specialized care to patients of all ages.

I gained exposure to ENT during a surgical elective that was part of my third-year surgery clerkship. I had just completed my internal medicine rotation and was considering a career in medicine when I was introduced to otolaryngology. The ENT physicians I had the pleasure of working with demonstrated great knowledge of general medicine combined with excellent surgical skills. They had very good rapport with their patients, and they appeared to be some of the most satisfied physicians I had seen in my years as a medical student. They gave me hands-on experience in both the clinic and the operating room. By the end of my surgery rotation, I knew that I would be happiest pursuing ENT as my specialty.

I have worked hard during medical school to put myself in a position to be competitive for residency training in the specialty of my choice. I believe my work ethic stems from being raised on a dry-land cotton farm in West Texas. I was taught that people are judged by their integrity and their hard work, and any effort I made was expected to be the best I could muster. These values have served me well in all aspects of my life. They have provided me academic success at all levels, and they have been reflected in my clinical evaluations in each rotation. I also believe that my success in medical school is due in large part to my balance between my family and school. I am married to a terrific woman, who has encouraged me at each turn, and I have a wonderful four-year-old daughter who keeps my world and priorities in perspective.

Outside of school and family, I enjoy golfing, hunting, fishing, and exercising. I have recently taken an interest in photography, and I plan to concentrate this hobby on wildlife and nature photography. My wife and I are expecting our second child, and we are all eagerly anticipating the arrival of the next addition to our family. This is an exciting, changing time in our lives, made all the more so by the prospect of a career in otolaryngology.

## PATHOLOGY

"To Dr. Karen, with love, Timmy and family." This was the inscription on the inside cover of an 1899 edition of *The Merck Manual* that Timmy's mom gave me on the last day of my pediatrics rotation. At the bottom of the page, in royal blue marker, was the scribbled signature of a three-and-a-half-year-old, "Tim."

Timmy had mitochondrial encephalomyopathy. The clinical picture of his illness early on was that of failure to thrive, and he continued to have waxing and waning episodes of muscle weakness and neurological deficits, including a significant degree of hearing loss. He taught me to sign "lion" and "tiger" because these were two of his favorite stuffed animals; the reason he taught me to sign "see ya later, alligator" is self-evident. He and his family struggled through several misdiagnoses, including cerebral palsy, until the presence of "ragged red fibers" on a muscle biopsy led to the correct diagnosis. I remember wondering at the time what ragged red fibers looked like under the microscope, and wishing that I could see them myself.

Then there was Chase. He was six months old, an ex-23-week preemie, third of triplets. He had spent all but four days of his life in the hospital, suffering from multiple complications stemming from his birth history and necrotizing enterocolitis in his perinatal period. His last night was also my last on-call during my pediatrics rotation. I wept after watching my attending stand stoically with his hand on the shoulder of Chase's mother as she held her dying boy. The next day, after just 15 minutes of sleep, I was working in a primary care clinic that was about 25 miles away. I drove 70 miles an hour back to the hospital after receiving a call that the pathologist wanted me to attend the autopsy. Nothing unexpected was found on the gross, but I was strangely excited a few days later when the pathologist showed me the micro, which revealed gut bacteria in nearly every organ system.

Before entering medical school, I decided to be a pediatrician. As pathology continued to intrigue me during clinical rotations, I faced a dilemma. Pathology was exciting, interesting, and fun, but the lack of patient contact gave me serious doubts. Would I feel like less of a doctor if I never met another Timmy or held another Chase? I was born to blue-collar parents, grew up in a blue-collar neighborhood in Chicago, and had blue-collar friends. I wanted to make my parents—especially my father—feel proud. My mom trained my nephew to say "Auntie Doctor" any time he saw a woman with a stethoscope. Friends pledged to bring their sick children to me someday. Would they all be less proud of me if I never wrote a prescription, never again used my stethoscope, if they couldn't see that I too would help heal people because they didn't understand what I did?

So I delayed the decision. I started my fourth year still answering "I'm not sure" to questions about my specialty choice. Then I began a pathology elective and sought the advice of my attendings. They were offended when I asked questions like "Were you ever disappointed that you won't ever make anyone better?" They reminded me that their work makes a difference every time one of them calls the results of a frozen section back to the OR, or determines whether a lesion was merely dysplasia or carcinoma in situ, or looks at a bone marrow to see if chemotherapy has been effective. I was ashamed at having asked the question.

It is possible that no one will ever again call me "Dr. Karen." It is probable that I will never again receive a gift from a patient. And I am not holding my breath for Christmas cards. But I will make patients better. I will make a difference in their lives by giving them the peace of mind of knowing what caused their loved one's death, or perhaps by finding what everyone else missed to provide a diagnosis. I will be excited and challenged and I will have fun as a pathologist. Whether or not my dad will ever understand what ragged red fibers are remains to be seen.

## PEDIATRICS

When I was in kindergarten and got asked the question, "What do you want to be when you grow up?," there were really only two acceptable answers. I could choose a life of either fighting crime as a policeman or extinguishing blazing infernos as a fireman. I chose fireman. As I got older, the same question became more difficult to answer because the choices became more varied and the decision held more gravity. The question wasn't so simple to answer anymore. I went through third-year rotations in a quandary about this decision when it suddenly became so simple: I want to do something where I wake up in the morning and can't wait to get to work, and at the end of the day I am sad to leave. This is pediatrics for me. Some say that children are just little half-sized adults, but I choose to differ. They are their own individuals. Children possess an honesty about them that adults have lost somewhere along the way, and they will openly share with you this honesty. I still remember Maria, the two-year-old with acute gastroenteritis who hugged me and planted on my cheek the biggest, wettest kiss I have ever had the pleasure to receive. She was convinced I was the one who had made her feel better. Of course, there was also Mikey, a four-year-old with a sprained wrist who was very verbally profound in how much distaste he had toward me after I attempted to manipulate the wounded wrist. Then there are the difficult cases that eternally remain etched in your brain. Karen, an eight-year-old with eczema herpeticum that had spread to cover both eyes and eventually sealed both her eyes shut. It is experiences like these that can cause a person to hesitantly leave the floor at the end of a hectic day and want to come back in the morning hopeful to see what a new day has in store.

Several other experiences also shaped my decision to enter into pediatrics and work with children. During my undergraduate years at a large public university, I was involved in a study of methylphenidate in children with attention deficit disorder. Being a psychology major, I found the research extremely intriguing and found myself enjoying spending time with the "difficult" children. While in medical school I worked with the Department of Child and Adolescent Psychiatry at Westchester Medical Center developing an alternative method of therapy for reaching children and adolescents diagnosed with a history of both substance abuse and physical abuse. This was based on previous studies, which demonstrated that traditional "talk" therapies are not as effective for children who have suffered severe emotional distress. For these types of patients, other modalities of creative expression had to be developed. This proved to be one of the most challenging yet rewarding projects I ever had the opportunity to be involved in.

For my current project, I have chosen to explore a different venue in child care. I am currently in the process of compiling the research for my master's thesis in public health. I chose to pursue a joint MD/MPH degree after being inspired by other physicians with MPH degrees that I worked with at the National Institutes of Health. My thesis centers on the topic of pediatric emergency room utilization in a metropolitan area. I hope to provide evidence of incorrect utilization of the emergency room for nonemergent health issues and underutilization of the primary care physician for these nonemergent situations. In addition, I will attempt to establish that incorrect utilization of the emergency room may have indirectly contributed to the rising cost of health care. In the future, I plan to use my MPH as a tool to create positive changes not only in ER pediatrics but also in the field of pediatrics in general. Whether it is in the area of maternal-child health or even policy for prevention of pediatric disease, my goal is to make a difference in the realm of child health care.

So what do I want to be when I grow up? I want to be challenged every single day of my life. I want to feel the satisfaction that what I do improves the lives of children in big and small ways. Most importantly, I want to be enamored by the work I do … I want to be a pediatrician.

## PHYSICAL MEDICINE AND REHABILITATION

"A very good one!" That's the way I answer people when they ask me what kind of doctor I am going to be. This has been my answer since I started medical school. Growing up in a family of six, with two educators as parents, I was taught to strive for excellence in whatever I do. Although the start of my medical career was somewhat turbulent, over the last two years I have demonstrated this attribute in all of my medical school activities. I must say that taking a leave of absence from my medical education was one of the best things I could have done. It enabled me to refocus my life and rededicate myself to medicine. Never has my determination to become a physician been stronger.

I have chosen to pursue a career in physical medicine and rehabilitation for three main reasons. First, I am intrigued by the area of study. Throughout my medical education, I have been very interested in neuromuscular medicine. I can remember back to anatomy lab, when I was amazed at the way our neurological system was "wired" to the rest of our bodies. Never during my basic science education was I more curious; an elective rotation in PM&R solidified this interest even more. I look forward to the challenges of treating patients in this field.

The multidisciplinary approach to patient care is another reason I like PM&R; I have always felt that the team approach to almost anything was the best way to go about things. I see myself as a "team player." My interpersonal skills are very good, and my abilities to lead a group have been demonstrated as the director of a summer camp. Sitting in on "team rounds," I found a great sense of accomplishment in seeing that all of these people were working toward a common cause. I can see how the ultimate goal of helping the patient is better met in this setting.

The last reason I have chosen PM&R as a specialty is my appreciation of the way that this field approaches the patient. I have always felt that patients should be seen as individuals, not cases. I have found that PM&R, unlike most other fields, pays very close attention to the psychosocial aspects of medicine. Patients are seen as mothers, husbands, students, and workers, etc. I feel that this is the only way to truly deal with the care of patients. It is relatively easy to "treat" a disease, but only through a holistic approach can one hope to "heal" a patient. As a candidate for residencies, I feel that I possess traits that many programs are seeking: enthusiasm, a strong work ethic, and a positive attitude. I have often been told that the vigor with which I approach life is contagious, and that my upbeat attitude is appreciated by many of the patients I have seen. I work hard at whatever I am doing yet have the ability to put life into perspective. I believe that these aspects of my personality will make me an asset to any residency program.

In summary, I am an enthusiastic, hardworking individual with a positive attitude who is dedicated to the field of physical medicine and rehabilitation. I hope that I will be given the chance to elaborate these thoughts in an interview with your program.

## PSYCHIATRY

The story is told of the late Wilfred Bion that another analyst once consulted with him regarding the case of a schizophrenic who would wake up in the middle of the night to see if he was really there. Bion thought for a moment and then commented, "Well, everyone deserves a second opinion." Indeed, when I informed my family and friends of my choice to go into psychiatry, I found myself with more "second opinions" than I had ever bargained for. One resident told me he was surprised, since he thought I was very motivated and interested in medicine. Other medical students commented enthusiastically that they admired me for choosing such a difficult field. Invariably, this was followed by a story about a person they had heard about who had left surgery—or obstetrics, or medicine—to become a psychiatry resident, after a psychotic episode in which he or she had almost killed several patients. Strangely enough, no one could tell me which program the resident was in. My interest in psychiatry comes from several different perspectives, which is probably why I find the various biological, social, and psychodynamic aspects of psychiatry so interesting. As a psychology major at Princeton, my courses were mainly biologically and pharmacologically oriented. I wrote my sophomore and junior papers on the psychobiology of seasonal affective disorder (SAD), and then spent two summers in Oxford studying the epidemiology of SAD. Yet, driven by a deeper desire to be able to understand and communicate with as many people as I could, I also studied three different languages at Princeton, was a peer counselor, and sang with three choruses. After college, I taught mentally retarded and emotionally disturbed adolescents, where I learned how to talk to and work with children who had problems ranging from autism to severe hyperactivity, and also spent much of my free time in the deaf community, where I learned about cultural values and the responses to societal pressures in closed communities.

Upon my arrival at medical school, I didn't know if I would go into psychiatry. I was fascinated with how the human body worked, and thought that the cerebral challenge of diagnosing physical disease might be more compelling than the gentle and creative exploration toward understanding the origins of a woman's depression or personality disorder. However, my unconscious betrayed me—I spent much of the time with my medical inpatients talking about what their illnesses meant to them or how their families dealt with their hospitalization. Throughout my third year, I found myself sitting with patients like the young woman at the OB/GYN clinic who admitted with shame that she was being hit by her boyfriend; a gigantic nightclub bouncer at the ambulatory clinic complaining of fatigue, who was just starting to adjust to regular life again after being in jail for 11 years; and a middle-aged woman with unexplained chest pain in the ICU, who cried and held my hand as she told me about months of insomnia and sadness following her painful divorce. I knew this was what I wanted to do.

As for the future, I still love research and will be doing a few months of research this year on the topic of memory in survivors of childhood trauma, but I also have a strong leaning toward psychotherapy and am giving serious consideration to becoming trained as a psychoanalyst. Eventually, I would like to have a career in an academic setting, where I can focus on patient care using both psychodynamic and psychopharmacologic techniques, and also teach and do some writing or research. Yet, wherever my future lies in these changing times, I know that as long as I have the unique opportunity and privilege to sit with people, listen to them, and help them tell their stories, I will always be satisfied.

# RADIATION ONCOLOGY

My decision to become a physician was influenced by several factors that led me to pursue a career in an oncologic subspecialty. My grandmother was diagnosed with breast cancer that later metastasized. My grandfather was diagnosed with lung cancer after having smoked for over 30 years. Recently, my cousin was diagnosed with melanoma, which later spread throughout his body. He was treated with advanced oncologic treatment, including radiation therapy, before passing away a few months ago. These experiences, along with a family friend who is a radiation oncologist, solidified my goals to become a radiation oncologist. Helping my family has given me an understanding and sensitivity for treating cancer patients.

Before learning about cancer through firsthand experience, I worked with cancer patients while volunteering at local hospitals while at the university. Volunteering was invaluable because the patients were very eager to share their experiences with me. I was fascinated in biochemistry classes and research by the interactions of genes, normal and mutated, that lead to neoplastic growth.

While working toward my MD degree at the State University of Medicine, my interests were again fueled by classes and conferences concerning oncology. I started my third year with a surgical oncology rotation under Dr. Johnson and Dr. Smith, who challenged me and taught me the surgical aspects of treatment. Dr. Galvez, my preceptor for gynecologic oncology, allowed me to participate in Tumor Board conferences. These increased my awareness of the risks and benefits of the numerous gynecologic treatment modalities.

Radiation therapy engages my interest because of the chance to cure and offer palliation in a minimally invasive to noninvasive manner. I am gratified to be involved in a treatment modality that offers relatively immediate and anatomically directed results. I am amazed by the wide spectrum of clinical cases one sees as a radiation oncologist. I also saw patients treated for heterotrophic bone growth and management of cardiac transplant rejection. Through research, I am involved in two projects at S. Cancer Center with the Radiation Oncology Department. One project entails biliary duct carcinoma and the other involves spinal cord carcinomas and gliomas. I am also comfortable offering palliation to terminally ill patients because I know that advances will shift to an increasing improvement in treatment and hopefully cure.

I have discovered many things about myself. Clinically, I can easily establish rapport with my patients. My evaluations consistently commend my ability to form strong patient-physician relationships. If I do not know the answer to a patient's question, taking the time to learn from and consult with an attending or resident allows me to answer the patient. There is no greater tool for learning than teaching someone else, and in that light I hope to remain in an academic setting as my career progresses. I am a diligent worker and an excellent time manager. I will happily spend extra time with a patient because as Dr. Khan, my preceptor in radiation oncology, says, "When I am with you, YOU are my only patient."

During my residency I wish to obtain excellent clinical and academic training that will provide a strong foundation for a successful and fulfilling career in both an academic and community setting. A quote I found in a book reminds me of the difference I hope to make in people's lives:

"A hundred years from now it will not matter what my bank account was, the sort of house I lived in, or the car I drove … but the world may be different because I was important in the life of a patient."

## RADIOLOGY

Sure, I will become a doctor. But what field of medicine will I choose? To find the answer to this ever-present question, I entered my clinical clerkships with an open mind, looking to discover my strengths and interests. As I went through my third-year clerkships I saw appeal in each experience; however, as the year came to a close I still had not found a niche. I began to look beyond the core clerkships I took as a third-year student. The vast number of career options for aspiring physicians can be quite overwhelming. So I decided to persevere in the manner in which I undertake most tasks. I stood back and thought, evaluating positives and negatives, and evaluating myself. I realized that perhaps the best fit for me was possibly something that I had exposure to during every third-year clerkship, yet its intricacies and true definition were still very foreign. This field was radiology.

Radiology can easily be taken for granted by an inexperienced medical student such as myself. It is ingrained in our heads that to rule in or rule out certain diagnoses on our differential often requires a visual study. The patient goes off to another place and receives this visual study, and soon thereafter a report is made revealing the medical situation that is occurring beyond the human eye. What this place is like and what the people do there began to capture my interest. It seemed quite ideal for a person such as myself who found interest in each clerkship I was exposed to during my third year. It allowed diagnosis in the medically ill, in the young child and infant, in the psychiatric patient with mental status changes that cannot be ruled out by history and physical alone—and of course it allowed diagnosis in the surgical candidate. Radiology in a sense allows exposure to the entire potpourri of medical specialties, therefore allowing continuing diversity but from a specialized viewpoint.

Realizing the specialty that appeals to you is one step; deciding whether you feel you can succeed and contribute in that area is the second. As an incoming resident I feel I have many attributes that suit me to be successful in radiology. First, I feel that the old adage that all radiologists sit in a dark room away from all other human contacts is incorrect. Interpersonal skills are essential for a successful radiologist. Patient contact does occur, although on a limited basis, and interaction with other physicians, whether as a consult or as a fellow radiologist, occurs on a daily basis. I enjoy interacting with others and feel that my personal skills will provide a comfortable environment for patients and colleagues. Second, I enjoy variety but at the same time realize that I prefer to focus within a specialty. I enjoy anatomy and anatomic relationships, which is also applicable in the field of radiology. Third, I have come to learn that I am quite visual both in my approach to learning and in my everyday tasks. The field of radiology allows me to take advantage of this ability. I have also always enjoyed solving mind puzzles and games. Radiology allows me to take these visual puzzles, if you will, and put the pieces together to make a differential.

A career in radiology provides the challenges and intellectual interests that I desire in my chosen field of medicine. I feel that by not making a career choice until after evaluating every clinical experience with an open mind, I have made the correct decision. Given the opportunity, I feel I have the abilities and determination to succeed and develop into a competent radiologist. My success throughout medical school helps to demonstrate my drive and self-motivation. I have confidence in my abilities, enjoy working as a member of a team, and feel I can be a strong advocate for my patients. With my skills and motivation I feel I will be a valuable member to the field of radiology.

## UROLOGY

I performed my first surgery at the age of 12 during a Boy Scout campout. My surgical staff, the other members of Troop 148, watched around the operating/picnic table as my attempts to clean the only fish caught that day developed into an exploration of fish anatomy. I was fascinated by the intricate anatomy of living things. I eventually realized that surgery was not only an exploration but also a chance to heal.

During my high school years, my mother was diagnosed with a rare cancer of the kidney. Despite a nephrectomy and short periods of hope, the cancer eventually metastasized to her liver. Surgery was no longer an option for her, and she began a difficult path of chemotherapy. She died a few years later, but her death did not dim my surgical aspirations. Rather, it made me determined to become a surgeon who strives to improve surgical treatments while maintaining empathy for the suffering of my patients. My research, teaching, and clinical experiences have strengthened this resolve and have helped me choose urology as my future career.

My research experience began during my undergraduate education. Intrigued by the challenges and complexities of basic science research, I continued my research endeavors during my first and second years of medical school. I worked with Dr. Durbin investigating the use of antigen cytokine fusion proteins as a means of achieving antigen-specific alterations of the immune response. I also participated in clinical research during my final two years of medical school. I worked with Dr. Perry on a retrospective study to evaluate the utility of preoperative CT scan in staging patients with colon cancer. I enjoyed the intellectual challenge of laboratory and clinical research and realized its potential to improve patient care. The field of urology is rich in research opportunities, and I look forward to continued involvement in research both in residency and beyond.

I was given unique teaching opportunities in medical school, being selected as a teaching assistant for human anatomy and as a USMLE review course instructor. As an anatomy teaching assistant, I led daily small-group discussions and cadaveric dissections. I gained a deeper appreciation of the complexity and variability of the human body while increasing my communication and teaching skills. I enjoy teaching and helping my peers learn. I look forward to the opportunity to both teach and learn from my patients and colleagues as an academic urologist.

My clinical rotations were especially influential in my decision to become a urologist. I enjoyed all of my clinical rotations and hoped to find a surgical specialty that would offer a similar diversity of clinical experiences. To me, urology provides an ideal blend of surgical precision and medical management and a wide spectrum of patients and problems. In the future, I would like to specialize in one of the many available subspecialties in urology. I am especially interested in urologic oncology.

Surgery, whether on a picnic table or in a sterile room, still inspires me as it did as a child. My research, teaching, and clinical experiences in medical school have been instrumental in focusing that interest to the surgical specialty of urology. My knowledge has grown since my first fish surgery, but I still feel the awe at the complexity of anatomy and how much more there is to learn. I look forward to the ongoing opportunities to learn and contribute as I strive to advance treatment and patient care within the field of urology.

# 10

# Gearing Up for Interviews

Once you've completed your ERAS application, take time to plan for interview season. Good preparation for interviews is essential to making the best impression. Being overtired, disorganized, inappropriately dressed, or upset about travel glitches can only hurt your chances. Generally speaking, the timeline for interviewing begins with preparation in the late fall, invitations being offered in late October through November, interviews occurring from mid-November into February, and follow-up opportunities with programs—in the form of second looks or e-mail/phone conversations with program directors—lasting through February. You can breathe a small sigh of relief when invitations for interviews start coming in. You have cleared the first major hurdle in the Match process, and your foot is in the door at several programs. Now, however, you need to maneuver the rest of yourself through the doorway. In this chapter, we will walk you through the stages of interview preparation so that you can hit the ground running by the time your first interview day arrives.

## HOW DO I PREPARE FOR THE INTERVIEW?

### SCHEDULING INTERVIEWS

If you get your ERAS application in early, you will likely be invited to interview early as well. Some programs invite applicants to interview before seeing their Dean's Letters, which arrive on November 1, but this varies a great deal between specialties. For most specialties, the vast majority of invitations will go out after November 1. Most programs have an administrative assistant who is in charge of scheduling. Once you are selected, he or she will e-mail you a list of available interview dates from which you can choose.

At this point, you will have to sit down with a calendar and draw up a few possible scenarios in order to maximize the efficiency of your interview trip and prevent overcrowding of your interview schedule. Once you receive an invitation, you should call or e-mail the program's administrative assistant and select an interview date as soon as possible. This is particularly important in the more competitive specialties. The schedules usually fill quickly, and the longer you wait, the less likely you'll be to get your first choice for an interview date. If you later find that your desired interview date has changed, it is always okay to try and reschedule an interview. For some of the specialties with fewer spots, such as plastic surgery, a program may only have two interview dates. So it is not uncommon for two programs to interview on the same days, requiring you to choose which one to interview with.

> Remember that you are always being evaluated, so be polite to administrative assistants when scheduling or rescheduling interviews.

Many program directors will tell you that the date of your interview should not make a difference. Certain programs, especially those with fewer applicants and residency positions, will offer only a few interview dates, which may be concentrated early or late in the season. Others may have many interview dates extending over the traditional interview season from mid-November through the first week of February. Conventional wisdom may favor choosing the latter half of the interview season so that committee members will better recall your application during ranking sessions, but what is most important is that you schedule interviews so that you are able to interview at every program in which you are truly interested and so that you are able to complete any required medical student rotations that may be scheduled for December or January. It is also advisable to try to interview at your home medical institution earlier in the season. This allows you the opportunity to gain confidence in a safer, more familiar interview environment and may also provide your home department the chance to give you feedback before you hit the road for interviews elsewhere.

Try to arrange interviews in geographical clusters so that you can easily drive between sites or take advantage of cheaper regional travel options (see "Planes, Trains, and Automobiles" below). It is okay to politely request an interview at a specific program if you will be traveling to that general area for other interviews. A tactful way of approaching this issue is to e-mail the program's administrative assistant explaining that you are planning to travel to their particular region or city and asking if they would be able to notify you whether you'll have an opportunity to interview at that time. Ask if rounds or a morning conference is a scheduled part of the day's activities. If not, ask if you can attend one or the other as part of the interview day or on the following day if you are able to stay an additional night. Rounds and conferences are often one of the easiest and most useful ways to judge the style and caliber of a program because you are directly exposed to the faculty and to resident education. For specialties such as emergency medicine or anesthesiology, having an opportunity to spend an hour or two in the ED or OR is the best way to see what kind of supervision and teaching the residents receive and what type of patients are treated in that hospital. Asking if there is opportunity to shadow or observe after your interview can be critical, especially at your top choice programs.

The interview process can be more grueling than you think. **Don't schedule interviews too close together.** Many programs will offer applicants the opportunity to attend a social event with residents either the night before or after the interview, so by spacing your interviews and arranging your travel accordingly you can maximize your chance to attend these sessions. In addition, by scheduling interviews at least two days apart, you'll have time to travel, recuperate, and digest information from the previous interview. You should also visit the most competitive and desirable programs in the middle of your interview schedule. By then you should have reached peak interview form without having lost your enthusiasm and energy (see Figure 10-1). In fact, many applicants end up canceling interviews near the end of the season out of apathy and fatigue. Before canceling an interview, review your reasons for selecting the program in the first place and try to avoid declining to interview at a program that was high on your interest list for good reasons because of "interview fatigue." Students often comment, in fact, that it was the last program they visited that ended up being their ideal Match.

If you decide that you do not want to make an interview appointment or cannot do so, inform the program as far in advance as possible so that they can fill your interview slot with another applicant. Generally, giving programs at least two weeks' notice of your cancellation is considered appropriate. Whatever the time course, always e-mail or call the program as soon as you decide to cancel your interview. Reports of bad manners travel far in the small circle of residency program directors, so **you should never just not show up!** This will be seen as unprofes-

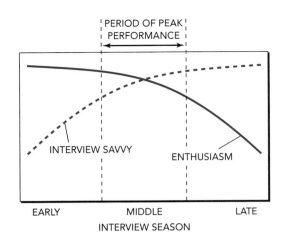

**FIGURE 10-1.** Performance during interview season.

sional, and will not only reflect poorly on you, but also on your medical school colleagues and deans. Occasionally, emergencies or travel delays may occur. Even in these cases, you should always call the program immediately, leaving a voicemail message if necessary, to apologize for not making the interview, explaining the situation, and asking politely whether there is room to reschedule.

## MOCK INTERVIEWS

After four years in medical school, anyone can lose his or her interviewing finesse. Get a little practice before the real thing and set up a mock interview early in the fall with your career advisor or another faculty member. The best time to complete a mock interview is in September or October, after you've made your specialty choice and completed your ERAS application. When you hit the interview trail, you want to be in fine shape. Real interviews are time consuming and take serious effort to set up. You should also remember **never** to treat a real interview as a practice session, even if it is at one of your less desirable programs. You never know how a visit might affect your rank-order list, especially if you end up bumping one of your lower-ranked choices to the top of your "most wanted" list.

    Ideally, you should complete the mock interview with a faculty member who is a veteran interviewer and who is in a separate but related department. For example, if you are interested in emergency medicine, you may choose to practice interviewing with a surgeon or an anesthesiologist; or if you are interested in internal medicine, you may choose to be interviewed by someone in primary care or family medicine. If you choose to interview with a member of the selection committee in your desired specialty—especially if you are interested in remaining at your home institution—be cautious! This information may be used when you are discussed during intern selection. If you are unsure of how to set up a mock interview or which faculty member to ask, you might seek help by contacting your dean of students or a career-planning office at your school. For the truly obsessive-compulsive, interview coaches can play the interviewer, videotape the session, and coach you toward a fine-tuned performance.

> Practice with mock interviews before you hit the road.

Before you go for your mock interview, review Chapter 11. Then have your "interviewer" conduct a realistic interview with hard questions. These tough conditions will give you the confidence you need to get through a difficult interview when the time comes. You should treat your mock interview just as you would the real one. Once you've selected an "interviewer," send that person a copy of your CV and/or ERAS application so that he or she can prepare realistic, tailored questions. Arrive five to ten minutes early for the interview dressed professionally in full interview garb, with a folder containing the materials you would bring to a real interview. Introduce yourself to the faculty member's administrative assistant and wait politely until you are ushered into the interview.

Afterward, your "interviewer" should give you detailed feedback on the ease and confidence with which you handled the questions, the quality of your answers, and other personal characteristics that you projected during the interview (eg, maturity, thoughtfulness, intelligence, ability to think quickly). It is especially important that your interviewer is honest and provides constructive criticism regarding your performance and your ability to maintain a conversation. If you want to squeeze even more feedback out of your practice interview, you can have it videotaped or audiotaped and then review it with your "interviewer." Try to evaluate yourself from his or her perspective. Finally, do not get overwhelmed by negative feedback from this mock interviewer. If you have a nasty habit of interrupting someone midsentence, it is better to know now and to keep it in the back of your mind when the real interviewer walks into the room. When all is said and done, be sure to send your mock interviewer a thank-you e-mail/card within the next day or two; this will get you in the habit for your real interviews.

## DOING YOUR HOMEWORK AND PREPARING FOR THE INTERVIEW TRAIL

One week before an actual interview, call or e-mail the institution to confirm the date, time, and location. Some programs may send you a confirmation automatically. Researching information about your interviewers is not generally considered necessary. Most often, you will not find out who your interviewers will be until the morning of the interview. If you call the administrative assistant, you can find out if your interviewers have been assigned. If you have any of your interviewers' names, try to build on this knowledge. Is your interviewer a researcher, a clinician, a house officer, or an administrator? Once you've found out this basic information, get to work. You might try and call up local contacts (eg, graduates from your school who are currently in the program) to ask about the interviewer's research interests, personality, etc. Often, major academic institutions will provide physician profiles, which may allow you to determine where your interviewers attended medical school and completed residency, as they may know people at your home institution. Second, run a MEDLINE search on the interviewer and read his or her abstracts, Google the interviewer's name, and check out the program's departmental Web site (if applicable) to learn more about the faculty. Your goal here is not to appear political or "calculated" but rather to be prepared to highlight any strengths or mutual interests you have that might appeal to the interviewer. Even if what you learn does not come up in conversation, you will gain confidence just from know-

> Level the interview playing field by learning about your interviewers.

ing something about the interviewer. Remember, he or she already knows a great deal about you, so doing your homework offers you a chance to level the playing field a bit. Do not worry if you are unable to find out who your specific interviewer will be. In this case, you can still peruse information about program directors, codirectors, prominent faculty, and department chairs, as these individuals often interview or meet with applicants during the interview day.

While researching the interests of individual interviewers is optional, researching the program itself is not. Look at program Web sites to obtain basic information about the residency, including information on program length, number of residents in each class, the curriculum, required rotations, elective opportunities, and whether research is required and available to residents. Review this material, printing out relevant parts of the Web site, and be sure to jot down questions and concerns that come to mind for that program. Interviewers will expect you to know about their program and to ask questions. This demonstrates a true interest in the program. In preparation for the interview, you will want to organize the information you have obtained (see Figure 10-2). To do so, place all the material you have gathered in a labeled folder that you can easily take with you to the interview. You should also include your own application materials in this folder. Of course, residency directors will also have this information—plus your application—in front of them when they interview you, all of which is fair game. However, by having the information with you, you can quickly review it before your interviews begin and also supplement it. For example, if you are asked about a publication, you could provide a copy of the article. However, do not offer your interviewer any articles or paperwork if he or she does not ask about it.

In preparation for the interview season, you should gather a set of basic travel items, which you can pack ahead of time and use for all your interviews (see Figure 10-3). As part of your homework, you'll also want to gather information about the cities you'll be visiting. It is imperative that you find out about weather patterns

## ✅ checklist

- ○ The *First Aid for the Match* Program Evaluation Worksheet and Worksheet of Application Requirements (from the end of this book)
- ○ The full FREIDA printout
- ○ The interview information packet from the residency program
- ○ Photocopies of your application or CV and personal statement
- ○ Any notes that you picked up from faculty house staff or fellow students
- ○ For the research minded, copies of your manuscripts to give to the interviewer and a MEDLINE search of your interviewer's work, if known
- ○ A color photograph of yourself if one was not sent to the program
- ○ Information from the program's departmental Web site

FIGURE 10-2. Checklist for materials to take to an interview.

## ✓ checklist

- ○ Interview day attire and a change of clothes for the social event
- ○ Lodging information, including hotel reservations or name of host
- ○ Map of the city, including public transit options
- ○ Weather-related items, including an umbrella, raincoat, and boots if needed
- ○ Map and directions to the hospital campus
- ○ A list (on paper or programmed into your phone) of important numbers: the residency program secretary, the office of student affairs at your own institution, any friends, family, or contacts you have in the city you are visiting in case of emergency

**FIGURE 10-3** Checklist of materials for interview traveling.

for particular destinations so that you will know whether to pack a raincoat or snow boots if needed. In addition, you might want to print out local maps or make copies of a city guidebook from the library, all of which you can include in your travel folder. If you'd like to create and print a custom packing list, check out the Packing List Online Web site (www.packinglistonline.com). After entering in some basic information about your travel itinerary, planned activities, and modes of transportation, the Web site populates a list of essential items and allows you to add or subtract other suggested items to your virtual packing list.

> You never get a second chance to make a first impression. Now is the time to splurge on quality interview attire.

## INTERVIEW ATTIRE AND PRESENTATION

First impressions are important! Even before you smile and say hello, your interviewers are evaluating what they see. Dress the part! Look at yourself in a full-length mirror. Give yourself some candid feedback. Do you look business-like and polished? If not, you may want to reassess your choices. This is definitely not the time to try out exciting new colors, experiment with some edgy fashions, or acquire new piercings. Also try asking someone whose opinion you value about your appearance. By dressing in your interview attire at your mock interview, you can receive honest feedback from a veteran interviewer. Remember, too, to check the weather projection for the city you are visiting and dress appropriately. Most interviews occur in late fall and winter, so dress for warmth and comfort. Clothes are not the only factor, however; proper grooming is essential. In general, it is unlikely that your interviewer will pay much attention to your appearance as long as there is nothing that stands out as unusual or inappropriate. However, you can be sure they will notice if your hair is a mess, your clothes are wrinkled, your nail polish is chipping, you are not clean shaven, or if they can smell your aftershave or perfume from down the hall!

Many programs will offer coffee, lunch, or snacks throughout the day, so stash some breath mints in your bag if you're worried. Do not use chewing gum as an al-

> Your outfit should not only be professional, but should help make you feel confident.

> Avoid lethal doses of aftershave or perfume on interview day.

ternative. Choose meals wisely—give the pasta or lasagna a pass, as stains at lunch could haunt you for the rest of the afternoon.

The following section contains tips for men and women regarding the specifics of what makes up a great interview outfit. Take these to heart, and remember— the goal is for you to wear clothes that are professional and comfortable, and that help you step out with confidence. And no matter what you wear, always put on a smile!

**Just for men.** Attire for men is rather straightforward: business suit, tie, and dress shoes. There is no single "right" color for a suit, but once you have chosen your color, remember that your shoes, tie, and shirt should coordinate. The most popular colors for suits are black, charcoal, and navy. Black, charcoal, and navy suits look best with black shoes. Dark brown suits look better with dark brown shoes. Speaking of shoes, give them a shine before you hit the road!

When choosing a tie, stick with a classic, conservative style. For instance, a tie with cartoon characters may be fun on your pediatrics rotation, or a tie with beer cans on it may be great for a party, but a solid or simply patterned tie is best for interviewing.

If in doubt, choose a white shirt. Remember, however, that while a white shirt is a good choice, white socks are not. Choose socks that match or are darker than your pants or shoes. Jewelry is another aspect of attire. A watch—preferably a dress watch—is acceptable. Earrings and visible body piercing are not. Light aftershave or none at all is best.

Two suits should suffice for the interview season. Alterations are a must if you are not a standard size, so make sure they are well tailored. Each suit may be used for two to three interviews if no spots or spills occur. Have your suits dry-cleaned during a break in the interview schedule. Pack a portable iron and a lint brush for trips, and inspect your suit closely before packing for any spots, lint, loose threads, or holes.

**Just for women.** The motto for women should be "professional yet simple." This is the time to splurge on good-quality clothing. A well-made, classically cut suit will serve you well. Skirts or pantsuits are both acceptable. You need to be comfortable in your interview day clothing. If you will be uncomfortable in a skirt (especially in the middle of winter), a tailored pantsuit may serve you better. If you opt for the traditional skirt suit, remember to choose the right length for your height. The length of your skirt should be no shorter than the top of the knee and no longer than two inches below the knee. This is largely an issue of practicality, as a skirt that is too short will show too much leg when you are sitting, while a skirt that is too long will hamper mobility when you are walking. You should also wear stockings. Choose something close to your skin tone in a color that complements your suit. Always pack an extra pair of stockings, as stockings invariably seem to run when you are most hoping they won't.

You may need two solid-colored suits, depending on the number and timing of your interviews. Wool and cotton-blend fabrics travel best and wrinkle least. Linen wrinkles easily and is not warm, so it is probably not a good choice. Women tend to know what color looks best on them. On the interview trail, basic black, navy, and dark gray are the most popular. Classic colors such as evergreen, dark brown, or maroon can serve as alternatives.

For the blouse or button-down shirt, choose a color that complements your skin tone. Stick with understated, professional colors. Magenta would definitely make an impression, but so would showing up in your underwear (both of which should be avoided)! A patterned blouse is acceptable if properly chosen. However, no matter what color you choose, make sure it is conservatively cut. Cleavage has no place in the interview room, or in the hospital for that matter!

Shoes should be sensible and stylish, but most of all comfortable. Remember that most interview days will involve tours, walking to interviews, and going to lunch, so low-heeled shoes that complement your suit will be the most comfortable and appear professional. Jewelry is an accessory that should not distract from your finished appearance; simple studs, small hoops, or pearl earrings work well with most suits. Depending on the blouse, a strand of pearls or a simple chain is optional. A dress watch and a simple ring are also acceptable. Multiple earrings and visible body piercing are not. If you choose to wear makeup, use it to enhance your appearance. Remember that, like perfume, less is more.

If possible, do not carry a handbag. A leather attaché case or bag that can accommodate paper, pens, keys, and a comb or brush is a better alternative.

**Clothing emergencies.** Occasionally during the interview season, luggage is lost on flights, shoes may be misplaced, or other unforeseen events may occur. If this happens to you, stay calm and do not stress out. Program directors and interviewers realize that these situations arise and in general will be very understanding. As soon as you realize your luggage is lost, call the program's administrative assistant; if you do not reach that individual by phone, leave a message and follow-up with an e-mail. This will help to put your attire in context and will notify the program to expect you without your über-professional clothing. Just as with canceling interviews, by calling ahead and politely explaining the situation, you will appear professional and receive compassionate understanding from your prospective employer.

> Always use carry-on luggage to prevent lost luggage situations.

In order to avoid these clothing disasters, it is advisable that you always use carry-on luggage for air travel. Not only will this ensure that your all-important interview suit remains in your control, but it will allow you to exit the airport faster. Always be sure to follow FAA/TSA security guidelines for carrying liquids, toothpaste, and razors when packing your carry-on luggage. In addition, when traveling, you should wear clothing that might be useful as a backup should your luggage or suit get lost. For example, men may choose to wear khaki pants, a button-down shirt, and a pair of dark shoes on the plane, rather than jeans, a sweatshirt, and flip-flops; this will ensure that should you lose your suit, you can at least go to the interview wearing business casual attire.

## HOW CAN I TRAVEL INEXPENSIVELY?

Unfortunately, interviews will cost you a lot of time and money. During the 1999–2000 interview season, students reported spending an average of 20 days away from medical school at their program interviews and paid $2000 for application fees and travel expenses (see Figures 10-4 and 10-5). Plan to spend more money and more

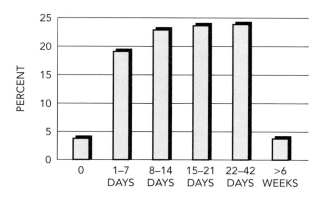

FIGURE 10-4. Days spent interviewing away from school.

time away from school if you are applying in a competitive specialty or if you desire matching in a particular geographic location that is far from your medical school.

In most cases, it is possible to make travel arrangements for your interviews without razing your bank account. To some extent, the most cost-efficient means of transportation depends on your geographic location. Some parts of the United States have better rail service than others. In some areas, a rented car may be your best option. The next section will introduce you to some ways to minimize your travel expenses.

## PLANES, TRAINS, AND AUTOMOBILES

**All-in-one travel resources for residency applicants.** There are a few travel resources that are available specifically to help medical students who are traveling for residency interviews. These "all-in-one" Web sites provide links and information for discount air travel, car rental information, and lodging. SmartMedTravel (www.smartmedtravel.com) is a resource created by graduates of Vanderbilt's School of Medicine that contains information organized by city; it includes infor-

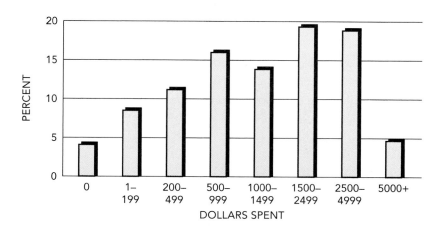

FIGURE 10-5. Amount in U.S. dollars spent applying and interviewing for residency positions.

mation on local accommodations; local air, rail, and bus options; rental car services for the city; and current weather. InterviewTrail.com (www.interviewtrail.com) is a social utility program that requires registration with the Web site and allows medical students to share travel trips and review programs they have visited. It also includes links to calendars that you can use to plan your interview schedule and book travel. You can also share your interview path, and if your schedule overlaps with other applicants, arrange to share costs for hotel rooms, taxis, etc.

**American Airlines Meeting Saver Fares for the AAMC Student Residency Interview Program.** Discounts of 5% off the lowest coach fare on American Airlines fares are available only to senior students in AAMC member institutions during the interview season through this program with the Association of American Medical Colleges (AAMC). For more information, call:

American Airlines Meeting Services Desk
(800) 433-1790

For questions and to access the AAMC Discount Code, contact Denine Hales, dhales@aamc.org.

**Low-cost and discount regional airlines.** There are also several upstart airlines (see Table 10-1) that generally provide a price break when compared to the major airlines. Often, however, they will not appear in travel agents' computers or on some Web sites, so you may need to go to each airline's Web page directly. In light of recent competition from low-fare airlines such as Southwest, you can obtain very reasonable airfares when traveling regionally (see Table 10-1). As with other airlines, tickets are cheapest with a 21-day advance purchase and a Saturday night stay. With discount airlines, you may have less choice in flight times and more stopovers.

Southwest Airlines (800-I-FLY-SWA, www.iflyswa.com) is a regional airline that takes pride in its low fares and customer service, and its Web site is extremely user friendly. Another perk is Southwest's cancellation policy. If your plans change and you need to cancel or reschedule, you can apply the original purchase price of your travel toward future bookings (within one year) without penalty. Other airlines charge $100 or more in penalties for canceled reservations.

**Amtrak.** Amtrak offers deals on multiride tickets for short distance travel within the Northeast, Midwest, West, and South. The California Rail Pass offers 7 days of travel in a 21-day period for $159. Student Advantage members ($22.50 annual fee, www.studentadvantage.com, 877-2-JOIN-SA) and AAA members are eligible for discounts. See the Amtrak Web site for weekly specials and advertised specials. For more information, call or visit:

Amtrak
(800) USA-RAIL [(800) 872-7245]
www.amtrak.com

**Metro-North and Long Island Rail Road.** Because the entire Eastern Seaboard is well connected with light rail, rail is a viable alternative to driving, especially given distances of 200 miles or greater. Reasonable fares are available even with little or no advance reservation. In general, rail travel may be a more useful option than you think; you can use the time to review interview materials, rest, or catch up on other reading, none of which is possible when you drive. It's also harder to get lost!

## TABLE 10-1

**Discount and Regional Airlines**

| Airline | Phone Number | Web Site |
|---|---|---|
| AirTran Airways | (800) AIR-TRAN<br>(800) 247-8726 | www.airtran.com |
| Alaska Airlines/Horizon Air | (800) 252-7522 | www.alaskair.com |
| America West Airlines/<br>US Airways | (800) 428-4322 | www.usairways.com |
| Frontier Airlines | (800) 432-1FLY<br>(800) 432-1359 | www.frontierairlines.com |
| Jet Blue | (800) JET-BLUE<br>(800) 538-2583 | www.jetblue.com |
| Midwest Airlines | (800) 452-2022 | www.midwestairlines.com |
| Southwest Airlines | (800) I-FLY-SWA<br>(800) 435-9792 | www.southwest.com |
| Spirit Airlines | (800) 772-7177 | www.spiritair.com |
| Sun Country Airlines | (800) 359-6786 | www.suncountry.com |
| Virgin America | (877) FLY-VIRGIN<br>(877) 359-8474 | www.virginamerica.com |

> Some airlines will charge a service fee for booking over the phone, so buy your tickets online if possible.

To receive general rail schedules for the New York metropolitan area, Long Island, and Connecticut, call or visit:

Metro-North Railroad
(800) METROINFO
www.mta.info/mnr/index.html

Long Island Rail Road
(718) 217-LIRR
www.mta.info/lirr

**Super shuttle.** This door-to-door van service is available at several airports and offers shared rides from the airport to your lodging destination. Some airports require advance reservations, and others do not. The shuttle is a great way to get to your lodging if you are staying with a recent graduate, friend in the area, a hotel that does not have an airport shuttle, or a current resident in the program. It offers a much cheaper alternative than taking a taxi from the airport. For more information, visit or call:

Super Shuttle
(800) 258-3826
www.supershuttle.com

**Travel agencies.** You can purchase a ticket directly through the airlines described earlier, or you can visit your local travel agency. One student-oriented discount travel agency is STA Travel at (800) 781-4040 or www.statravel.com; they also have several local branches around major universities and sell student fares for rail and air travel as well as some lodging. Travel agents have access to information about the lowest available airfares on all major airlines. Unfortunately, however, some discount airlines, such as Southwest, are not listed on their computers. Travel agents' services are free to you, since their commissions are paid by the airlines. In general, try to purchase tickets three weeks in advance for the cheapest fares. You should also make sure that the airport you fly into is the best one in terms of price and distance from your program destination. You must balance the airfare with the time and cost of a taxi or shuttle to your lodging.

Internet travel agencies have proliferated because of their usability and cheap prices. While they are most popular for air travel, several also provide options to rent cars and hotel rooms, sometimes providing bundled deals. When using the Internet agencies, be sure to shop around at multiple sites, as booking fees and taxes may vary from site to site. The following are some of the more popular sites:

- **Priceline** (www.priceline.com). Priceline's Web site allows you to search for affordable fares or to name your own price for your airfare. After you enter in your desired travel plans, Priceline will search for any airline with the lowest fares, similar to other Internet travel sites. You can then select the carrier and flight times best suited to your needs. Priceline also offers "Name Your Own Price," which can often yield a better deal. You choose your desired airport, the amount you wish to pay, and your credit card number. If an available fare matches your criteria, your card is charged automatically. Once you have purchased your ticket, you cannot change, transfer, or cancel it. You should also be aware that although you choose your travel dates with the "Name Your Own Price" option, the airline will choose the travel times (which will range between 6 A.M. and 10 P.M.). Priceline will search for nonstop flights first, but there is a chance that you will have to make a stop or a connection.

- **Cheap Tickets** (www.cheaptickets.com). Cheap Tickets has been providing discount airfares on major airlines since 1986. Finding fares is easy; the site will lead you through a series of questions regarding airport, dates, and number of travelers. Using your search parameters, the site will list available itineraries. Click on the "Fare Rules" button to view the restrictions for the lowest fare. A Visa, MasterCard, or American Express credit card can be used to purchase flights. Cheap Tickets has recently removed booking fees from their orders, but this, of course, is always subject to change. Be sure to check their "Specials" page, as well as their hotel discount and rental car pages.

- **Expedia** (www.expedia.com). Expedia has a variety of features you can use to check for airfares. Expedia's basic fare search is similar to that of other Web sites in that it will search for the lowest airfare once you have typed in your search parameters. For some fares, Expedia allows you to reserve your flight itinerary until midnight of the following day, but the fare is not guaranteed; most discount fares will not allow this option and require immediate purchase. Some hints for getting your fare are as follows: (1) travel on a Tuesday, Wednesday, or Saturday; (2) plan a Saturday night stay-over; and (3) be flexible about your travel times and connecting flights. As with other sites, Expedia.com has hotel discount and rental car pages.

- **Orbitz** (www.orbitz.com). This is another Web-based service that surveys multiple carriers. Orbitz also offers hotel and rental car reservations.

- **Travelocity** (www.travelocity.com). Travelocity has the basic airfare, hotel, and rental car search engines. It also has a "FareWatcher Plus" feature that allows you to pick certain cities for which the Web site will continually check for low fares. You will need to register before you can use any of Travelocity's advanced features, such as FareWatcher.

- **Lowest Fare** (www.lowestfare.com). Be sure to check their specials, which are on their home page. Lowestfare.com also links to a "City Guide," giving you access to maps and weather information in a selected city.

- **Kayak** (www.kayak.com). Many airline and hotel Web sites offer exclusive deals or low fare guarantees. Kayak allows you to search most of the sites for the best deals. You then book directly with the airline or hotel Web site to avoid fees charged by travel agency Web sites.

- **SeatGuru** (www.seatguru.com). This site, which links with a flight search engine called TripAdvisor, contains detailed seat maps and recommendations so that you can find the best seat on the flight. This information is great for tall travelers who want to know which emergency exit row is ideal, or those who are trying to avoid being seated next to the bathroom!

## WHERE TO STAY

You will need to account for overnight housing in your travel plans. It isn't always necessary to figure big bucks into your budget for this item, so consider the following possibilities.

**Free or low-cost accommodations arranged by the program.** Some programs—especially primary care programs in the Midwest and East—will provide complimentary or discounted lodging at a nearby hotel or guest house. If your program does not volunteer information about such arrangements, ask the administrative assistant if any are available. Many programs will provide a list of current residents who offer their apartment or home to prospective applicants. Taking advantage of this option will give you added time with a resident from the program and guarantee that you'll have help finding the hospital the morning of your interview! If you use this option, you may consider taking the resident a small gift, such as a bottle of wine or box of chocolates, to thank him or her for providing your lodging.

**For women: AMWA Bed and Breakfast Program.** The American Medical Women's Association (AMWA) has a "Bed and Breakfast Program" for members traveling to residency interviews. A member calls AMWA and specifies her destination. AMWA then supplies her with a list of members in the area, mostly physicians who have agreed to provide short-term (one to three days') lodging for other members. The student is then responsible for making arrangements with the host. There is an administrative fee of $10 for students and $15 for physicians. To use the service or for more information, contact Mare Glanz at:

American Medical Women's Association
801 North Fairfax Street, Suite 400
Alexandria, VA 22314
(703) 838-0500
www.amwa-doc.org
E-mail: mglanz@amwa-doc.org

**Recent graduates from your school.** Some student affairs offices maintain lists of recent graduates and their residency programs. Not only are recent graduates at your target programs an invaluable source of honest information about the program, but they might offer to put you up for a night when you visit.

**Other applicants.** On the interview trail, you often meet applicants from the schools and institutions you will later be visiting. They may be friendly enough to offer you housing when you visit their home institution or just show you around the evening before the interview. If they will also be visiting your school at some point, consider extending them the same courtesy. In addition, if you find that you'll be interviewing with another applicant on the same day in a different city, you might consider splitting the cost of a hotel room for that interview date.

**Accommodations recommended by the program.** If you are stumped for housing options or prefer more luxurious surroundings, you can always check out local hotels recommended by the program. Residency programs often make arrangements with a hotel to offer discounts if you mention that you are interviewing with them. This information is frequently included with written invitations for interviews. If you don't get the official word, you can ask the administrative assistant for suggestions.

**Budget-priced chains.** Finally, you can simply go with a budget hotel/motel chain. If the residency program is not helpful with names and numbers of nearby lodging, you can call any of these major chains (see Table 10-2). Many have a AAA discount. When you make your reservation, ask about the room. Common concerns include a nonsmoking room, location in a quiet part of the hotel/motel, and a phone connection.

**University dorms.** Many residency programs are located at colleges and universities that rent out empty dormitory rooms for $15 to $30 per night. Unfortunately, programs sometimes neglect to mention such accommodations in their brochures. Again, you can ask the administrative assistant if he or she knows whether this option is available.

> Lodging can cost you more than airfare, so plan ahead. Hostels and some hotels may lack amenities like ironing boards.

> Arrive early; leave late.

> Check in and print your boarding pass off the airline's Web site the night before or after your interview to save time.

## HANDY TRAVEL TIPS

Finally, we offer a few additional pointers to make your interview trip as smooth as possible:

1. Plan to arrive at your accommodations no later than the afternoon of the day before your interview. This will give you a chance to get oriented, adjust to time-zone differences, shower and clean up after a long flight, and handle any unexpected mishaps (eg, lost luggage). If you are planning to leave on the day

## TABLE 10-2

**Major Budget Hotel/Motel Chains**

| Hotel Chain | Number | Web Site |
|---|---|---|
| Baymont Inns | (800) 4-BUDGET | www.baymontinns.com |
| Club House Inns | (800) CLUB-INN | www.clubhouseinn.com |
| Comfort Inns | (800) 4-CHOICE | www.comfortinn.com |
| Country Inns and Suites | (800) 456-4000 | www.countryinns.com |
| Courtyard Marriott | (800) 321-2211 | www. courtyard.com |
| Days Inns | (800) 325-2525 | www.daysinn.com |
| EconoLodge | (800) 4-CHOICE | www.hotelchoice.com |
| Fairfield Inn | (800) 228-2800 | www.marriotthotels.com |
| Hampton Inn | (800) HAMPTON | www.hampton-inn.com |
| HoJo Inn | (800) 654-2000 | www.hojo.com |
| Holiday Inn Express | (800) HOLIDAY | www.ichotelsgroup.com |
| La Quinta Inns | (800) 531-5900 | www.laquinta.com |
| Motel 6 | (800) 4-MOTEL6 | www.motel6.com |
| Ramada Ltd. | (800) 2-RAMADA | www.ramada.com |
| Red Roof Inns | (800) THE-ROOF | www.redroof.com |
| Rodeway Inns | (800) 4-CHOICE | www.rodeway.com |
| Super 8 | (800) 800-8000 | www.super8.com |
| Travelodge | (800) 255-3050 | www.travelodge.com |

of the interview, check with the departmental secretary to make sure there are no events scheduled for later that day. In general, it is better to leave later in the day so that you can have extra time to talk to house staff and faculty or to see more of the hospital and facilities.

2. When flying, try to take everything as a carry-on. You can bypass the crowded airport counter for a gate check-in and eliminate the chance that the airline will lose your luggage. We suggest a durable garment bag or a roll-aboard suit carrier for your interview clothing. If you must travel heavy, at least pack your interview essentials (eg, program interview materials, application materials, and interview suit) in a carry-on.

3. If you plan on driving to most of your destinations, get a good U.S. map/road atlas for trip planning, or a global positioning system (GPS) for your car. Carry a pocket local map for each city you visit, or tear out the detail pages from an inexpensive road atlas. If you belong to the American Automobile Association (AAA), call or visit your local office once you know your itinerary. Member-

ship privileges usually include free road maps. These can be requested through their Web site. It's also worth inquiring about discounts on car rentals and lodging; many AAA clubs offer coupons for these services. And if you should have car problems en route, a AAA card can often save you much more than the cost of the annual membership fee. Before you set off, have your car properly winterized and tuned; ask the service station attendant to check your fluids and tire pressure and to replace your windshield wipers if necessary. Be sure to keep your car registration, inspection and insurance papers, and auto club materials in the glove compartment. If you don't already have one for your car, buy a flashlight and batteries—particularly if you will be driving at night.

4. If you rent a car, be sure to check for any available discounts, either through AAA rates, rates associated with your own university, or sometimes discount rates through your frequent flier mile programs or credit cards. In addition, check your credit card policy to determine if it will cover your liability insurance when you pay for a rental car using the credit card—several credit cards, including MasterCard and American Express, offer this as part of the fine print, and it will save you money if you can decline the company's insurance and use your credit card's coverage instead.

5. If you have the time, the interview season can be a great way to mix business and pleasure. You can squeeze in some sightseeing if you have more than a day between interviews. That way, you'll get to unwind between interviews and learn more about the local attractions in the vicinity of the program.

6. Be sure to check local weather conditions in the city where you will be interviewing before you set off. This is especially important if you are traveling to an unfamiliar part of the country or if you are flying to a region with an extreme climate.

> Give yourself plenty of time to get through increased airport security.

## REFERENCES

AirTran Airways Web site (www.airtran.com).

Alaska Airlines Web site (www.alaskair.com).

America West Airlines/US Airways Website (www.usairways.com).

American Medical Women's Association Web site (www.amwa-doc.org).

Amtrak Web site (www.amtrak.com).

Baymont Inns Web site (www.baymontinns.com).

Cheap Tickets Web site (www.cheaptickets.com).

ClubHouse Inns Web site (www.clubhouseinn.com).

Comfort Inns Web site (www.comfortinn.com).

Country Inns and Suites Web site (www.countryinns.com).

Courtyard Marriott Web site (www.courtyard.com).

Days Inns Web site (www.daysinn.com).

EconoLodge Web site (www.hotelchoice.com).

Entertainment Publications Web site (www.entertainment.com).

Expedia Web site (www.expedia.com).

Fairfield Inn Web site (www.marriotthotels.com).

Frontier Airlines Website (www.frontierairlines.com).

Hampton Inn Web site (www.hampton-inn.com).

Holiday Inn Web site (www.ichotelsgroup.com).

Hotel Discounts.com Network Web site (www.hoteldiscount.com).

Howard Johnson Hotels and Inns Web site (www.hojo.com).

InterviewTrail.com Web site (www.interviewtrail.com).

JetBlue Airways Web site (www.jetblue.com).

La Quinta Inns Web site (www.laquinta.com).

LowestFare.com Web site (www.lowestfare.com).

Midwest Express Web site (www.midwestexpress.com).

Motel 6 Web site (www.motel6.com).

Orbitz Web site (www.orbitz.com).

Packing List Online Web site (www.packinglistonline.com).

Priceline.com Web site (www.priceline.com).

Quikbook Web site (www.quikbook.com).

Ramada Ltd. Web site (www.ramada.com).

Red Roof Inns Web site (www.redroof.com).

Rodeway Inns Web site (www.rodeway.com).

Southwest Airlines Web site (www.southwest.com).

SeatGuru Web site (www.seatguru.com).

SmartMedTravel Web site (www.smartmedtravel.com).

Spirit Airlines Web site (www.spiritair.com).

Sun Country Airlines Web site (www.suncountry.com).

Super 8 Web site (www.super8.com).

Travelocity Web site (www.travelocity.com).

Travelodge Web site (www.travelodge.com).

University of California at San Francisco School of Medicine. *The Next Step: Your Guide to Residency. San Francisco.* University of California at San Francisco, 1995.

Virgin America Airlines Web site (www.virginamerica.com).

# Interview Day

## INTERVIEW PREPARATION

> Be prepared by reading up on the program.

The interview process enables you to come to life in the minds of program directors and faculty. So if you have a strong record and good letters of recommendation, you are likely to receive a "halo effect" during the interview process—you will generally be seen in a favorable light. If your record is weaker than you would like, however, the interview may allow you to showcase your personal qualities and commitment to do better.

It may be useful to think of the interview day as offering you the chance to highlight certain aspects of your application as well as your personal interest in a program. The possibilities include:

- An opportunity to express enthusiasm for the specialty to which you have committed.

- An opportunity to express enthusiasm for the specific program to which you are applying and to gain a deeper understanding of the strengths of that program.

- A chance to express important character traits that are valued by programs, such as hard work, endurance, and teamwork.

- A way to provide evidence that you have been well trained with good faculty mentors and role models—ie, that your medical school has provided an environment of excellence.

The advice given below applies to all specialties. When you are interviewing for highly competitive positions, however—such as those in dermatology and ophthalmology—questions and processes may become more discriminating as program directors try to distinguish one outstanding student from another.

## REVIEW ALL PROGRAM INFORMATION

If you are interviewing with several programs over a few days, be sure you don't mix facts about one program with those of another. One very common interview question—"Why have you chosen to apply to this program?"—requires knowledge of the strengths of the particular program. Always prepare an answer for this question in advance. Good answers to this question might be: the excellent variety of clinical experiences; the fact that the program is affiliated with a university, VA, community, or county hospital; the breadth of electives offered; the research opportunities available; the opportunities for international work; or the outstanding specialty divisions. You are visiting the program to learn about it and to assess its strengths and weaknesses, but be prepared to demonstrate your favorable impression of the program even early on in the interview day. You can make up your own mind about the program later, but during the interview, always keep it positive.

You should also make sure you are familiar with the basic structure of the program, including the length of the residency, the number of residents, and the names of at least the program director(s) and the administrative assistant. In addition, you might choose to familiarize yourself with the basic curriculum at that program, including the names and types of hospitals affiliated with the program. Much of this information is readily available on Web sites, and although the program directors will likely review this information with you during the interview day, it's always best to have a basic understanding of the program before you arrive.

## REVIEW ALL INFORMATION YOU HAVE SUBMITTED

A lack of knowledge or understanding about one's own activities and personal statement is a common shortcoming that is frequently observed in student interviews. Be familiar with every detail of what you have said about yourself. Review the file you have prepared. Think of your CV as a menu of topics that your interviewer might choose to discuss. If your CV says that you participated in a research study that was published, be prepared to discuss that research in a polished manner. If you were a member of the internal medicine interest group, be prepared to describe what that group actually did. Look over the copies of your CV, personal statement, board scores, and literature about the residency program that you have brought with you on the interview day. (Review Figure 10-2 as a reminder of key documents to bring to the interview.) You never know when you might have some down time, and refreshing your knowledge of the program demonstrates interest and enthusiasm. Or if you've published a manuscript, it may be nice to leave a copy with an interviewer if they asked you about the research topic during the interview. Before the big day, you should also get in touch with residents or faculty with ties to your home institution and ask if they will be available to talk with you during the interview day, the social event, or before or after your visit. They may be more open with you about the virtues of the program than people with whom you don't share a common link.

## TYPICAL EVENTS IN AN INTERVIEW VISIT

Each program you visit may organize its interview day differently. Much of the tone of the day will also depend on the competitiveness of the situation. For example, many primary care residency programs will use their time to attract you to their programs and make you feel good about yourself and your opportunities. Obviously, a program that matches with just the right number of applicants will not want to risk turning applicants off by asking difficult patient management questions. On the other hand, a competitive program in neurosurgery or plastic surgery may design their interview day in a manner that will help sort one applicant from another as efficiently as possible. During all interview activities, applicants must balance making a good impression with finding out everything they can about the program in a short period of time. Also, remember that the evaluation process is occurring at every event, not just within an interview itself; so be polite, courteous, and enthusiastic with whomever you meet during your interview day and during the social event. Get contact information from helpful residents whom you met during the day, so you can ask more questions later if needed. Find out if "second looks" or revisits are welcomed, as these often cement favorable impressions. Usual activities for all specialties typically include at least the following:

- **Preinterview social events.** Some programs may arrange dinner the night before the interview with one or more members of the house staff. These dinners

> Stay away from alcohol! You need to be in your best form at preinterview social events.

are usually casual but do vary from one program to another. Informal conversation and frank questions about resident satisfaction with the program are appropriate, but bear in mind that you are potentially being evaluated by the house staff. This is a time when everyone tends to be positive; more objective evaluation will come later. That being said, use common sense. Stay away from excessive amounts of alcohol, mind your table manners, and don't order the most expensive items on the menu. These events may be social (residents only) or more formal extensions of the interview visit (faculty-sponsored). Find out ahead of time and be prepared. Also make an effort to know the dress code. For some affairs, jeans are appropriate; for others, more formal attire may be required. The dress code will usually be outlined in your interview invitation, or you can contact the program's administrative assistant to find out what to wear. The social events are often the best chance to hear candidly from the residents and ask challenging questions. In addition, they often provide applicants the best chance to get a gestalt feeling for a residency program's members.

- **Introduction and orientation.** Larger programs in particular may have interviewees start out together to be addressed by the department chair or the residency program director. This is a time to get a feel for the overall tone and philosophy of the program. Consider it a plus when the department chair shows an interest in the recruitment effort. The department chair controls the budget, faculty, and resources of a program, and some are more interested in residents than others. The general orientation meeting is usually a time to keep a low profile and listen. This is the time when program directors will review basic information about a residency, the curriculum, hospital sites, as well as salary and benefits. While some of this information may be provided on handouts, it never hurts to have your pen ready to jot down a few notes or reminders to yourself during the presentation. Often, what is emphasized in these presentations is an indication of what the leadership considers to be key features of the residency so they can be helpful in identifying programs where the emphasis and resources "match" yours.

- **Morning rounds and conferences.** Applicants are usually invited to attend morning report or other conferences. Again, this can be an excellent learning experience. Such conferences go on just as they would if guests were not attending. You can therefore judge the value of morning report as a learning experience, see how faculty and residents interact, and assess the spirit of the house staff in an important activity. On rare occasions, if you are appropriately encouraged and have a valid point to make, you may also participate as you would as a student in your own conferences. As a general rule, however, a low profile is the best approach. Do not fall asleep during the conference session, as program directors and current house staff will take notice!

- **A tour.** Most programs will incorporate a tour of the hospital and main areas where you will be working. Table 11-1 lists commonly included tour sights. If there is a part of the hospital that you did not tour but are interested in seeing, be sure to ask if you can visit at the end of the interview day. As you move through the interview season, every hospital will start to look the same, but you can take advantage of the tour, usually led by a resident, as another op-

## TABLE 11-1

### Sights to See on a Program Tour

| Highest Priority | Possible Areas to See | Extras |
|---|---|---|
| Wards (or emergency room for Emergency Medicine interviews) | Emergency room | Surrounding city |
| | Cafeteria | Fitness facilities |
| ICU | Library/computer resources | Child care facilities |
| Surgical suites (for surgical fields) | | |
| Call rooms or resident lounges | | |

portunity to ask questions and expect more candid, realistic responses from a current house officer.

- **Lunch with residents or faculty.** For those who may have missed the preinterview social events, lunch can be a chance to get to know the residents and get a better feel for the program. Use proper table manners and don't eat too much. You don't want to suffer a postmeal crash in the middle of afternoon activities.

> Watch what you say to whom. Assume everyone you meet will have a hand in ranking applicants.

## INTERVIEWING

In almost all studies on resident selection, the interview is judged to be one of the most important factors influencing house staff selection. Indeed, specific studies from most disciplines rank the interview at the top of the list or second only to grade point average. Applicant characteristics felt to be important in the interview include compatibility with the program, the ability to articulate thoughts and goals, the ability to work with a team, maturity, and hard work. It should also be noted that medical students find the interview process to be an extremely important element figuring in their selection decisions. "Perceived happiness of current residents" is one of the most important considerations for students, and this assessment is generally made during the interview day.

Try to arrive 10 to 15 minutes early on the day of the interview. If possible, make a trial run to the interview location the night before so that you don't get lost or delayed the next day. Punctuality is critical as a resident, and you don't want to make a bad impression to start off your interview day. If there is an interview social event the night before, ask the current residents in attendance about the best way to reach the interview location; they will give you great pearls on how not to get lost. If you drink coffee regularly in the morning, help yourself to your usual cup (most programs will provide breakfast); but be careful not to over-caffeinate, especially if you are jet-lagged. Your interview day is no time to make yourself more jittery or to find yourself needing to use the bathroom continuously.

You should also recognize that programs seldom attempt to standardize interviewing techniques from one faculty member to another or even to ask similar questions. Instead, interviews are usually quite informal. However, most will result in some type of quantitative rating that will be included in an overall point score.

Generally, during the interview day the entire group of applicants gathers in a conference room and then waits to be called into individual interviews. This is a good time to learn the pronunciation of your interviewer's name from the departmental secretary or the interviewer's administrative assistant. It may help allay anxiety to remember that interviews often run behind schedule and that experienced interviewers are aware of this tendency. If you are running late, your subsequent interviewer will understand when you explain that your previous interview has just concluded. When you meet your interviewer, introduce yourself and offer a firm, confident handshake. Remember to smile and conduct yourself with confidence and poise. After you are invited into the office, do not sit down until the interviewer takes a seat or invites you to do so.

During the interview, maintain fairly constant eye contact with the interviewer. Do not let your gaze or attention wander, especially when the interviewer is speaking directly to you. Do not take notes during the interview; instead, remember to write them down later. Try to project a high energy level even if this is your fifteenth interview. Lack of enthusiasm is the most common mistake students make. Many students complain that the most difficult interviews are those with faculty members who lack enthusiasm. In fact, this will be the student's greatest challenge. Answer questions fully, but do not ramble; if the interviewer wants to know more about a particular subject, he or she will ask. Speak clearly and use proper grammar. If you can, steer the interview toward your strong points, but do not pressure the interviewer or dominate the dialogue. Never look at your watch even if you know that the interview is running overtime. When the interview is finished, thank the interviewer, shake hands again, and leave gracefully.

> Table Manners 101: Always place your napkin in your lap, don't talk with your mouth full, and use utensils, not your fingers.

> Apathy is the kiss of death at interview time.

## POPULAR INTEVIEW QUESTIONS AND THE RIGHT ANSWERS!

While the interview conversation could wind its way through many topics, there are certain questions that are relatively universal across specialties. It is a good idea to jot down some notes on how you would answer these questions. In doing so you will be more prepared and feel confident, avoiding any momentary deer-in-the-headlights look when these questions are asked.

### 1. TELL ME ABOUT YOURSELF.

This is perhaps the most common and most universal opening question during residency interviews. It is an opportunity for you to tell the interviewer what you feel is important to know. It is also a way for the interviewer to understand what excites you and what experiences have shaped you. Do not simply share historic or biographical data. The key is to focus your answer, be succinct, and use the opportunity to share something unique or expand upon what the interviewer already knows. One way to answer this question, is to briefly outline the motivation that

Should you have a case presented to you, see if it is intended to test a basic lesson. For example, that lesson might be to not believe every lab test, to ask the patient a question that was missed, to check the physical exam again, or to take the history and do the physical yourself. We do know of some cases that have been presented to students with the goal of testing basic approaches to a patient. If you're put in the position of discussing a very specific disease or treatment modality that you are unfamiliar with, don't panic and instead take a moment to think through the problem presented. As with most parts of medicine, there will not always be one correct answer to a case presentation. Instead, it's important that you can explain your approach to a patient and demonstrate your reasoning using evidence-based medicine.

## 2. DISCUSS THE POLITICS OF HEALTH CARE.

Although we have not found this topic to be a significant area for student interviews, it is important to be aware of the challenges health care providers face today.

Department chairs and residency program directors will be concerned about how medical education, especially as it pertains to their specialty of interest, will change in the future. They will be concerned about how faculty can generate their own salaries while still finding the time to teach effectively and do research. They will want to provide indigent care but will recognize that academic medical centers cannot care for all patients who lack health insurance. They will seek reform in the medical malpractice process. Be engaging but not overly political in your discussion of these topics. In general, expect interviewers to stay away from topics that require you to reveal partisan leanings or that test your own political affiliations. If you find an issue to be overly polarizing, take the judicious route of explaining both sides of the argument and your understanding of the reasoning for each side. If you feel very comfortable and knowledgeable on the topic, you may choose to take sides, but always acknowledge and be understanding of the fact that your opinion is not shared by all.

## 3. DESCRIBE A CHALLENGING SITUATION OR ETHICAL DILEMMA YOU FACED ON THE WARDS AND HOW YOU DEALT WITH IT.

Interviewers will sometimes be interested in learning about how you approach challenges and what problem-solving skills you use. Inevitably during third year you've had to deal with difficult patients or been placed on teams where the dynamics did not work well. These are perfect examples to use when answering the question. Interviewers will not be interested in learning about all the details of why the situation is challenging or hearing you complain about what problems you encountered. Instead, they will be more interested in hearing a short summary of the situation and what you did to overcome it. For example, if you had to deal with a patient who exhibited drug-seeking behavior, focus on the fact that you were able to treat the patient's pain at the same time as working with a social worker to help the patient discuss issues of addiction.

Interviewers will be interested to learn that you understand what resources are available in both the hospital and outpatient settings. They will want to understand your approach to a situation and what teamwork skills you employ during those encounters. Focus on specific examples, rather than generalities. Describe situations that ended positively and in which you were able to bring your team together to truly improve the situation.

## 4. WHERE ELSE HAVE YOU APPLIED?

Applicants are sometimes thrown off when program directors or other interviewers inquire about where they have applied. Most often, this question is asked as a general conversation topic, as a way to learn more about the applicant, or as a way to gauge the types of programs an applicant is interested in. It is not asked in order to find what programs the director might contact to gossip about you, and it should not be used by an interviewer to highlight negatives of other programs. If that occurs, you should be somewhat skeptical.

You should feel comfortable answering the question honestly and may choose to answer by naming specific programs or by being more vague and describing the geographic regions to which you have applied. Sometimes, this question can be a great segue into explaining what you are looking for in a program. By giving examples of the types of programs you applied to, you can describe what common themes led you to apply—perhaps the programs all include research opportunities or they are all associated with county hospitals seeing urban populations—and it allows you to highlight how the program at which you are interviewing is particularly attractive to you. However, do not use this as an opportunity to be overly negative and bash other programs. You should instead highlight the positives of the program you are visiting.

## 5. DISCUSS CONCERNS OR AN INCONSISTENCY IN YOUR APPLICATION (EG, DIFFICULTY WITH A SPECIFIC COURSE, ROTATION, EXAM).

Rarely, a faculty member or program director may bring up a specific issue with your application. If this occurs, you should stay calm and consider it as an opportunity for a clear explanation. Your immediate response may be to become emotional or overly defensive; instead, you should not take the question personally, and you should try to take full responsibility for any specific difficulty that you had. Identify what the confounding situation was (eg, family member illness) and state what you learned from this that will help you the next time a similar situation arises.

In addition to the common questions discussed in detail above, below are a list of questions gleaned from residency directors, departmental chairs, and interviewers in a number of fields. Some are straightforward, some are off the wall, and others require some thought, preferably forethought!

1. Describe a patient with whom you had a particularly meaningful interaction.

2. What was the first job or the most interesting job you have had?

3. What is your favorite activity outside of the hospital? Or what do you do for fun?

4. Do you feel comfortable working with patients of all ages?

5. What is your leadership style?

6. What will you be considering or thinking about when you make your rank list?

7. What would you do if you did not go into this particular specialty?

8. If the field of medicine did not exist, what profession would you have chosen?

9. Do you enjoy working under pressure?

10. What is the last specialty you would choose, and why?

11. What would you choose as your personal theme song?

12. What will be most important to you in ten years?

13. What is it that separates you from the other interviewees and applicants?

14. At the end of your life, what would you like to be able to say about yourself and your life?

15. What do you think is an important unanswered question in medicine, and how would you design a research project to address it?

16. What would you like to talk about?

There are also numerous Web sites and online resources that contain common interview questions, tips and techniques, and examples of how to answer the "hardball" questions. Many of these resources are not tailored specifically to residency interviewing, or the field of medicine for that matter, but they do often contain useful general principles and answers for general questions. One large database can be found at Answers.com, a Wiki site, which catalogs common job interview questions and "answers" (wiki.answers.com/Q/FAQ/1869). Keep in mind, however, that this is a public site that contains unverified information, so take answers with a grain of salt.

Student Doctor Network also contains a useful column (www.studentdoctor.net/category/medical/interview-secrets/) about common interview questions and pitfalls. This resource is more tailored to the Match.

## ILLEGAL QUESTIONS

Questions considered illegal in employment screening are those that deal with race, sex, age, body habitus, marital status, family plans, or physical disability. If you are asked an illegal question, don't be defensive. Many faculty may be new to interviewing and may not realize that their question is inappropriate.

In response to an illegal question, you may choose to:

1. **Answer.** This is the safest course. You may be open or vague. For example, if asked about plans to start a family, you might answer, "I have no plans to do so until after I complete my training." Another answer could be, "My education is my priority right now."

2. **Deflect.** You can sidestep the question by saying something like, "That is an interesting question. I haven't really thought about it." Or "I would have to think about that more before I could answer."

3. **Decline to answer.** You could remind the interviewer that his or her question is illegal and politely refuse to comment. This is a high-risk tactic.

If you find yourself feeling uncomfortable during an interview because of an obvious or egregious "illegal question," and you feel that it may affect your overall review during the selection process, it is permissible to discuss the situation with the program director after the interview. Be sure to recall the name of the interviewer and the specific situation that made you uncomfortable. While it is often difficult to approach your potential employer about the incident, the process should be made fair for everyone. After the interview day is over or during a break in interviews, politely ask the administrative assistant to talk with the program director. Alternatively, you can call the program director after the interview day is over—often, it isn't until a day or two later that you truly feel that your performance may have been affected. Explain the situation and ask if there is anything you can do to rectify what happened. The program director may simply make note of the situation and take that particular interview with a grain of salt, or may offer you another chance to interview. More often than not, you'll find that the interviewer will not have realized that anything was wrong and that your review would not have been affected either way.

## INTERVIEW PITFALLS

Given all the time, expense, and adrenaline that enter into your program interviews, you don't want to hurt your chances for success with an ill-considered answer or comment. Some of the problems that students face during the interview day are as follows:

- **Underestimating the importance of first impressions.** Before you ever open your mouth to answer a question, you are sending a message to your interviewer. Proper appearance, confident posture, a smile, and a firm handshake are key. You may be nervous, but this is not the time to let it show.

- **Blurting out responses.** If you are blindsided by a difficult question, it's okay to pause for a moment and think before you answer. Silence during an interview may feel long and awkward, but taking a few moments to collect yourself can pay off with a smooth answer.

- **Rambling.** Interviewers probably hear enough poorly constructed medical student presentations as it is, so try to focus your responses. If rambling is just a nervous habit for you, the problem should dissipate as you gain experience and become more comfortable with the interview process. If this is not the case, however, you should make a conscious effort to provide complete yet focused answers. You may find that practice sessions with a friendly classmate can help you overcome this tendency.

- **Not knowing anything about the program.** No one will ever expect you to know their program through and through, but you should at least know the basics of each one. Interviewers do not want to waste the time allotted for the interview going over information that is already available in their printed materials.

- **Focusing on the program's weaknesses.** It's true in a philosophical sense that you are interviewing the program as much as they are interviewing you. But be practical; don't put the interviewer on the defensive by concentrating on the program's weaknesses. If these problem spots are of paramount importance to you, save your concerns for the house staff or raise the issue in a friendly, nonconfrontational manner.

- **Inconsistent/evasive answers.** Answers that don't match up with what you wrote on your application will place interviewers on the alert, as will answers that are incomplete. Emphasize your strengths as well as the clinical and academic interests you share with the interviewer. At the same time, do not exaggerate, lie, or otherwise distort facts. Interviewers expect applicants to be open and honest.

- **Displaying an eccentric personality.** The interviewer is trying to picture you as a junior colleague with whom daily interaction will be necessary. So if you come across as domineering, uncooperative, or temperamental, you will hurt your chances of selection even if your grades and other scores are good.

- **Pejorative comments about other programs.** Negative statements (especially unsolicited or unsupported digs) about other programs or your own school will be noted as indiscretions and will reflect badly on you. Interviewers will wonder what you might say about their program at the next stop on your tour. You should also remember that the academic community is tight, and the interviewer may have colleagues and friends at the programs you just put down.

- **Poor interactions with administrative staff or current residents.** Rudeness or lack of consideration for administrative personnel will be relayed to the residency selection committee and will end up as a strike against you. Always be on your best behavior and remember your manners in all of your interactions throughout the interview day. It's important to be polite to everyone, not just your interviewers.

- **Not rehearsing answers.** As discussed earlier in this chapter, several interview questions are quite common, and you should have practiced the right answers before the big day. Avoid fumbling by participating in a mock interview session (speak with your advisor). However, try to vary the structure of your answers a little so that you don't come across as rehearsed.

- **Not promoting key assets.** Before you begin interviewing, you should prepare a list of key points that you would like to get across during the course of your interview. You will not have complete control over what is asked of you during the interview, but by knowing beforehand what information you would like to convey, you can work it into your answers.

- **Zoning out.** Now is the time to focus and show that you have good listening skills. If you have adequately prepared for your interview, you won't need to think of how you are going to answer a question while the interviewer is still speaking. Avoid the embarrassment of not addressing a question properly by concentrating on what your interviewer is saying.

- **Selling yourself short.** You should avoid rambling, but never give a "yes" or "no" answer to an interviewer's questions. Always follow up with something that emphasizes your strengths as an applicant. When in doubt, you can always lead the interviewer back to some aspect of your application, whether it is an activity, research, or your personal statement.

- **Sticking your foot in your mouth.** A little silence is okay during the interview. If you finish answering a question and are met with a blank stare, don't panic. The interviewer may be taking a mental note or thinking of what to ask you next, or he or she may be trying to make you nervous. Avoid the temptation to change your answer or say something stupid.

- **Minding your manners—to the extreme.** It is important to be polite and formal, but not to the point that you avoid making a connection with your interviewer. Don't be so focused on professionalism that you come across as rigid and distant. Relax a little and enjoy getting to know your interviewer.

- **Being apathetic.** People who volunteer to interview do so because they are excited about their program and their specialty. They are looking for applicants who share the same enthusiasm. If you are jet-lagged, feeling blue, or having a slow morning, put that aside and focus on being the animated, energetic person that they might want to work with some day.

- **Lacking confidence.** If you have made it to the interview, you are past the hurdle of being considered acceptable. Don't let the stress of the interview day or the competition get the best of you. Remind yourself of how far you have come, and go on your selling points. Projecting poise requires more than speaking confidently. Remember nonverbal cues as well: be certain to stand tall, smile, offer a firm handshake, don't fidget, and maintain eye contact.

- **Lacking interest.** Even if all your questions have been answered a hundred times over, never say no when an interviewer asks if you have any questions. It is always of benefit to get different perspectives on aspects of the program, and not asking a question could lead the interviewer to think that you are not very interested in the program. You can always turn the tables a bit and let the interviewer do the talking by asking something like: "What made you choose this particular field/program/city/?"

- **Ending on a low note.** The end to the interview should mirror the beginning. Eye contact, a smile, and a firm handshake, together with thanking the interviewer for his or her time, are critical for a memorable finish.

> You have put a lot of work into interviewing. Don't cut yourself short by being unprepared.

> Don't get lured into criticizing other programs.

## WHAT DO I ASK THE INTERVIEWER?

Toward the middle or the end of the session, your interviewer will invariably ask you, "Do you have any questions?" As the interview season rolls on, you will begin to get tired of this repetitive question. However, on every interview you attend, be prepared in advance with at least one or two questions that demonstrate your interest, as long as they are appropriate to the interviewer and to the program. Faculty members can field more philosophical and broad-based questions such as the ones listed below.

An ideal question to ask is one that the interviewer will enjoy answering, thus lending a positive tone to the encounter. Remember that you are still the person under observation and evaluation, so do not harp on the program's weaknesses. Also avoid asking questions about salaries and benefits, vacation, moonlighting, call schedules, and other aspects of day-to-day program operations. These questions will be answered by the program director during the presentation portion of the interview day. Also, you can save these practical concerns for the house staff, and keep your interview questions friendly and benign. Appropriate questions for faculty interviewers are as follows:

> The questions you ask can be revealing to the interviewer.

1. Where have your residents gone after graduation?

2. What process do you have for improving the residency? For evaluating rotations? Do you anticipate any changes in the residency program?

3. Have you ever done surveys of your graduates? What do they tell you?

4. What research opportunities are available? What is the availability of funding for research? What kind of mentor support is available from the faculty?

5. In what direction do you see the chair (or residency director) taking the program? Do you believe that he or she will remain here during my residency training?

6. What opportunities are available to attend regional and national conferences and seminars?

7. How well do residents perform on board certification exams?

8. What is the structure of the last years of residency? Does the program offer elective time? Mini-fellowships? Time and opportunity to work abroad?

9. Is there training relating to the business and legal aspects of the specialty?

10. How does the faculty support residents, and is there a formal mentorship program within the residency?

11. What attracted you to join the faculty of this program, and what changes have you seen during your time here?

## WHAT TYPES OF QUESTIONS SHOULD I ASK THE HOUSE STAFF?

We have compiled a list of questions that you might ask house staff while you are visiting the program. Most of these questions deal with the daily operation of the residency. A few questions, however, are sensitive ones that you might not feel comfortable asking all house staff members you encounter (eg, chief residents steeped in the program's "party line"). These are ideal questions to ask at interview day social events, lunch with residents, or during the tour. Given that any question you ask could potentially make it back to the selection committee, always exercise discretion, especially with touchy topics.

### GENERAL QUESTIONS

1. Are the residents happy? What features of the program do they like or dislike?
2. Would the residents choose the same program again?

### LOCATION

1. Is the program located in a safe part of the city? If not, what is the security system like?
2. What do residents do for fun around here?
3. What advantages are specific to the location (eg, unusual patient population, cultural opportunities, climate, low cost of living)?
4. How do residents commute to the hospital? Is there a useful public transit system in the city?
5. Where do most residents live? Do they rent or buy housing?

### REPUTATION

1. Do graduates of the program have problems finding jobs?
2. How difficult is it for residents to get a good fellowship?

### EDUCATION

1. Is the program fully accredited? For how long?
2. How are the residents evaluated? By whom?
3. Is there an organized curriculum? What is its emphasis?
4. How many conferences are there per week? Do conferences emphasize practical knowledge or state-of-the-art research?
5. What is the quality of the attendings? What are their responsibilities? Do they get along?

6.  How interested are the faculty in the education and welfare of the house staff?

7.  What proportion of attendings are private?

8.  Are there medical students on the wards? What school(s) do they represent? What are the residents' teaching responsibilities to the students?

9.  What research opportunities are there? Are faculty research preceptors readily available?

## WORK ENVIRONMENT

1.  What is the patient load like?

2.  What are the typical admissions diagnoses?

3.  How many cases are treated by the average resident?

4.  Is the caseload sufficiently varied?

5.  How much autonomy do residents have to manage patients?

6.  What is the patient population like? Ethnicity/language? Socioeconomic status?

7.  Is there continuity of care for patients after discharge?

8.  What is the extent and quality of the ambulatory experience?

9.  How strong is nursing support? Consult services? Radiology? Pathology? Emergency services?

10. How much "scut work" is done by house staff? Are there blood-drawing/IV teams?

11. What is the typical call schedule?

12. How does the work environment vary from service to service? From hospital to hospital?

13. How busy are call nights? How much sleep do you usually get?

14. How available are the attendings? Can you call them at night?

15. Is there backup available when you're on call? Is there a night float system?

16. How many hours do you work each week? Do the residents ever exceed the 80-hour workweek cap?

17. How much time do you get off each week?

18. Is there a fair backup or "jeopardy" system in case a resident is ill or has a family emergency? How often is this system used?

## SALARY

1.  What is the starting salary for an intern? For an R2?

2.  What about cost of living in the area?

3.  Is moonlighting permitted? If so, how does it work around here?

## BENEFITS

1. What health benefits are available (eg, medical insurance, dental plan, vision plan)? Are spouses covered?

2. What is the maternity/paternity leave policy?

3. Is life insurance available? Disability insurance?

4. Is parking provided? Is subsidized housing available? What is the vacation schedule setup?

If you have a chance, you may also want to speak with senior medical students at the institution you are visiting. They can provide additional insight and perspective into the institution and area.

## QUESTIONS FOR THE DEPARTMENT CHAIR AND THE PROGRAM DIRECTOR

Department chairs see the residency program as lying somewhere in a list of priorities. They are also responsible for the overall budget, and their generosity may make the difference between going to a conference or staying home; whether or not an away elective is possible on the basis of funding issues; or whether start-up funds are available for a resident research project. Similarly, chairmen will know what changes may be imminent in a program or whether a program is likely to grow or get smaller. They will also be responsible for helping recruit the best possible teaching faculty. Questions about these objectives—eg, whether additional faculty are being recruited or whether residents are encouraged to do research—will give the chair an opportunity to discuss his or her role in the residency program.

The residency program director is the most important person with whom you will interview. It is therefore key to determine if he or she appears to have a genuine concern for residents. If the program director does not demonstrate the personal qualities to treat you well on the interview, the situation will be worse when you arrive for work. Ask about the director's plans for the future, ideas about curricular change, assessment of the quality of the graduating residents, and approach to board preparation.

## WRAPPING UP THE INTERVIEW DAY

If you are serious about a program and want to learn more about it, speak to the departmental secretary or a house staff member and get the contact information for one or two of the residents with whom you developed a good connection. This may be helpful if you have additional questions or need advice. You can also ask about whether the institution allows or recommends second visits. A second visit allows you to spend more time on rounds, in clinic or surgery, in conferences, and in the surrounding neighborhood. It also gives you an opportunity to confirm or modify your initial impressions of the program. However, do not feel obligated to return to a program, and do so only if you are truly interested in learning more. Many institutions discourage it, as it takes a great deal of work to set up shadowing opportunities and second-look visits. Also, returning for a second visit will have no bearing on your rank position with the program.

Be sure to jot down your impressions of each program while they are still fresh in your mind. After you have visited four or five programs, the details will start to blur. To help keep your facts and impressions straight, write down all your thoughts about a program as soon as you can at the end of the day. Use the Program Evaluation Worksheet provided in Appendix B if you need help organizing your thoughts. You will thank yourself later when you can rank your programs with detailed notes while your classmates are banging their heads against the wall trying to remember which program had the deluxe call rooms with the well-stocked refrigerators and HBO.

Also make a point of evaluating your own performance during the interview. If you were surprised by a question, review how you might give a more polished answer. If you had any difficulties, review the "Interview Pitfalls" section and take steps to ensure a better interview at the next program.

## FOLLOW-UP LETTERS

Unless your interviewer explicitly tells you not to do so, write a letter to thank the program for its hospitality as well as to express your continued interest. In general, you can write one letter addressed to the program director who invited you to interview. This letter should be composed and mailed no more than a few days after the interview, while memories of the interview (both on your part and theirs) are still fresh. A sincere follow-up letter can help solidify the impression you left on the interviewer before it is washed away by subsequent interviews. If you also happened to click individually with one or more interviewers, you might choose to write them a brief thank-you note as well. Alternatively, you can mention that you enjoyed interviewing with those particular faculty members, and ask the program director to whom you are writing to extend your thanks to the other faculty.

Personalize your letter by mentioning a specific topic that was discussed during the interview. If you recently received any honors or awards, it is perfectly okay to use your letter to update your application file. Do not be shy in describing why you liked the program and in stating that you will be ranking it highly, but only if you plan to do so (see Figure 11-1). It should be noted, however, that follow-up letters carry limited weight, as many applicants choose to follow up on all the programs in which they interviewed and will often tell every program they will be ranked highly. It should be reiterated that program directors do not take follow-up letters into consideration when making their rank lists.

> Have follow-up letters in the mail within 1–2 days of the interview.

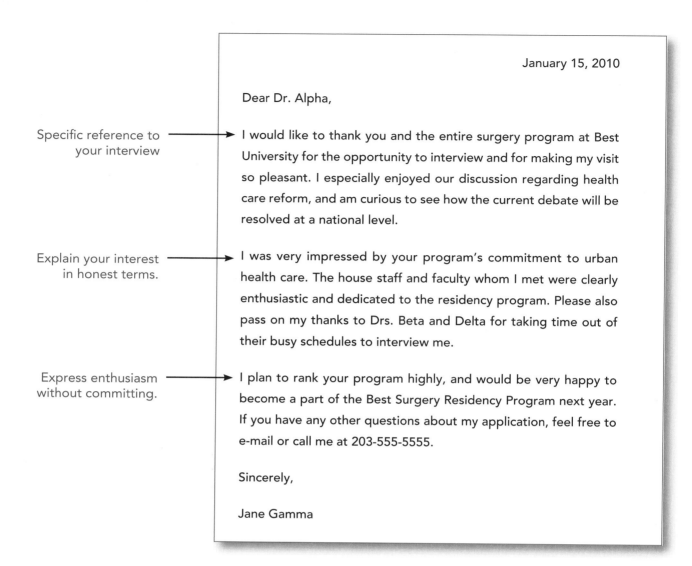

Specific reference to your interview

Explain your interest in honest terms.

Express enthusiasm without committing.

January 15, 2010

Dear Dr. Alpha,

I would like to thank you and the entire surgery program at Best University for the opportunity to interview and for making my visit so pleasant. I especially enjoyed our discussion regarding health care reform, and am curious to see how the current debate will be resolved at a national level.

I was very impressed by your program's commitment to urban health care. The house staff and faculty whom I met were clearly enthusiastic and dedicated to the residency program. Please also pass on my thanks to Drs. Beta and Delta for taking time out of their busy schedules to interview me.

I plan to rank your program highly, and would be very happy to become a part of the Best Surgery Residency Program next year. If you have any other questions about my application, feel free to e-mail or call me at 203-555-5555.

Sincerely,

Jane Gamma

**FIGURE 11-1.** Example of a follow-up note.

# REFERENCES

Answers.com "Job Interview Questions" Web site (wiki.answers.com/Q/FAQ/1869).

Crane JT, Ferraro CM. Selection criteria for emergency medicine residency applicants. *Acad Emerg Med* 7(1):54–60, 2000.

Delisa JA, Jain SS, Campagnolo DI. Factors used by physical medicine and rehabilitation residency training directors to select their residents. *Am J Phys Med Rehabil* 73(3):152–156, 1994.

Koscove EM. An applicant's evaluation of an emergency medicine internship and residency. *Ann Emerg Med* 19(7):774-780, 1990.

Pretorius ES, Hrung J. Factors that affect National Resident Matching Program rankings of medical students applying for radiology residency. *Acad Radiol* 9(1):75–81, 2002.

Student Doctor Network "Interview Secrets" Web site (www.studentdoctor.net/category/medical/interview-secrets).

Taylor CA, Weinstein L, Mayhew HE. The process of resident selection: a view from the residency director's desk. *Obstet Gynecol* 85(2):299–303, 1995.

Wagoner NE, Suriano JR. Program directors' responses to a survey on variables used to select residents in a time of change. *Acad Med* 74(1):51–58, 1999.

Wagoner NE, Suriano JR, Stoner JA. Factors used by program directors to select residents. *J Med Educ* 61(1):10–21, 1986.

# 12

# The Rank List and Match Day

## HOW DO I RANK THE PROGRAMS?

Before the dust even settles from the whirlwind of interview season, you will be faced with a still more challenging task: creating your rank-order list (ROL). The ROL and Match process is one of the most peculiar ways to find a job, but if completed properly, most find that everything works out as it should. Year after year, however, really smart applicants make regrettable mistakes when it comes to ranking programs. These missteps can only shortchange the applicant. To clarify the ranking process, we have developed two absolute rules to remember when you create your ROL.

**Rule #1: Rank programs in order of their desirability to you.** Desirability combines what you, the applicant, consider to be your true preference for residency with the strength of an individual program as it relates to your residency training. Since you have already deeply scrutinized all the programs across the country while determining where to apply and subsequently interview, the process now focuses on your interpretation of the desirability of each program using the information you've gathered on the interview trail.

Generally, most applicants are able to group programs into certain categories of desirability: the perfect match; programs that you would love; programs that are acceptable; and programs that you wouldn't ever want to attend. One strategy is to write the name of each program you are considering on a note card and then put the note cards into piles for each of the aforementioned categories. It may be that several programs fall into one of these categories, so the next step is to tease apart which program is more desirable within the particular category. Once you've sorted the note cards, you've found at least a preliminary ROL!

When trying to sort programs into the various categories and rank one program above another, you should take into account the core characteristics of the programs you are considering. Look back through the notes you took along the interview trail, remembering your gut feeling at each place and your interactions with residents and faculty. While some people need only a few minutes of reflection to solidify the "best" order, others may find it helpful to make a list of pros and cons when faced with close ranking decisions. Remember, your ROL need not mirror the "Top 10" from any source other than your own head. The object is to match with your most desirable program, not to match with the choice ranked first by your peers, your mentors, or by *US News and World Report*. The major factors that may affect where a program ranks in desirability include (in no particular order):

- Geographic location, surrounding activities, and associated cost of living.

- Program structure—are there additional years of research or elective opportunities?

- Program setting—academic, private, or county.

- Program curriculum or specific training experiences that are offered.

- Administration and faculty, including related research opportunities.

- Benefits and salary.

- Job opportunities for a spouse/partner.

- An overall gut feeling about a program and how well you "connected." This factor is frequently cited as the most important.

> Do not rush the rank. It is a decision you'll have to live with for a long time.

Ideally, the programs at the bottom of your ROL will serve as backups—acceptable programs that are a sure bet. **Do not rank a program lower because you believe your chances of attaining that program are slim.** The Match process favors the applicant's choice, so be sure to rank programs in the order that you would want to attend. Do not try to "play the game" and overthink how a program will rank you, because you may miss your opportunity to go to a more desirable program. For example, if you guess that your third-choice program will definitely rank you at the top of their list, and you then rank that program first, you could miss out on the opportunity to attend your true first- or second-choice program if they rank you highly.

Remember, the ROLs for both applicants and programs are private. You don't have to show yours to anyone, and once the Match is over, it will never be seen again. So this is the time to shoot high—don't sell yourself short, but be prepared for the unexpected as well. This caveat brings us to the second rule.

**Rule #2: Rank all acceptable programs.** Do not rank any programs in which you would not be willing to work. Remember that you are under contract to report to the program in which you match. If the program is on your ROL at all, you're telling the National Residency Matching Program (NRMP) that you are willing to go to that program if you match there. You are under no obligation to rank every program that you visit. However, you must decide whether it is better to match at a less-than-ideal program or take your chances in the Scramble if you do not match. The latter option, while highly undesirable, is certainly viable in specialties that often have a large number of unfilled positions on Match Day, such as family medicine or internal medicine. As you near the bottom of your rank list, it is important to ask yourself for each of the programs: "Would I rather attend this program than go unmatched and have to scramble?" If the answer is no, then do not rank the program.

The actual number of programs to rank depends on several factors, including the competitiveness of the specialty, the competitiveness of the specific programs being ranked, and the applicant's qualifications. In most instances, the issue is not the actual number of programs on the ROL, but whether to add one or more programs to the list in order to reduce the likelihood of being unmatched. Both applicants and programs are well advised to include all acceptable choices on their ROLs. A long ROL in no way affects the chances of being matched to choices higher on the ROL. It is interesting to note, however, that U.S. seniors consistently have the highest Match rate and the longest average ROLs. Data from 2008 suggest that for those applicants who matched, the ROL contained an average of about 8 programs, almost twice the number of programs listed compared to those who went unmatched. Although there are small year-to-year variations, about 94% of U.S. seniors match each year. The upshot: ranking more programs improves your chances of matching.

> A common reason for going unmatched is ranking too few programs.

For students applying in extremely competitive fields such as plastic surgery or dermatology, following these rules too strictly can lead to heartbreak. The intense competition in some specialties means that unless you walk on water, it is possible that you will not get a match. To prepare for such a competitive match, students should carefully consider the value of applying to positions outside their specialty of choice. If not matching is unacceptable, it would be wise to have a backup

## TABLE 12-1

**Ways to Improve Your Chances of Matching**

Build a strong foundation through your CV and a solid interview performance.

Realistically assess your competitiveness and the competitiveness of the programs.

Apply and interview at a sufficient number of programs.

Rank all programs acceptable to you.

If you aim for a tough specialty, have a backup plan.

plan in another field, whether this includes scrambling for a different residency specialty, choosing to do a preliminary or transitional year, or applying for a year of postdoctoral research.

The two rules above do not guarantee a match; they guarantee only that you will do the best you can with the tools you have at your disposal. If you are having a tough time putting all your information together, walk through your ROL with your significant other, friend, or career advisor. See Table 12-1 for a summary of ways to improve your chances of matching.

## THE NRMP MATCHING ALGORITHM

The NRMP and the Canadian Resident Matching Service use the same matching algorithm. Outlined below is a simplified explanation of the NRMP algorithm. For details (or to view a sample match between five students and five programs), visit the NRMP Web site (www.nrmp.org/res_ match/about_res/algorithms.html).

1. The process begins with an attempt to place an applicant into his or her first-choice program. If a match cannot be made because the program is already filled (with more desirable applicants) or the applicant was not ranked by that program, an attempt is then made to match with the next program on his or her ROL. Note that the second program on the ROL is now treated as that applicant's first choice in the Match. This process continues until a tentative match has been made or the applicant is left unmatched.

2. In the next round, an attempt is made to place the next applicant into his or her first-choice program. If this new applicant is more attractive to a program than another applicant who is already tentatively matched, the least preferred applicant is removed to make room for the more desirable applicant, and a new tentative match is made. The process will be repeated for the candidate who was removed from the Match.

3. The process is carried out for all applicants until each has been tentatively matched to the most preferred choice possible or until all choices have been exhausted.

4. When all applicants have been considered, the tentative matches become final and the process is complete.

In short, each applicant moves "down" his or her ROL until a tentative match has been made or all choices have been exhausted, while each program moves "up" its ROL. Note that no applicant can be bypassed by a lower-ranked applicant for a given program. If the higher-ranked applicant did not match there, it's because the applicant already had a more desirable offer in hand. Since the algorithm was computerized in 1974, the process takes only minutes to run each year—but we still wait weeks to find out the results!

## HOW DO COUPLES RANK PROGRAMS?

The NRMP Web site (www.nrmp.org/res_match/special_part/us_seniors/couples. html) includes a step-by-step guide for creating a couples ROL that is quite extensive and sound. In general, the goal of the Couples Match is for you and your partner to stay geographically close to one another. This is a good time to reiterate that any two people can register in the Couples Match. Marriage, sexual orientation, medical school attended, and field of interest are not considered by the computer algorithm in the couples match.

That said, you and your partner should first rank programs as if you were matching on your own. Read the section "How Do I Rank the Programs?" for guidelines (see above). You should then list the possible program pairs if you are ranking more than one program in the same city. In addition to program pairs in the same city/area (Type 1), there are two other types of program pairs to consider: pairs of programs not in the same city/area (Type 2) and combinations in which one partner goes unmatched (Type 3). Consider creating and ranking Type 2 pairings if separation is tolerable. These pairs allow both partners to match semi-independently. Because Type 2 pairings are not restricted by geography, the number of possible permutations is large. Consider creating and ranking Type 3 pairings only if it is acceptable for one of you to match and the other to enter the Scramble. This is usually preferable to both of you going unmatched.

Ranking program pairs is a classic process of give and take. Fortunately, the process can be less painful if you and your partner have communicated well during the application process and thus have an understanding of one another's preferences. Couples must decide how much weight to give to location as opposed to programs. Regardless, the process may take a few evenings and some honest conversations. After all, your ROL can easily be more than 100 pairs long. Staying organized through the process is also important. The NRMP Couples Match Web site contains useful Excel spreadsheets that can be used as a template for tracking and ranking all possible iterations couples are considering. When ranking Type 3 pairings, you should also factor in the location, as it will be easier for the unmatched partner to scramble in a large city where there are many training programs. You can register for the Couples Match when both of you enter your ROLs. You must have your partner's Association of American Medical Colleges (AAMC) ID number, and he or she will appear as a "linked" Match list.

As with the regular Match, you should keep in mind that it is possible that you, your partner, or both may not match at any of your ranked programs. Remember to always hope for the best, but prepare for the worst. Discuss the possibility of not matching and think through the different scenarios if the worst comes to pass. Coordination, communication, and a good action plan are critical for a couple in the Scramble (see below).

> Ranking programs as a couple is an exercise in communication and compromise.

## SUPPLEMENTAL RANK-ORDER LISTS

When an applicant ranks an advanced position, one that begins during the second postgraduate year (PGY-2), he or she also submits a ranking of PGY-1 (transitional or preliminary) programs on a supplemental rank-order list (SROL). The applicant can submit more than one SROL, thus tailoring PGY-1 preferences to the location of the advanced training. So, for each advanced position, you will submit a list of PGY-1 positions in the order of your preference. If you do not match into an advanced position, your SROLs will not be used. If you go unmatched on your SROL, your advanced Match result still holds. You can rank up to 15 programs on your SROLs combined at no charge. See the NRMP Web site for more information on how to create and link individual SROLs to programs on your ROL.

Remember that if you rank a program on your SROL and match at it, you are under contract to attend; therefore, continue to follow the same two rules that were discussed with regard to the ROL—rank programs based on desirability and rank only acceptable programs! Most applicants will rank programs for the SROL based on two main factors: program style/strength and location. A common consideration for the SROL is to rank strong programs that are in the same geographic location as your medical school or the same location as the advanced position.

## COMMUNICATING WITH PROGRAM DIRECTORS BEFORE THE MATCH

Programs often call candidates or send follow-up letters after an interview to confirm or feel out their interest in the program. Some program directors call every single applicant they have interviewed with the genuine purpose of answering any last-minute questions. While applicants and program directors may express a high degree of interest in each other and try to influence a decision in their favor, they should be careful not to make statements implying a commitment that is contingent upon any rank order or other requirement. This type of communication is a clear Match violation. Follow-up letters often contain statements that can be misinterpreted by either party. Sometimes program directors may even assure you that you will be ranked at the top of their list. While such information may be flattering, do not count on it, and do not let it affect your ROL. Remember that you should rank programs based on their desirability to you, not based on where they claim they will rank you on their list. If a program says that you will be ranked first, all it means is that you can match no lower than that program. Some applicants have an instinctive but unfortunate tendency to favor programs that they believe are more likely to accept them. Others allow these follow-up letters to limit the length of their ROL inappropriately. Again, all acceptable programs should be on your ROL.

You may sometimes find conversations with program directors or phone calls slightly awkward, especially when your interest in a program may be less than the program's interest in you. Whatever the situation, the first rule when speaking with program faculty or administration is to be honest and tactful. If a program director calls you expressing interest, politely thank the individual and highlight what you liked about their program. Do not tell a program they are your number one choice unless this is the absolute truth! At the same time, do not tell a program they are seventh on your list. Simply discuss the strengths of the program, ask any remaining questions you have, and thank the program director or faculty member for taking the time to call you. Remember, your ROL is private and personal; you are under no obligation to reveal it to anyone.

Once you've narrowed down your rank list, it is perfectly okay to communicate your interest in a program so long as it does not involve bartering of any kind (ie, suggesting that you will rank a program only if they rank you highly). The Match Participation Agreement does not prohibit either party from making statements that volunteer ROL information, but asking the other party for this information is not permitted. In some of the more competitive fields, program directors or department chairmen may call applicants after the interview but before Match Day to ask about their ranking of the program. It is a violation of Match rules for programs to ask you (or vice versa) for this information. If this occurs, you can politely inform them that you are considering their program, but cannot make any definitive statements about your rank order. You might consider reporting the incident to your dean of students, the NRMP, or the appropriate specialty board after the Match. It is by no means required to communicate with programs before the Match, and in fact this practice is often frowned upon by advisors and deans because of the amount of miscommunication that can occur.

Contacting your single top-choice program is, however, a good idea. Telling your first-choice program they are at the top of your list in no way guarantees a match at that program. However, expressing interest in a program never hurts and may affect how a program views your enthusiasm about their residency. If you choose to notify your number one program of your interest, you should **communicate to only your one, top-choice program that it is your first choice!** Telling multiple programs that you will rank them first may come back to haunt you; program directors often talk to each other, and your credibility rating will soon be in the dumpster if word gets out that you have told more than one location they are your "number one pick." It is important to remember that the faculty who help choose the ROL for the program you match with will ultimately be your colleagues, and breaking trust among work partners across the country is a poor way to start any business.

A great way to communicate with programs is through advisors and deans. In some fields, especially smaller ones such as neurosurgery, faculty and program directors know each other quite well. If your advisor at your home department feels comfortable, he or she can communicate your interest in a program. Politely ask if he or she would be willing to call your top-choice program and speak with the program director or chair about your interest. Some department faculty may automatically offer to do this if you discuss your ROL with them.

Occasionally, students will select a first-choice program and then change their minds later; while this is perfectly okay to do, it becomes a little tricky once you've already told a particular program they are your number one choice. Therefore, it is advisable not to notify your first choice program until you have certified your ROL and to do so no earlier than at least a week before the ROL deadline (as last minute changes can and often do occur). If you do change your mind after you have already called or contacted a program, it is courteous to call and inform them of the change.

## UNDER-THE-TABLE DEALS

It has been noted that several programs—especially those in less competitive specialties—are increasingly using "under-the-table" negotiating to recruit international medical graduates (IMGs). They see these applicants as less choosy than U.S. medical graduates and therefore think they can "lock in" a good applicant from abroad by offering him or her a deal outside the Match. If you find yourself in this situation, carefully consider what is to be gained and lost from such an agreement. On the one hand, it is nice to have a guaranteed position in the United States. On the other hand, if you are being offered a position outside the Match, it is likely that other programs will find you equally desirable, so you might fare well at a higher choice if you went through the Match. In the end, the final decision is yours—but without a contract and a discussion of visa and licensure issues (see Chapter 5), you should not even consider withdrawing from the main Match.

## ENTERING YOUR ROL

All ROLs for specialties participating in the NRMP Match must be submitted electronically through the Internet using the NRMP Registration, Ranking, and Results (R3) system, which is separate from the ERAS application system. The first step to entering an ROL is to make sure that you have appropriately registered with the NRMP and paid the associated fees. Registration with the NRMP should be done before November 30 to avoid a late fee—so register early and save a few bucks. Once you log into the R3 system, you will indicate your preferences from among the programs at which you interviewed, which are each identified by a specific program code. Be sure to double check the program name and code number as you enter them into the system, as some programs have similar names. Programs entered into the R3 system may include preliminary or transitional, categorical, or advanced programs or a combination of these. Make sure you double check that the code you list on the R3 system completely matches your desired program. You can also list several different specialty types (eg, internal medicine, family practice, surgery). If you rank advanced (PGY-2) positions on your ROL and wish to secure a first-year (PGY-1) position as well, you will also be required to submit an SROL (see previous section on SROL). Note that you will be charged additional fees for ranking more than 20 programs on your primary ROL and more than 15 programs on your SROL.

More detailed information can be found on the NRMP Web site. The site also includes a link to a spreadsheet that can be used to create an ROL before entering ranks into the system: www.nrmp.org/res_match/special_part/us_seniors/order_list.html.

Students applying to specialties that have their own Match, such as urology, must send their ROL to their specific matching program. Contact information for these specialties is provided in Chapter 1.

Only certified lists are used in the Match. When applicants have finished entering their lists, they must certify them by clicking on a button and entering their NRMP password to confirm it. Changes can be made to the ROL after it has been certified. This gives applicants a way to "try out" a ranking order for a few days while retaining the option of changing it in the future—as long as the deadline has not passed. However, **once the list has been changed, the new version must be certified in order to be used in the Match.** Changes include adding a program to the list, deleting a program from the list, and changing the order of the programs. A common error made by applicants is changing the list and forgetting to recertify it; if this occurs, the program will default to using the previously certified list. Also note that the system does not retain previous versions of the rank

> Certify your list well ahead of the ROL deadline! Computer and Internet errors occur at inopportune moments.

list, so the list displayed on the screen upon logging in is the only version on file with the NRMP.

Finalizing or turning in your ROL can feel like asking someone to marry you. You're absolutely sure until the moment you turn in that piece of paper. Then you start thinking, "Wait a minute ... did I do the right thing?" Most of the soul searching and turmoil you experience will focus on the ordering of your top two or three choices, which are most likely those programs that fell into your "dream match" category. Discuss the strengths and weaknesses of these three programs with your significant other or close friend. Most advisors and deans over the years have found that students who second-guess their lists and make changes during the final days and hours before the ROL deadline often make rash decisions that they end up regretting. It is human nature to make emotional decisions under pressure, so when in doubt think back to the careful logic that went into making your initial list and go with that instinct! Last minute changes, although they feel right at the time, may not represent your best interests.

Once the deadline, usually occurring at 9 P.M. EST, has passed, the NRMP will not accept or make any changes to your ROL. Therefore, it behooves you to enter and certify your ROL well in advance of this deadline. In addition, it is important to note that if you are actively making changes in the R3 system during the deadline, you will not be allowed to complete the session and will be forced off the server. If you have not certified any list by the ROL deadline, you will not match because the NRMP R3 system will have no record of your desired programs.

## GETTING OUT OF THE MATCH

While all applicants and programs who enter into the Match agree to a binding commitment, there are extenuating circumstances of serious hardship wherein a waiver may be granted. For specific information about the process, read the NRMP policy, which is posted on their Web site (www.nrmp.org/res_match/policies/waivers.html).

"Serious hardship" refers to the occurrence of a highly unusual, unexpected, and unpredictable situation or circumstance that renders the fulfillment of the Match obligation impossible or would result in irreparable harm to any one of the committed Match participants. Examples of serious hardship include an applicant who failed to graduate on time; the closing of a program or institution; the death or serious illness of a family member that requires the applicant to alter the choice of residency location; or the loss of accreditation by a program or institution. It does not include taking advantage of a more desirable program or applicant after the ROLs are submitted. If the waiver is not granted, individuals will be expected to complete the match process and attend the program to which he or she has matched, just as stipulated in the original Match Agreement.

## MARCH MATCHNESS ("IT'S AWESOME, BABY!")

The NRMP Match itself is run in late February, but Match Week does not arrive until the third week of March, with Match Day generally occurring on that

Thursday. The Monday before Match Day at 12 noon is the moment of truth for most applicants because information on whether you have matched or not matched is released. Dean's offices often find out this information earlier in the morning of that Monday, so if you do not hear from your dean's office during this period, you can assume that you matched. For all applicants, including independent applicants, the NRMP R3 system will also send you an e-mail stating that you have either matched fully, matched to an advanced but not a first-year position, matched to a first-year position only, or not matched at all. In addition, you can check this status on the R3 Web site itself. If you did match, pat yourself on the back and then settle in for the continued wait until Match Day, when you will find out where you matched. If you learn that you have not matched, read on for information about the Scramble.

At medical schools on Match Day, the results are announced simultaneously across the nation at noon EST. Many schools organize ceremonies or more casual breakfasts around this event; applicants often bring their significant others to provide moral support and to share in the anticipation. The atmosphere is usually electric by the time the signal is given to open the envelope. If this is a moment you'd rather not share with your entire medical school or if you find yourself traveling away from your medical school on Match Day, you can log into the R3 system at 1 P.M. EST to find the results of your match and where you will be spending the next few years in residency. The R3 system will also send you an e-mail with this information.

> Prank calls pretending to be the dean's office on Unmatch Day are not funny.

## WHAT HAPPENS IF I DON'T MATCH? THE SCRAMBLE

> Now is not the time to panic. Relax and focus. The Scramble begins at noon EST on Tuesday of Match Week.

If you did not match, keep in mind that this does not amount to a personal rejection from the entire medical profession. It might help your bruised ego to recognize that failure to match most often results simply from either applying to or ranking a small number of programs, particularly within a highly competitive specialty. It might also be comforting to know that you are not alone; approximately 1000 U.S. medical students and several thousand non-U.S. applicants enter the Scramble each year, and most find good-quality residency positions immediately.

You will have to postpone your moping and self-pity until later. First, you will be apprised of your situation by your dean on Unmatch Day, or you may find out from your account on the NRMP site. It is likely that on the Monday afternoon of Match Week, you will meet with your advisor or your department chairman to devise a strategy for the Scramble. Your two main options are to enter the Scramble the following day and try to gain a residency position in your selected specialty, a backup specialty, or simply a transitional or preliminary year; or to delay matching for another year and instead opt for a year of research, extra electives, or a different backup plan.

Things will begin to happen very quickly if you decide to enter the "Scramble" period, which lasts from 12 noon EST (no earlier!) on the third Tuesday in March, until 12 noon on the third Thursday in March each year. When the Scramble begins on the Tuesday of Match Week at noon, the NRMP releases the Dynamic List of Unfilled Positions, accessible through the NRMP R3 system and updated every hour to reflect the number of remaining unfilled positions. Only students who have not matched in a particular category can see the unfilled positions related to that category. For example, if you matched in an advanced position but not a preliminary/transitional year, you will only have access to the unfilled position list for preliminary/transitional years.

During the scramble, applicants must use ERAS to apply for unfilled positions. ERAS is available to all applicants who have participated in the ERAS application during the regular season and who have paid their account in full no less than two weeks prior to the Scramble period. These applicants can use ERAS to apply to a maximum of 30 programs free of charge, including up to 15 programs that they may have already applied to during the regular season. If your advisor is unavailable or if you are not a U.S. medical student, you may have to contact the programs directly. After you make your list of programs in order of interest, track down the program phone numbers in AMA-FREIDA or by using the program's Web site. There are some commercially available services and companies that offer to communicate and fax application materials on behalf of unmatched applicants. You should approach these companies cautiously and realize that the NRMP does not endorse or support the use of such services. Remember to always be vigilant for identity theft schemes. The advantage of using ERAS during the scramble is avoiding jammed fax machines and busy phone lines. Electronic transmission of documents through ERAS is immediate and allows program directors to access your information immediately and conveniently. However, if you choose to transmit paper copies of your information during the scramble, you will need to assemble the following documents for a faxable application file:

- Dean's letter

- Transcript

- A copy of the NRMP Universal Application/ERAS application

- Your CV (ERAS provides a printable CV)

- Any letters of recommendation that you may have

You are not restricted to programs in a previously selected specialty. Many applicants decide to pursue additional programs in another specialty because there are too few Scramble positions available in their initial specialty selection. For example, a student who originally applied in plastic surgery, but did not match, might try to scramble into a general surgery position.

Begin your quest by calling programs in the order in which they appear on your hot list. The day will be hectic and stressful, so prepare yourself for busy signals and harried program secretaries, and make a conscious effort to remain calm and friendly. You will need to fax your application file to interested programs. Your dean's office or the department in your specialty should give you full access to their phones and fax machines. Positions will be offered by phone. If you are offered a position at a program that is low on your hot list, ask them how long they are willing to hold that position for you. Otherwise, be prepared to wrap up your acceptance over the phone. Most unmatched seniors are placed within a day, many within the first hour.

Beware of programs that stall on making a commitment to you. Remember that this is as difficult a time for program directors as it is for you. Many programs hope to find the best unmatched resident they can, and they may be waiting on someone else. If you wait too long on them for a confirmation, it could cost you a spot at a program you would be perfectly happy with. If you are in the Scramble, don't do anything desperate—but at the same time, don't be too picky. Sometimes you have to take what you can get if you really want to be an intern the next year. On the other hand, you are not obligated to enter any residency program if you don't want to. If you really had your heart set on a certain city or specialty and it didn't work out, consider taking a year off, bolstering your application, and trying again next year. After all the years of schooling you've put into medicine, one year off will not kill you.

Finally, you should be aware that the NRMP and AAMC have commissioned a task force to study the fairness and effectiveness of the current Scramble process. The task force has proposed changes that could occur as early as the Match process for year 2011 and might delay Match Day until Friday, thus allowing a more calm, thoughtful process for the Scramble. The primary change is to create a "managed" Scramble that would contain oversight from a specific organization. Other changes that have been proposed include not allowing programs to make rolling offers during the Scramble, instead opting for a specific time period after which offers would be made, and allowing applicants at least two hours to consider a position they are offered, thus avoiding rushed and rash decision making during the Scramble. Also, ERAS may be the only permissible method for applying to unfilled programs in the future. Always be sure to check the NRMP Web site and read important e-mails regarding the Match Agreement and policies so that you are up-to-date on the latest rules and regulations for the Match and Scramble processes.

## REFERENCES

AMA FREIDA Online Database Web site (freida.ama-assn.org/Freida/user/viewProgramSearch.do).

ECFMG ERAS: Resources for Applicants Web site (www.ecfmg.org/eras/resources.html).

ERAS for Residency Applicants Web site (www.aamc.org/students/eras/start.htm).

Freedman, Jessica. "The Scramble: How it works and how it can be improved." Studentdoctor.net Web site (www.studentdoctor.net/2009/03/the-scramble-how-it-works-and-how-it-can-be-improved/).

National Residency Matching Program Web site (www.nrmp.org/).

NRMP Proposed Match Changes Web site (www.nrmp.org/scramblechanges.pdf).

# After the Match

289

> Thank-you notes to those who helped you are polite and preserve productive relationships.

## THE DAY AFTER

Congratulations! The Match is over, and a new day is beginning. The day after the Match may be a time of celebration, introspection, or planning. You now know where you will be for the next several years and perhaps for much longer. For most students, this day will also signal the need to start thinking about moving, finding a house or an apartment, and saying one's good-byes.

Although relatively few students think about thank-you messages so soon after the Match, now is the appropriate time to personally thank all your advisors and letter writers. Some busy faculty and community physicians may not even be aware that Match Day has passed, but they are likely to be interested in what happened to you. Others may not be able find out where you matched even if they tried to get Match Day results. Therefore, it is your obligation to tell them. At the very least, a thank-you note is in order. Continuing to maintain a positive relationship with your medical school and your mentors will serve as a foundation for your career.

Many program directors will contact you within a day or two after you Match. Often, they will have prepared an e-mail to be sent out shortly after Match results are available, and some might even choose to call (so be careful about becoming inebriated during Match parties). If the program doesn't contact you right away, it may be nice for you to send an e-mail or give the program director a phone call. However, it would be advisable to wait a day or two for things to settle down in the residency program office. A list of first-year matched residents is usually available shortly after Match Day. This list is often where the picture you submitted to ERAS will come back and haunt you, as it is the first impression of you that your co-interns will see. So spend the time to get a good picture for your application!

> Second thoughts about your match are normal. Just remember not to act on them.

## WHAT IF I'M NOT HAPPY WITH MY MATCH RESULT?

The good news is that based on the NRMP Match data from 2009, more than 80% of U.S. seniors get one of their first three choices in the Match. Even if you did not match at one of your top choices, you should have few regrets if you followed the two cardinal matching rules outlined in Chapter 12.

Now that success has been achieved, you might feel as though you are in over your head, particularly if you have chosen to enter a highly prestigious (or infamous) program. Rest assured that the vast majority of students complete residency training successfully. Furthermore, if a residency program judged that you were capable and qualified by accepting you in the Match, they are very likely to have been correct. So this should be a time to relax—not to spend another month in an ICU or take an ECG book to the beach in June. Taking some time off (especially right after the Match) can be a great idea. You will certainly be busy enough once residency starts! It's also the best time to travel or visit family members that you may not see so often during residency.

Although it is rarely appropriate to switch to a different program within the same specialty, students may have second thoughts about the program to which they have matched. This might occur because a family member has become ill and the student needs to return home. Alternatively, a student may become convinced that he or she has chosen the wrong specialty and wants to forestall a multiyear mistake. Should you find yourself in one of these situations, you must go see your new program director in person and explain your circumstances. Although you are legally obligated to remain in the program to which you have matched for at least one year, most program directors have students' best interests at heart and are sympathetic to extraordinary circumstances that may arise.

If you begin having second thoughts about your chosen specialty, you should discuss these feelings with your mentors at your medical school and potentially your new program director. Remember, you hopefully already went through a thorough heart-to-heart with yourself when choosing the specialty you've matched in. Refocus on the reasons you chose this specialty, and gear up to start residency and give it a try. While the Match is binding, there are mechanisms to switch specialties after the first year if you truly feel it is not the right fit for you. If the feelings of displeasure and angst about your matched specialty continue, you can talk to your program director after the first few months and make plans to enter the Match again and switch specialties. You may or may not be allowed to count your intern year toward your new specialty. You should never plan to break your contract with your residency by leaving in the middle of the year! This can be seen as an illegal breach of contract and/or a Match violation, and it is unprofessional and insulting to your program and its faculty.

## THE RESIDENCY CONTRACT

After the Match, you will receive a residency contract that you must sign and return to your program. The Accreditation Council for Graduate Medical Education (ACGME) recommends that certain terms and conditions be clearly addressed in the contract and policies provided to newly hired employees. Every contract should clearly outline the residents' responsibilities, length of employment, and terms for renewal, and it should specify the salary. Before you sign your contract, understand the definitions of all essential terms. In addition, your contract will often be supplemented with the program's policies, including those on extended leave, benefits, sexual harassment, wellness, and resident expectations and corrective processes. Be sure to read the entire contract and supplemental packets carefully.

> If you will be traveling out of the country after the Match, immediately contact your residency office with an address where paperwork can be faxed/sent while away.

You will also begin to receive a large number of forms from your residency program. As obvious as it may sound, open your mail as soon as it is received! Try to stay on top of these forms to help ensure a smooth transition into your internship. You will likely receive a vacation request form and an elective request form. Remember that your vacation weeks will usually fall during your elective or outpatient rotations, so think about when you might want to schedule a lighter month or be required to travel (eg, for weddings or graduation ceremonies). You might also want to organize essential documents such as proof of citizenship (eg, birth certificate, passport, or Social Security card), and you may need to address your visa status. In addition, Advanced Cardiac Life Support/Advanced Trauma

Life Support (ACLS/ATLS) and Basic Life Support (BLS) training dates and certificates are useful to have on hand. Be sure to ask your doctor or school's health service for your vaccination records, including any tuberculosis testing or antibody titers you may have on file. You are also likely to need a head shot (you can use your ERAS application picture) for your residency program's composite. It is a good idea to print a hard copy of all your application materials (from ERAS and the NRMP site) after the Match, as this information will disappear when the new applicants come along. Some programs and hospitals will also require you to obtain a physical examination from employee or occupational health, and this will potentially involve blood tests and drug screening.

The program coordinator and chief residents will likely send you either an e-mail or a packet of information with important dates and information. The months between the Match and residency move quickly, and there is a lot of paperwork and preparation that the program will need in order to have everything ready for you to start. If absolutely critical, specific scheduling issues, such as your upcoming wedding, should be discussed shortly after the Match. In addition, ask your program what information or credentials it needs to receive from you. Some of the more academic programs have prerequisite reading that must be completed before the program begins. It's also important to ask about your program's ACLS/ATLS and/or Pediatric Advanced Life Support/Advanced Pediatric Life Support (PALS/APLS) training policy. Some programs expect you to arrive with certification in hand; others will put you through an ACLS course when you start. Some U.S. medical schools offer this training after the Match, while others do not. If either your residency or medical school will offer the course, arrange attendance through them because they will often pay for it completely or offer you a great discount.

## LOANS

It is a good idea to get a handle on your student loans now so that you will not have to spend as much time thinking about them during your busy internship year. Most U.S. medical schools' financial aid offices will conduct exit interviews in which they will provide information, resources, and strategies for dealing with your loans. Be sure to come to this exit interview prepared— know your loan type and amount, lender, interest rates, and loan features (eg, grace period, deferment, capitalization). Also, bring a permanent or family home address where your loan paperwork can be sent if you are in the process of moving. The better prepared you are, the easier it will be for you to understand your repayment options and arrange them with your financial aid officer.

> The period before starting residency can be a good time to organize your finances.

It is very important that the demands of the intern year do not result in missing due dates for deferment or forbearance applications or overlooking the end of your grace period for your loans. Mark a date a month in advance on your calendar or PDA to remind yourself of the upcoming deadlines. Forms often take up to three weeks for delivery and processing, so simply meeting a postmark deadline won't always be adequate.

## GETTING SET UP

Moving right along, your next priority is relocating. Nobody enjoys this process, but it doesn't have to be horrible. Some choice pointers follow.

### HOUSING TIPS

Housing should be arranged before graduation if at all possible. Your first step should be to explore the pros and cons of renting versus buying, since housing costs vary widely across the United States, and a good deal for one area may not be your best bet in another. Often, the best approach is to talk to members of the current house staff at your program to get their impressions of the local market. As long as you can afford the payments, buying a small home or a condo may make investment sense if you plan to stay in the area for several years. On the other hand, renting will give you the flexibility to look for bigger and better places after you have had a chance to size up the area. For the first year, it's important to focus on finding a short commute and a hassle-free situation, as every hour is precious during internship.

If you are moving with a partner, you might consider making a list of housing options and features, and prioritizing the list into "must haves" and "can live without." For example, knowing that you couldn't live without a dishwasher but can compromise with a small yard is important for narrowing your search. If you've couples matched with a partner and will be working at two different hospitals within the same geographic area, location, commute times, and available public transit may be important considerations in choosing housing.

There are many ways to find housing opportunities: You can call up friends who live near the program for housing tips; ask the residency office about housing options; visit a realtor or a professional rental service (ask your program or other residents for referrals); go to the local library to look at the classifieds section in local newspapers; or use the Internet to search for available housing in your new city. Consider classmates who may have matched in the same hospital or city as possible moving buddies and/or potential housemates. Craigslist is a Web site that provides local classified listings and is a great resource for finding roommates and rental options. However, the listings are not screened, so be alert for possible scams. Listings available through rental and roommate agencies tend to be of higher quality, since the listing fee is self-selecting. Unless it's a huge hassle, plan to visit the city for at least two to four days to find and finalize housing arrangements. If the market is really hot, it is best to come prepared to settle or sign a lease during your visit. During this time, check with a second- or third-year resident to get a local opinion about your choice. The current residents may also provide you a place to stay while you are visiting and looking for housing. Also, in some housing markets, renters may require you to pay first and last month's rent in addition to a security deposit, so make sure you have enough funding available to sign the lease.

### MOVING TIPS

In anticipation of your move, prepare change-of-address cards and arrange mail forwarding with your local post office. Keep a list of bills you receive during

## TABLE 13-1

### Packing Essentials Checklist

- Packing boxes
- Newspapers
- Plastic/bubble wrap
- Cord/rope
- Packing tape
- Scissors
- Utility knife
- Markers
- Labels

the last few months before you move, and fill out the change-of-address form (or call) when you make your payments. Remember that if your move is job related, you may be eligible for federal tax deductions of up to $3000 for moving expenses, so keep track of your receipts carefully. For tracking and insurance purposes, you should catalog your belongings (if you have a lot of material, you might organize it by room) and photograph valuable items. Selling or donating all nonessential belongings will streamline both your move and your life in the long run. In addition, make sure you have adequate packing materials before you start the job (see Table 13-1). Many grocery stores, bookstores, or liquor stores will donate large cardboard boxes that are sturdy enough for packing books. Furniture stores are typically more than happy to supply you with boxes or large sheets of leftover plastic and bubble wrap.

You have several options for moving your belongings once you have packed. If you have little or no furniture (or none worth taking), one option is to mail your boxes; just pack your unbreakable belongings and call UPS at (800) PICK-UPS for a pickup. UPS does have a limit on the maximum size and weight per box, so call for details. The company automatically insures goods for up to $100 per box and sells insurance for belongings of greater value. The U.S. Postal Service also offers shipping services, and they are especially useful if there are particular textbooks, personal reading, or CD/DVD collections that you need to ship. You can ship boxes containing only these items at a discounted rate, called "Media Mail." The rate is cheaper, the time for shipment is longer, and there is no option to insure the items, but overall it will save you money on the move. Call (800) ASK-USPS for details, or visit www.usps.com.

Move your valuable and fragile items personally. If you have furniture worth keeping, you might want to consider moving it yourself. There are a number of self-moving companies with one-way moving vans, including Ryder and U-Haul. If you contact a local branch of such a company rather than the central office, you can often bargain for the truck/van rental. This is the cheaper way to move, but beware of the hassle factor. Another option is PODS (portable on-demand storage), where you pack and unpack your belongings, but delivery is provided. This service is not provided in all areas; for a complete listing and more information, visit their Web site (www.pods.com). It's also worth considering hiring professional movers to do the job. Although it will cost more, you won't be adding the stress of moving to the stress associated with starting your internship. Just be sure to carefully look over any contract you sign for all the terms and conditions (especially about delivery). Research the company you plan to use beforehand. Movingscam.com is a Web site that contains information about and customer reviews of many of the major moving companies.

UPS and PODS are alternatives to U-Haul and traditional movers.

## SETTLING DOWN

By all means, take a vacation, but give yourself at least one or two weeks to settle into your new home before your internship starts. You will need this block of time to set up your household, open bank accounts, transfer your driver's license and car license plates, turn on utilities, and install a telephone line or cable. If you show up two days before a busy internship begins, it may take you the next two months just to unpack. Also, you and your future co-interns may want time for informal get-togethers before orientation officially starts. In fact, this is a great time to have barbeques and get to know your class before the business of the intern year sets in. Extra time will also give you a chance to explore your new neighborhood and city before internship takes over your life. You won't want to waste time later locating grocery stores, affordable restaurants, 24-hour gas stations, and the like. Try to streamline all nonmedical aspects of your life (eg, bill paying, shopping) so that what little time off you have during internship is "quality time."

> There is no better time to simplify your life.

## STEP 3 AND LICENSING

The Match is over, and you've moved into a nice apartment five minutes from the hospital. Now all you have to do is brace for internship, right?

Well ... almost. At some point during your residency, you will have to register for and pass the USMLE Step 3, apply for licensure, and obtain a Drug Enforcement Agency (DEA) registration number. For most new physicians, licensure is most often left until the last months of training, but having your documents in order before residency starts is always a good idea—and keeps your vacation time free from frenzied searches for important credentials. (See below for more information on licensure.) Some states, such as California, require full licensure by the start of the third postgraduate training year. Also, if you plan to moonlight during residency, you will need to pursue full licensure. The applications require that you fill out a mountain of paperwork and will involve notarized documents, fingerprints, and birth certificates. Thus, the preparation you begin before starting your internship will minimize your stress and vastly enhance your ability to become licensed when you want or are required to be. All of the requirements for each state can be found on the state's medical board Web site or on the Web site of the Federation of State Medical Boards (www.fsmb.org).

## THE USMLE STEP 3

To apply for Step 3, you must meet the following requirements before submitting an application:

1. Meet the Step 3 requirements set by the medical licensing authority to which you are applying.

2. Obtain your MD degree (or the equivalent) or DO degree.

3. Receive a passing score on Step 1, Step 2 CK, and Step 2 CS.

4. If you are an IMG, obtain certification by the Educational Commission for Foreign Medical Graduates (ECFMG).

Because the requirements for Step 3 vary by state, it is imperative that you carefully read your state's requirements. For example, some states will require that you have completed one year of postgraduate training in a residency program accredited by the ACGME, others may only require that you have started the program, and still others might require that you've completed at least six months of a program.

> Schedule Step 3 early, and at least three months ahead of your medical licensure application deadline.

When you send in your application for Step 3, you will not be given the option to select a time period of three months over which you wish to take the exam (as was the case for Steps 1 and 2 CK). Instead, once your application is approved, your eligibility period of 90 days begins immediately. Therefore, you should allow one to three weeks for the processing of your application. When this is completed, a scheduling permit will be sent to you by e-mail. You may then schedule a test date. The Step 3 exam is available throughout the year except for two weeks in January. Because Step 3 is a two-day exam that must be taken on consecutive business days, it is important both to schedule your test date as soon as you receive your scheduling permit and to keep your appointment. You should discuss with your program director and chief residents when the best time to take the exam is, as you will not be able to work. Rotations such as elective time, research, or ambulatory rotations may be best, but be mindful that in some residencies, vacation and elective time is assigned and not flexible. As with Steps 1 and 2 CK, Step 3 uses computer-based testing. For general information on licensure and Step 3, contact:

Federation of State Medical Boards of the United States, Inc.
P.O. Box 619850
Dallas, TX 75261-9850
Main phone: (817) 868-4000
Main fax: (817) 868-4099
www.fsmb.org

Plan ahead for the USMLE Step 3. Although the cost of taking the exam is $690 (for the year 2009), some states add administrative charges to the overall cost. Moreover, these extra charges can vary from state to state since some state medical boards conduct the Step 3 examination themselves, while others rely on the USMLE to do so. In addition, the cost usually increases from year to year.

The application for Step 3 also differs somewhat from those for the USMLE Steps 1 and 2. The application can be submitted online or by mail. The online application will result in faster processing of the application, but you are still required to submit by mail a proof-of-identity form and any other forms required by your state medical board. Faxed documents are unacceptable, but you can use Express Mail, Federal Express, or UPS to deliver your application. Be sure to make copies of all documents, and allow for the six to eight weeks required to score the exam. You may also choose to submit the application entirely by mail, but keep in mind the processing time for this format may take three to four weeks. The forms for the paper application and the online application are found online at the FSMB Web site (www.fsmb.org/m_usmlestep3.html). Listed below are some basic administrative guidelines to follow when preparing to take the USMLE Step 3:

- Contact the FSMB or call your state medical board for a USMLE Step 3 application, and read it carefully. Experience has taught that it is critical to verify when you are eligible to take the Step 3 exam, as this varies from state to state.

- Start the application process early. Begin pulling together your supporting documentation as soon as possible.

- Find out when your state requires you to be licensed and whether that date differs from that of your training program's requirement. To help you determine when to take Step 3, work backward from your state licensure deadline to determine when you should schedule the exam. Be sure to factor in the six to eight weeks that it will take for scoring and notification of results.

- Locate a photographic service for required application photos.

- Identify a notary public in your facility to obtain required notarizations.

- Oh, yeah—don't forget to study.

For more information, refer to *First Aid for the® USMLE Step 3*.

## WHAT IS LICENSURE?

*Licensure* is the legal term that denotes approval to practice medicine. It is granted by a governing body, which is often the state's medical board, on the basis of the laws in your jurisdiction. Some states offer several types of licensure—eg, training, military, inactive, locum tenens, temporary, or permanent. Periods of licensure also vary from state to state; some licenses are valid for only one year, others for two. Similarly, some licenses can be renewed after a set period of time that is based on your birth date, while others are renewable on an annual basis during a particular month of the year. All 50 states require applicants to have successfully passed the USMLE Step 1, 2 (CK and CS), and 3 exams in order to be eligible for licensure. Since each state has a different fee, the cost of the entire process varies, but plan on putting aside at least $2800 total for all three USMLE Steps, and around $1500 for the licensure application process.

You should also be aware that in some states, the medical board can fine residents and programs up to $2500 for failing to obtain licensure as defined by the law. In support of this legislation, some programs have been known to terminate the contracts of house staff who fail to become licensed by state-mandated deadlines. As a corollary, however, some programs also reimburse residents for the application fees associated with initial licensure and renewal of the license each year.

Medical boards process thousands of applications each year, usually on a first-come, first-served basis. They will not process files that are out of order for any reason whatsoever. So be courteous when discussing your application with licensing technicians, and allow for plenty of time. You should speak with residents from the classes ahead of you to ask when the best time to take Step 3 is and what the best timeline for licensure is. Your program's GME office can also help you plan.

## STEPS TOWARD LICENSURE

The following tips will help further your goal of obtaining licensure in a straightforward and timely manner. Once you have matched, we recommend that you obtain the regulations for licensure in the state where you will be training. Then carefully review those regulations, paying particular attention to when the USMLE Step 3 exam dates and deadlines are, when you are eligible for licensure, and when you are required to be licensed in your jurisdiction. Then start the licensure application process at least six months before the licensure deadline in your state. Before you frame your medical school diploma, be sure to make a few copies of it on 8.5-by-11-inch paper. Send all forms via certified, registered, or express mail, or enclose prepaid postcards to allow for acknowledgment of materials received.

When dealing with medical board personnel, be very courteous. (They're just like residency application secretaries: cross them and you're history.)

Armed with the correct information, you will be able to control all three of these critical processes so that you can become licensed in a timely fashion with a minimum number of surprises (eg, deadlines, exam dates, and required fees). Online, fee-based services that will help you with each step for licensure are also available and include www.physicianlicensing.com and www.healthcarelicensing.com.

## WHAT'S NEEDED

Table 13-2 summarizes the most common materials requested by state medical boards for licensure. Once you know what is required for licensure in your jurisdiction, you can prepare for the application process by doing some or all of the following, as appropriate:

- Identify the location and cost of photographic services. Be sure to find a photographic service near your place of work, as you may need to make a few visits there during work hours.

- Identify the location and cost of a notary public. If there is no notary public in your facility, try real-estate offices or banks. Be aware, however, that many notary publics have limited hours of availability. Also be sure to complete your application before obtaining notarization, but do not sign the application until you are in the presence of the notary. A valid picture ID will also be required—eg, a driver's license or a passport. Some banks offer free notary services if you have an account with them.

- Identify the location and cost of fingerprinting services.

- Identify potential personal references and contact them to discuss their willingness to serve as references on your behalf.

- Research the addresses for and costs of obtaining academic transcripts.

- List all hospitals and addresses where staff privileges have been granted.

- Order a certified copy of your birth certificate.

- If you have changed your name, locate and obtain documentation that will verify that change.

## OBSTACLES TO LICENSURE

Potential obstacles to licensure that both U.S. graduates and international medical graduates (IMGs) may face are as follows:

- **Missing critical deadlines** (eg, failure to apply for and take the USMLE Step 3 in conjunction with licensing deadlines). Since one of the primary requirements for licensure is successful passage of the USMLE Step 3 examination, you must time Step 3 so that you take it at least three months prior to your licensure deadline. This will allow for the scoring of your exam as well as for the reporting of your scores to the medical board. Another benefit of taking the

## TABLE 13-2

**Items Commonly Requested by State Medical Licensing Boards as Requirements for Medical Licensure**

Medical school diploma (either original diploma or an official copy with the registrar's signature and school seal)

Official medical school transcript

Official undergraduate school transcript

Two to three recently taken passport photographs

Two to three letters of recommendation

Letter from residency program director

Official USMLE Step 1, 2 CK, 2 CS, and 3 score reports

Fingerprints

Completed application with notarized signature

Application fee (usually around $600–$1000)

Letter of good standing from any other state licensing boards from which you were granted licensure exam early is that it allows you time to take it again should that prove necessary.

- **Failure to include correct licensure/exam fees along with your application.** Most medical boards will return your application if the fees you enclosed are incorrect. You should also be aware that most application fees are nonrefundable.

- **Failure to provide complete and accurate information on your application.** In reviewing your application, medical boards sometimes uncover discrepancies such as inconsistently reported attendance dates. If this is the case, the board must send you a letter explaining the discrepancy they found and what you must do to rectify it.

- **Incomplete documentation.** As is the case with all bureaucracies, forms are not always completed properly by other institutions. Unfortunately, however, incomplete forms sent to the medical board by your undergraduate school, medical school, or training program will be returned to you to correct. You may then need to call the facility where the error occurred to ensure that the forms are properly handled the second time around.

- **Submitting unrequested documentation to the medical board.** Documents that have not been requested but are enclosed with your application can confuse and frustrate licensing technicians. Moreover, the inclusion of such documents in your application package can raise troubling questions both about your application and about your ability to follow basic instructions.

- **Administrative holds on transcripts.** Transcripts can be held for a variety of reasons, including delinquent student loans, unpaid library fines, and the like.

- **Administrative holds by training programs.** Program directors may deny your request to complete your licensure form on the basis of factors such as incomplete patient chart dictations. (This is rare, but it has been known to occur.)

- **Disregarding requests for additional documentation.** Requests for additional documentation by the medical board are commonplace and should not be ignored, as some states consider a file closed if it has not been fully completed within a certain period of time. You should provide all documentation requested in a timely manner.

- **Failing to report a change of address to the medical board.** Most states will not forward licenses in the mail. Thus, if you have recently moved, be sure to notify your medical board of your new address in writing at the earliest possible time.

- **Failing to keep copies of documents that are submitted to the medical board.** It is always a good idea to keep extra copies of all forms and their addresses. This will help you track lost documents and will also help resolve questions the board might have about a particular document.

- **Exhibiting abusive behavior toward medical board personnel.** Medical board personnel typically have a very large workload. Thus, working cooperatively with them is clearly in your best interests. Remember, board personnel don't make the licensing laws; they're just chartered to uphold them.

- **Starting the application process too late.** If you are not licensed by the deadline set by your state medical board, you may be unable to continue your training program.

  The following potential obstacles to licensure apply to IMGs only:

- **Getting forms completed by a foreign medical school.** Documents sent to foreign medical schools often require additional processing time. It can thus be highly advantageous to have someone living near your medical school oversee the process of document completion, mailing, and the like.

- **Failure to complete sufficient hours in required clinical rotations.**

- **Lack of familiarity.** IMGs should carefully review licensing requirements for the state from which they are requesting licensure.

- **Inadequate documentation of individual clinical rotations.** Some states have their own individual forms to be used for documenting each rotation. Again, contact your medical board for details.

- **Failure to use medical-board-approved translators for documents written in other languages.** Some state medical boards have a list of translators whom they have deemed acceptable for translating application documents. Contact your medical board for more information.

## DON'T FORGET TO WRITE

> Contact us through our blog or by e-mail to let us know how this book helped you, along with any suggestions for future students.

Congratulations! You've made it to internship. We hope that the advice and information in this book was helpful. Much of what you have read comes from the experiences of students who have gone before you. We hope you'll share the lessons you have learned with those who follow by giving us feedback at www.firstaidteam.com or e-mailing us at firstaidteam@yahoo.com. As for internship, nothing can save you from that. But don't worry—in a year, you'll be done. Best of luck!

## REFERENCES

CraigsList Web site (www.craigslist.com).

Federal Express Web site (www.fedex.com).

Federation of State Medical Boards (FSMB) Web site (www.fsmb.org).

Healthcare Licensing Services Web site (www.healthcarelicensing.com).

Physician Licensing Service Web site (www.physicianlicensing.com).

Portable On-Demand Storage Web site (www.pods.com).

United States Postal Service Web site (www.usps.com).

UPS Web site (www.ups.com).

# 14

# Web Resources

> Be wary of becoming bogged down by the volume of online information. Stay on guard for redundancies and misinformation—especially on blogs and discussion boards.

Exploring all of the resources available on the Internet can be a daunting task, especially when you are in the midst of making plans associated with the next stage of your medical training. Very few of us have the time to carefully pick through the jumble of information available on the World Wide Web, which is why we bring you this chapter. The following Web resource list is by no means comprehensive or exhaustive; instead, we have selected what we believe to be the most helpful online tools while navigating the Match process. Many of these links are also listed in the preceding chapters and have been collected here for easier navigating. Finally, if you're tired of entering long URLs, you can find all these sites at www.firstaidteam.com. Surf's up!

## CHOOSING A SPECIALTY

### CAREERS IN MEDICINE (CIM)

*www.aamc.org/students/cim/*

This Web site has an immense number of resources to help you through the entire Match process, from choosing a specialty to your application and interview. It has data for each specialty, showing the average salary, the demographics of the patients they see, the five most common illnesses encountered, and a wealth of other features. It also has several career-planning exercises designed to help you identify the best medical specialty for you. This four-phase process will guide you through the elements of career planning, including self-understanding, exploring a variety of medical careers, and finally choosing a specialty to meet your career objectives.

> Don't forget to take advantage of links that are listed on Web sites that you already trust.

Don't miss out on the "Related Resources" links on the right-hand side of the page (see Table 14-1).

## TABLE 14-1

| Related Resources on Careers in Medicine Web Site | |
|---|---|
| *Choices* Newsletter (PDF) | A monthly newsletter from CiM that offers a variety of helpful reads—ranging from feature articles on specialty choices to postgraduate debt management strategies. |
| CiM Liaison List | If you are a student at a U.S. medical school, this link offers a listing of appointed career advisors from your school. |
| CiM Timeline | This timeline will give you insight as to the thought processes and decisions that you will encounter at each stage of your medical school training to arrive at an appropriate specialty. |
| Charting Outcomes in the Match (PDF) | What does it take to match in a given specialty? Organized alphabetically, this document provides statistics on specialties participating in the NRMP Match, such as the number of applicants and the number of spots, as well as the average USMLE Step 1 scores of applicants who matched. |

# PATHWAY EVALUATION PROGRAM FOR MEDICAL PROFESSIONALS

*http://medpathway.wustl.edu/main_menu.htm*

This Duke University resource provides a self-assessment of your interests and values and compares your demographics with those of participating physicians in listing compatible career options. Whether you like every single specialty out there, are trying to decided between a couple of career options, or are pretty much ready to roll, this interactive tool is worth checking out. It includes:

- A three-step process consisting entirely of multiple-choice questions

- Easy flow from the self assessment to the specialty compatibility profile

## SPECIALTY INFORMATION PAGES

*http://residency.wustl.edu/medadmin/resweb.nsf*

An extremely valuable resource for any applicant, this site gives a concise and comprehensive preview of what to expect when going into a given specialty. Click on the "Choosing a Specialty" link. From there, the "Length of Residencies" gives a table comparing the different residencies. The "Information about Specialties" section has detailed descriptions and information for each specialty, including:

- Overview, training requirements, matching program information and match statistics, and subspecialty/fellowship training

- "At a Glance" information about training, fellowships, and lifestyle

- U.S. Match statistics

## CAREER MD

*www.careermd.com/physicians/directories_overview.shtm*

CareerMD's directories include profiles and contact information for thousands of physician training programs. This comprehensive site enables you to run an advanced search on all postgraduate training programs by state, hospital name, and even program directors' names. Directories are listed in Table 14-2.

## TABLE 14-2

**Postgraduate Training Program Directories**

| | |
|---|---|
| ResidencyFIND | Directory for allopathic medical students: all ACGME-accredited residency programs |
| OsteoFIND | Directory for osteopathic medical students: all AOA-accredited internships and residency programs |
| FellowshipFIND | Directory for fellowship-seeking residents: more than 9000 fellowship programs, both ACGME- and non-ACGME-accredited |

## NATIONAL MEDICAL SPECIALTY SOCIETY WEBSITES (AMA)

*www.ama-assn.org/ama/pub/about-ama/our-people/the-federation-medicine/national-medical-specialty-society-websites.shtml*

Get a glimpse of what you are getting yourself into! This Web site provides a list of links to medical specialty society sites and is alphabetically arranged and comprehensive. It includes organizations' public faces, current affairs, and news related to your field of choice.

## AMERICAN OSTEOPATHIC ASSOCIATION SPECIALTY SOCIETIES (AOA)

*www.osteopathic.org/index.cfm?au=A&PageID=lcl_spclty*

This is the AOA equivalent of the AMA resource listed above. A number of organizations work to represent various osteopathic specialties and subspecialties. Contact any one of these specialty groups to learn more about how they promote the practice of osteopathic medicine.

## KEIRSEY PERSONALITY SORTER

*www.keirsey.com/sorter/register.aspx*

The Keirsey Temperament Sorter®-II is the most widely used personality instrument in the world. It is an easy but powerful 70-question personality instrument that helps individuals discover their personality type. Use this tool to get some ideas about what careers might suit you, but don't rely too heavily on it.

# THE APPLICATION AND MATCH

## FELLOWSHIP AND RESIDENCY ELECTRONIC INTERACTIVE (FREIDA)

*https://freida.ama-assn.org/Freida/user/viewProgramSearch.do*

This is the primary central search engine to find programs in your field and in the area or state of your choice. For most programs, it provides several pages of information, including the program Web site, number of residents, salary, average weekly work hours, call schedule, and benefits. It contains information on approximately 8600 graduate medical education programs accredited by the Accreditation Council for Graduate Medical Education and 200 combined specialty programs. Some features of the Web site are as follows:

- It includes expanded listings for those programs that provide data. Click on the links at the top of the program page to find the detailed information. Not all programs provide all the pertinent information. However, the information can often be found on the program's Web site.

- It is searchable by specialty or location.

- It offers specialty training statistics.

- You have the option to save programs you like and download program information in a spreadsheet format (available only with valid log-in and password).

## MATCH ROUNDS WEBSITE

*www.matchrounds.com*

     This is a Web site created by two Northwestern MS4's available to medical students across the country, providing a centralized place for match information. Some features are as follows:

- Interactive timeline which allows users to track interview dates and add thoughts about each program as the season progresses.

- Interactive rank list that allows users to rearrange their programs.

- Expense calculator created to estimate the costs of the entire process.

## ELECTRONIC RESIDENCY APPLICATION SERVICE (ERAS)

*www.aamc.org/audienceeras.htm*

     This is the page where you apply for most residencies. You will get to know it very well! It is described in detail in Chapter 1.

## NATIONAL RESIDENT MATCHING PROGRAM (NRMP)

*www.nrmp.org*

     The NRMP organizes the "Main Match" for all specialties except those participating in SF Match and urology match. You will need to register with the NRMP and then submit your rank list after you have interviewed. Read through the rules and regulations to ensure that you understand the legal contractual nature of the Match.

> Make sure you understand the ins and outs of the application process, especially the distinction between centralized application services (ERAS) and Match services (NRMP).

## SAN FRANCISCO MATCH (SF MATCH)

*www.sfmatch.org*

     This is the centralized application distribution service for child neurology and ophthalmology and the match service for child neurology, neurotology, and ophthalmology. (Those applying for neurotology must request applications from individual programs.) Don't forget to apply through ERAS and NRMP for preliminary training requirements.

## AMERICA UROLOGICAL ASSOCIATION (AUA)

*www.auanet.org*

     This site offers match services for participating urology residency programs. The application is handled through ERAS.

## AMERICAN OSTEOPATHIC ASSOCIATION (AOA)

*www.do-online.org*

This is the official AOA opportunities database of available internship and residency positions.

## CANADIAN RESIDENT MATCHING SERVICE (CARMS)

*www.carms.ca/eng/index.shtml*

This is the Canadian equivalent of ERAS and NRMP.

## INTERVIEWS

### INTERVIEW TRAIL

*www.interviewtrail.com*

Plan, book, and share stories about your residency interviews. This site offers a plethora of resources including a blog, personal interview planner, statistics from past Matches, and ways to connect with future co-residents. Log-in is required, and all information is as private or public as you wish to make it.

### "THE RESIDENCY INTERVIEW: MAKING THE MOST OF IT" (ARTICLE)

*www.ama-assn.org/ama/pub/about-ama/our-people/member-groups-sections/minority-affairs-consortium/transitioning-residency/the-residency-interview-making-most-it.shtml*

This is a "must read" for everyone going on the interview trail. Organized chronologically with insightful, bite-sized nuggets of information, this article will prep you on first impressions and trip planning and also addresses commonly asked questions and questions that you should be asking about each program when putting together a rank-order list.

### THE MEDICAL RESIDENCY INTERVIEW

*www.rushu.rush.edu/studentlife/career/medint.html*

With subsections like "Know Yourself" and "Looking the Part," this Rush University page offers bullet-pointed tips on how to put your best foot forward during your interviews.

### "DON'T FORGET TO ASK: ADVICE FROM RESIDENTS" (PDF)

*www.aamc.org/members/osr/residencyquestions.pdf*

The process of applying and interviewing for a residency position involves both selling yourself to a program and collecting the information that you will need to decide how to rank the various programs you visit. Look sharp and gather important information about each program by asking the questions listed here.

## TRAVEL AND LODGING

### SMART MED TRAVEL

*www.smartmedtravel.com*

This self-proclaimed "most comprehensive collection of budget airlines, rental cars, and second-option airports compiled in one place" is specifically tailored for medical and premed students. It is arranged geographically and includes every city that has a medical school or residency training program. Although this site is still relatively new, it has many offerings and is well maintained. Features include:

- Simple click-thru menu format
- Information on planes, trains, buses, and automobiles
- Links to hotels and other accommodations specific to each geographical area

### SEATGURU (BY TRIP ADVISOR)

*www.seatguru.com*

The self-proclaimed "ultimate source for airplane seating, in-flight amenities, and airline information," SeatGuru.com offers plane tickets, hotels, and car rentals at competitive rates. For the particularly picky, this site offers information on in-flight amenities as well as detailed seat-map graphics that provide:

- In-depth comments about seats with limited recline, reduced legroom, and misaligned windows
- Color-coding to help identify superior and substandard seats
- In-seat power port locations
- Galley, lavatory, exit row, and closet locations

Don't miss out on the helpful links on the left side: frequent flier tips, travel tips, and comparisons.

### AIRLINES

Following is a list of relatively cheap airlines arranged alphabetically:

- AirTran Airways Web site (*www.airtran.com*)
- Alaska Airlines Web site (*www.alaskair.com*)
- America West Airlines/US Airways Web site (*www.usairways.com*)
- Frontier Airlines Web site (*www.frontierairlines.com*)
- JetBlue Airways Web site (*www.jetblue.com*)
- Midwest Express Web site (*www.midwestexpress.com*)
- Southwest Airlines Web site (*www.southwest.com*)
- Spirit Airlines Web site (*www.spiritair.com*)
- Sun Country Airlines Web site (*www.suncountry.com*)
- Virgin America Airlines Web site (*www.virginamerica.com*)

## ROTATING ROOM (SUBLET)

*www.rotatingroom.com*

This sublet Web site is created for medical students, by medical students. Select a medical school and a hospital and then a list of available rooms will be generated for you in order of availability. Listing your apartment is just as easy. This is an amazing resource, especially for lodging during away rotations.

## LODGING

Free lodging is always the best lodging. However, if you don't have any friends or family in the area, a cheap motel can be your home away from home. Following is a list of relatively inexpensive motels and hotels arranged alphabetically:

- Baymont Inns Web site (*www.baymontinns.com*)
- ClubHouse Inns Web site (*www.clubhouseinn.com*)
- Comfort Inns Web site (*www.comfortinn.com*)
- Country Inns and Suites Web site (*www.countryinns.com*)
- Courtyard Marriott Web site (*www.courtyard.com*)
- Days Inns Web site (*www.daysinn.com*)
- EconoLodge Web site (*www.hotelchoice.com*)
- Fairfield Inn Web site (*www.marriotthotels.com*)
- Hampton Inn Web site (*www.hampton-inn.com*)
- Holiday Inn Web site (*www.ichotelsgroup.com*)
- Hotel Discounts.com Network Web site (*www.hoteldiscount.com*)
- Howard Johnsons Hotels and Inns Web site (*www.hojo.com*)
- La Quinta Inns Web site (*www.laquinta.com*)
- Motel 6 Web site (*www.motel6.com*)
- Quikbook Web site (*www.quikbook.com*)
- Ramada Ltd. Web site (*www.ramada.com*)
- Red Roof Inns Web site (*www.redroof.com*)
- Rodeway Inns Web site (*www.rodeway.com*)
- Super 8 Web site (*www.super8.com*)
- Travelodge Web site (*www.travelodge.com*)

## ONLINE TRAVEL AGENCIES

Following is a list of travel agencies that advertise having competitive rates:

- Cheap Tickets Web site (*www.cheaptickets.com*)
- Expedia Web site (*www.expedia.com*)
- LowestFare.com Web site (*www.lowestfare.com*)

- Orbitz Web site (*www.orbitz.com*)

- Priceline.com Web site (*www.priceline.com*)

- Travelocity Web site (*www.travelocity.com*)

## MATCH OUTCOMES

### CHARTING OUTCOMES IN THE MATCH

*http://aamc.org/programs/cim/chartingoutcomes.pdf*

This yearly publication from the NRMP charts the match rate for different specialties and correlates it with board scores, research experience, and a host of other factors. This is a great resource for getting a feel for how competitive you are compared to other applicants who matched in your field.

### NRMP RESULTS AND DATA

*www.nrmp.org/data*

The NRMP's data reporting and research activities seek to:

- Enhance the transparency of the matching process.

- Assist Match participants in making better-informed decisions.

According to the Web site, "These goals are met while preserving the confidentiality of applicants, schools, and programs with regard to their ranking choices

> Unfortunately, there is no SF Match equivalent to the NRMP's *Charting Outcomes* publication. We suggest consulting with your school's student affairs office for statistics specific to your institution.

## TABLE 14-3

**Helpful Publications from NRMP**

Results and Data: Main Residency Match (*PDF, 100 pages*)

"This report contains statistical tables and graphs for the NRMP Match and lists every participating program, the number of positions offered, and the number filled." Use this resource to judge the selectivity of programs.

Results of the NRMP Program Director Survey (*PDF, 144 pages*)

"This report presents the results of selected items from the 2008 NRMP Program Director Survey. Data are reported for 19 specialties and include: (1) factors used for granting interviews and ranking applicants; (2) use of USMLE exam scores; and (3) the percentage of interview slots filled prior to the November 1 release date of the MSPE." Use this resource to get an idea of how program directors make decisions.

Characteristics of Applicants Who Matched to Their Preferred Specialty in the NRMP Main Residency Match (3rd edition) (*PDF, 281 pages*)

"This report documents how applicant qualifications affect match success. This edition includes data for one additional specialty (neurological surgery) and two new measures (number of work and number of volunteer experiences)."

Use this resource to guesstimate your chances of matching into the specialty of your choice.

and match success." Table 14-3 presents names of helpful links from the front page, quotes about their content from the Web site, and notes regarding their utility to current applicants.

## RESEARCH FUNDING AND TRAINING OPPORTUNITIES

Carrying out research as a medical student can help deepen your understanding of a certain field and can also bolster your application. If you plan to do a short- or long-term research project, there are some funding options available. There may be additional funds from your medical school. Check with your office of student affairs or office of student research. Many of the awards listed below are highly competitive and prestigious.

### HOWARD HUGHES MEDICAL INSTITUTE (HHMI) MEDICAL FELLOWS PROGRAM

*www.hhmi.org/grants/individuals/medfellows.html*

"The Medical Fellows Program supports a year of full-time biomedical research training for medical, dental, and veterinary students. This includes new joint initiatives with the Ivy Foundation for student researchers in the neurosciences, particularly neuro-oncology, and the Burroughs Wellcome Fund (BWF) for veterinary students."

### HOWARD HUGHES MEDICAL INSTITUTE (HHMI) OPPORTUNITIES FOR INDIVIDUALS

*www.hhmi.org/grants/individuals*

"HHMI grants support promising biomedical research scientists working outside the United States, medical and dental students seeking research training, and leading research scientists who are developing new approaches to undergraduate science education. Please note that HHMI's grants for individuals are awarded through competitions that have specific objectives and eligibility criteria and that HHMI does not encourage and rarely funds unsolicited grant proposals." IMGs should not miss out on the Biomedical Research Grants for International Scientists.

### HOWARD HUGHES MEDICAL INSTITUTE/NATIONAL INSTITUTES OF HEALTH (HHMI/NIH) CLOISTER PROGRAM

*www.hhmi.org/research/cloister*

"Students in good standing at U.S. medical, dental, and veterinary schools are eligible to apply to the program. Research Scholars spend nine months to a year on the NIH campus, conducting basic, translational or applied biomedical research under the direct mentorship of senior NIH research scientists. The Howard Hughes Medical Institute provides the administration and funding for the program, including the salaries and benefits for the Research Scholars. The NIH provides advisors, mentors, laboratory space, and equipment and supplies for laboratory work."

## THE OFFICE OF CLINICAL RESEARCH TRAINING AND MEDICAL EDUCATION (CRTP) AT NIH

*www.cc.nih.gov/training/student_programs.html*

Funding is available for the following student research programs through the NIH. Open only to U.S. medical and dental students, awards are given on a competitive basis. Visit the site and click on one of the following links for more information:

- Clinical/Research Electives
- Summer Internships
- Clinical Research Training Program (CRTP) for Medical and Dental Students
- Clinical Investigator Student Trainee Forum

## RESEARCH AND TRAINING OPPORTUNITIES AT THE NATIONAL INSTITUTES OF HEALTH (NIH)

*www.training.nih.gov/student*

This site offers research training opportunities for those in high school through graduate school and runs the gamut of summer programs to yearlong fellowships. This is a great resource for those seeking funded, meaningful research opportunities.

## THE INTERNATIONAL HEALTHCARE OPPORTUNITIES CLEARINGHOUSE (IHOC)

*http://library.umassmed.edu/ihoc/index.cfm*

This Web site is designed for health care professionals and students who are interested in volunteer work with domestic and foreign underserved communities. Search the extensive database of opportunities by region and occupation.

## FOGARTY INTERNATIONAL CLINICAL RESEARCH SCHOLARS (FICRS) PROGRAM

*www.aamc.org/students/medstudents/overseasfellowship/start.htm*

"This program offers one year of mentored clinical research training at a site in the developing world. It expands upon international opportunities for new investigators seeking hands-on experience working in resource-limited and transitional countries. Such experiences during a formative period will hopefully encourage these young researchers to pursue careers in global health-related clinical research. The program also provides support for graduate-level clinical research activities at the international sites, as well as a stipend for an international graduate student to work alongside the U.S. trainee during the clinical research year." This is a great opportunity for both U.S. and foreign graduate students.

## SARNOFF CARDIOVASCULAR RESEARCH FOUNDATION

*www.sarnoffendowment.org/index.cfm*

"The Sarnoff Fellowship Program offers research opportunities for outstanding medical students to explore careers in cardiovascular research. Applicants must be enrolled in accredited U.S. medical schools. Sarnoff Fellows conduct intensive work in a research laboratory, located in the United States, for one year. Prior research experience is not a prerequisite." This is a great opportunity for those interested in cardiovascular surgery or cardiology, as the foundation considers all award recipients "Lifetime Fellows" and provides an expansive networking opportunity.

## ADDITIONAL RESOURCES FOR IMGS

## EDUCATIONAL COMMISSION FOR FOREIGN MEDICAL GRADUATES (ECFMG)

*www.ecfmg.org*

This resource is essential for any IMG because it has information on the application and a timeline of events, including application deadlines for United States Medical Licensing Examination (USMLE) Steps. Do not miss out on the links/resources offered on the left-hand column, which includes frequently asked questions, certification verification services, and visa sponsorship information.

## THE APPALACHIAN REGIONAL COMMISSION (ARC)

*www.arc.gov*

The ARC sponsors physicians in certain places in the eastern and southern United States. Since 1992, the ARC has sponsored approximately 200 primary care IMGs annually in counties within its jurisdiction. Contact information for each state can be found on this very helpful site.

## IMMIHELP

*www.immihelp.com*

"It is advisable for residents to apply for H-1B visas as soon as possible in the year (beginning October 1) when the new quota officially opens up, because there is a cap on the number of such visas offered." This site is very easy to navigate and provides in-depth information and well-organized resources for your immigration and employment needs. This site offers links and resources related to visa status tracking, forms, classifieds, and more.

## BUREAU OF CITIZENSHIP AND IMMIGRATION SERVICES

*www.immigration.gov*

This is the U.S. government's official immigration Web site. Go here for important legal forms and information related to your eligibility to work and live in the United States.

## AMERICAN MEDICAL ASSOCIATION, DEPARTMENT OF IMG SERVICES

*www.ama-assn.org/go/imgs*

This is a very useful site filled with contact information for IMG leadership and groups that support IMGs in the United States. Resources include:

- Frequently asked questions

- Information on immigration, certification, and licensing

- IMGs in the U.S. Physician Workforce Discussion Paper, 2008 edition

- Updates and news relevant to practicing medicine in the United States

# Appendix A

## WORKSHEETS FOR APPLICATION REQUIREMENTS

Feel free to make as many copies of this worksheet as you need. Additional copies are available for download at www.firstaidteam.com.

**Directions:** Fill in blanks below with requested numbers/names/dates. Under **Application Requirements,** list each requirement by name. Once you have assembled the item for that application, check it off.

| Program Name | Program Director | Program Administrator and Contact Info | App. Deadline | Application Requirements | Notes |
|---|---|---|---|---|---|
| | | | | ☐ ☐ ☐ ☐ ☐ | |
| | | | | ☐ ☐ ☐ ☐ ☐ | |
| | | | | ☐ ☐ ☐ ☐ ☐ | |
| | | | | ☐ ☐ ☐ ☐ ☐ | |
| | | | | ☐ ☐ ☐ ☐ | |

# Appendix B

Fill out this worksheet for each program right after your interview, while the information is still fresh in your mind.

Program Name _____

Date of Visit _____

| Factor | Comments |
|---|---|
| Location | |
| Setting | |
| Reputation | |
| Stability of program | |
| Subspecialty strengths | |
| **Education** | |
| Conferences/rounds | |
| Faculty teaching | |
| Postresidency plans of graduates | |
| Research/teaching opportunities | |
| **Work Environment** | |
| Patient population/load | |
| Patient responsibilities | |
| Call frequency/ hours per week | |
| Ancillary support (e.g., nursing) | |
| On-call support (e.g., night float, admission caps) | |
| Health benefits | |
| Non-health benefits | |
| Vacation/sick leave/ parenting leave | |

### Other Factors/Notes

|  |  |
|---|---|
| Gut feeling | |
| Advantages | Disadvantages |

### Preliminary Rank

☐ Top third          ☐ Middle third          ☐ Bottom third          ☐ Do not rank

### Interviewers and Addresses

| Name/Address | Topics discussed during interview |
|---|---|
| ☐ Thank-you card or follow-up letter sent | |
| ☐ Thank-you card or follow-up letter sent | |
| ☐ Thank-you card or follow-up letter sent | |
| ☐ Thank-you card or follow-up letter sent | |
| ☐ Thank-you card or follow-up letter sent | |
| ☐ Thank-you card or follow-up letter sent | |

# INDEX

# About the Authors

## TAO LE, MD, MHS

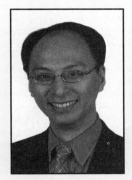

Tao has pursued his passion for medical education for the past 18 years. As senior editor, he has led the expansion of *First Aid* into a global educational series. In addition, he is the founder of the *USMLERx* online learning system as well as a cofounder of the *Underground Clinical Vignettes* series. As a medical student, he was editor-in-chief of the University of California, San Francisco *Synapse*, a university newspaper with a weekly circulation of 9000. Tao earned his medical degree from the University of California, San Francisco in 1996 and completed his residency training in internal medicine at Yale University and allergy and immunology fellowship training at Johns Hopkins University. At Yale, he was a regular guest lecturer on USMLE review and an adviser to the Yale University School of Medicine curriculum committee. Tao subsequently went on to cofound Medsn, a medical e-learning company, and served as its chief medical officer. He is currently section chief of adult allergy and immunology at the University of Louisville. He enjoys travel, movies, good food, and spending time with his family.

## VIKAS BHUSHAN, MD

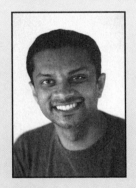

Vikas is an author, editor, entrepreneur, and teleradiologist. In 1990 he conceived and authored the original *First Aid for the USMLE Step 1*. His entrepreneurial adventures include a successful software company, a medical publishing enterprise (S2S), an e-learning company (Medsn), and an ER tele-radiology service (24/7 Radiology). His eclectic interests include medical informatics, independent film, humanism, Urdu poetry, world music, South Asian diasporic culture, and avoiding a day job. A dilettante at heart, he coproduced a music documentary on qawwali music and coproduced and edited *Shabash 2.0: The Hip Guide to All Things South Asian in North America*. Vikas completed a bachelor's degree in biochemistry from the University of California, Berkeley; an MD with thesis from the University of California, San Francisco; and a radiology residency from the University of California, Los Angeles.

## CHRISTINA SHENVI, PhD, MD

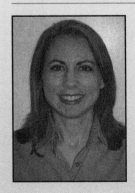

Christina completed her undergraduate studies in chemistry at Princeton University and then pursued what some may consider an excessive amount of postgraduate education, starting with a PhD in chemical biology from UC-Berkeley, followed by an MD from Yale Medical School. During medical school, Christina was a contributing author of two other *First Aid* books, held various tutoring and teaching positions, and spent a summer in Mozambique. However, the most rewarding part of her time in New Haven was the birth of her son, Adrian, who joined Christina, her husband Neil, and their overweight cat Emma in 2009. Christina is currently a resident in emergency medicine at UNC-Chapel Hill in 2010.

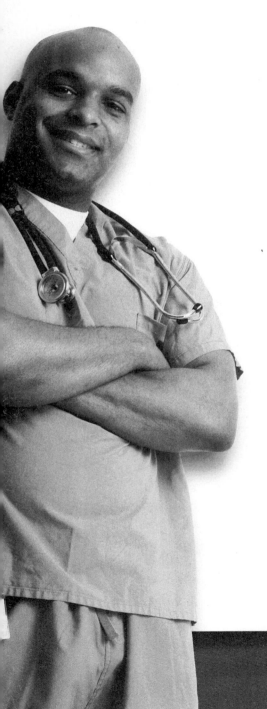